Pharmacology of cytokines

Contents

Preface

Interest in cytokines as tools and targets for therapeutic intervention has grown exponentially in the last two decades. While early cytokine-based, therapeutic efforts can be traced back to the early part of this century, the identification and therapeutic exploitation of interferons in the late 1970s to early 1980s marked a turning point in cytokine research (see Chapter 1). We may be witnessing a new and profound change of perspective in the cytokine world. Emphasis is more and more on antagonists (proteins or simple chemicals). Cytokine biology becomes more and more structural and structural analysis provides a basis for rational design of agonists and antagonists.

This book is aimed at providing the reader with an overview of pharmacological approaches to cytokines. The first part deals with the pharmacology of cytokines, while the second tries to put cytokines and cytokine-modulating agents in a context. In other words, the role of cytokines in the pathophysiology of selected organs, systems or diseases (e.g. the central nervous system, cancer, etc.) is reviewed in some detail. Chapter 1 is an attempt to provide an overview of the cytokine world because the pharmacology of cytokines is intimately connected with pathophysiology.

Chapter 7 is focused on the pharmacology of chemokines. This is an emerging area, characterized by intense efforts, rapid progress, and high expectations. Chemokines interact with 7-transmembrane spanning receptors. Classic pharmacology is largely centered on the development of selective agonists and antagonists for this class of receptors. This, together with the involvement of these molecules in diverse processes, from leukocyte recruitment to viral infections, has prompted intense efforts in this area.

Obviously the book suffers from bias and limitations. The authors are aware of some of them, as they result from their background and perspective, or from deliberate choice. The authors study inflammatory cytokines, and this may have resulted in an inflammation/innate immunity bias well above the actual relevance of this important area. The borders of the cytokine world (see Chapter 1) are ill-defined and we made arbitrary choices in the identification of limits. Finally, by choice, the book is not comprehensive. In particular, we chose not to include the pharmacology of agonistic cytokines, in particular of those that are already part of the clinical armamentarium (e.g. interleukin-2, colony stimulating factors, etc.). The Type I interferon chapter (Appendix) was designed to provide a paradigm for cytokines in clinical practice. We hope that, in spite of its limitations and bias, this book will represent a useful tool in a most active area of research, with implications in diverse human diseases.

Milan   A.M.
Colorado   C.A.D.
Milan   P.G.
June 2000

Acknowledgements

We wish to thank Antonella Palmiero for her help and patience in the preparation of this book, Felice De Ceglie for skillful assistance in the artwork, and Judy Baggott and Brie Romines for checking the style and grammar of many chapters; we are grateful to collegues and friends who read and criticized chapters of this book: Paola Allavena, Giampiero Girolomoni, Marta Muzio, Silvano Sozzani and Annunciata Vecchi.

Abbreviations recurrently used

ARDS, adult respiratory distress syndrome;
BCA-1, B cell-attracting chemokine 1;
CNTF, ciliary neurotrophic factor;
COX, cyclo-oxygenase;
CSF, colony stimulating factor;
EC, endothelial cell;
ELC, EBI (EBV-induced gene) 1-ligand chemokine (=MIP-3ß/CKß-11);
GC, glucocorticoid hormones;
GCP-2, granulocyte chemoattractant protein 2;
IP-10, interferon γ inducible protein 10;
GRO, growth-related oncogene;
IFN, interferon;
IL, interleukin;
IL-1ra, IL-1 receptor antagonist;
ITAC, interferon inducible T-cell α chemoattractant;
LARC, liver and activation-regulated chemokine (MIP-3α/Exodus);
LBP, LPS binding protein;
LO, lipo-oxygenase;
LPS, lipopolysaccharide;
MCP, monocyte chemotactic protein;
MDC, macrophage-derived chemokine;
MIG, monokine induced by interferon γ;
M, G, GM-CSF, macrophage, granulocyte, granulocyte/macrophage CSF;
MIP, macrophage inflammatory protein;
NF-κB, nuclear factor κB;
NOS, NO synthase;
NSAID, non-steroidal anti-inflammatory drug;
PAF, platelet activating factor;
PDGF, platelet derived growth factor;
PG, prostaglandin;
PLA2, phospholipase A2;
PMA, phorbol myristate acetate;
R, receptor;
RANTES, regulated on activation normal T cell expressed and secreted;

ROI, reactive oxygen intermediates;
SDF-1, stromal cell-derived factor 1;
SLC, secondary lymphoid tissue chemokine;
SMC, smooth muscle cell;
TARC, thymus and activation-regulated chemokine;
TECK, thymus-expressed chemokine;
TNF, tumor necrosis factor;
TGF, transforming growth factor;
Th, T helper;
TLR, Toll-like receptor.

1 Cytokines: a world apart?

Cytokines are secreted proteins that have pleiotropic regulatory effects on hematopoietic and non-hematopoietic cells. They are produced by virtually every nucleated cell in the body and encompass families of regulators including interleukins, tumor-necrosis factors, interferons and certain growth factors. The borders of the cytokine world are ill-defined and unstable. For instance, a 'growth factor', like transforming growth factor β (TGFβ), is perhaps better accommodated in the cytokine realm than among growth factors *sensu strictu*. Sometimes this sliding continent even includes hematopoietic and non-hematopoietic growth factors.

The focus of this book is on cytokines *sensu strictu*, as discussed in the Foreword and as largely dictated by the pharmacology of these mediators. While it is obviously impossible to provide a description, or even a detailed map, of the cytokine world in one chapter, here an attempt will be made to provide the reader with a general overview of cytokine classes and modes of action.

1.1 Historical perspective

The cytokine field as it exists today has evolved from several independent areas of research. Major contributors were immunology and lymphokine research, and the study of interferons, and of hemopoietic and non-hematopoietic growth factors.

Conventionally, the beginning of lymphokine research dates from the demonstration in the mid-1960s that products released by sensitized lymphocytes exposed to antigen inhibit macrophage migration. The development of a reliable *in vitro* lymphokine assay, for the putative factor termed macrophage migration inhibitory factor (MIF), represented a turning point in cytokine research.

Prior to this conventional starting date, a less well-defined 'prehistoric era' of cytokine research can be identified. In the early 1930s, Rich and Lewis (1932) observed that in cultures of sensitized tissues, the migration of phagocytes was impaired and macrophages died in the presence of antigen (Rich and Lewis, 1932). These experiments are usually taken as the early precursors of subsequent lymphokine research, and earlier studies by Zinsser and Tamiya (1926) are usually forgotten. They showed that products of activated leukocytes affected vessel-wall elements. These experiments can rightly be considered the forerunners of the whole field, particularly the demonstration in the mid-1980s that cytokines profoundly affect endothelial cell function (reviewed by Dinarello, 1996; Mantovani *et al.*, 1997). In 1958, Waksman and Matoltsy observed that tuberculin actually stimulated macrophage preparations. In this line of early cytokine research, George and Vaugham in 1962 developed a better method for assessing macrophage migration, using capillary tubes. This technical tool was put to use by David in 1966, and Bloom and Bennet (1966) who demonstrated that sensitized lymphocytes responded to antigen by producing MIF.

The line of development of early steps in cytokine/lymphokine research described so far is a current, accepted vulgata. It focuses on *in vitro* approaches to study the presence and function of antigen non-specific mediators of immunity. An equally important approach focused on *in vivo* reactions that are now known to be mediated by cytokines. Centanni, in the 1920s–1930s, injected cancer patients with pleural fluids from people exposed to bacterial toxins and observed regression (Centanni, 1921); thus, he brought Coley's toxin a step further, implying endogenous ultimate mediator(s) of tumor necrosis.

In a completely different field, researchers studying the pathogenesis of fever had focused on the role of soluble products derived from leukocytes as possible mediators of fever. Menkins in 1943 suggested that leukocytes released a pyrogenic substance, and called it pyrexin (for a review of the history of the discovery of endogenous pyrogens, see Dinarello and Wolff, 1982). In 1955, Atkins and Wood found a circulating pyrogenic factor in febrile rabbits that they called endogenous pyrogen (EP) (Atkins and Wood, 1955). In the same year these authors reported the antipyretic action of cortisone in pyrogen-induced fever (Atkins *et al.*, 1955). Later on, production of EP *in vitro* by human, murine, and rabbit mononuclear cells was demonstrated (Fessler *et al.*, 1961).

In 1977, it was suggested that EP was identical to another macrophage product then known as leukocytic endogenous mediator, responsible for the changes associated with the acute-phase inflammatory reponse, including hypoferremia, hypozincemia, and induction of hepatic acute-phase proteins like fibrinogen. Human EP was purified to apparent homogeneity by C. Dinarello (Dinarello *et al.*, 1977). Early biochemical characterization of lymphocyte-activating factor and EP revealed similarities between the two. The fact that all these mediators were the same became clear when the cloning of human interleukin-1β (IL-1β) was reported (Auron *et al.*, 1984).

Strangely enough, these *in vivo* studies on endogenous mediators of defense and toxicity, which were subsequently identified as cytokines, are generally not part of the conventional cytokine/lymphokine story. At a time when clinical exploitation and gene-modified mice show so strongly the importance of *in vivo* findings, we feel that these early *in vivo* studies should be an integral component of the historical background of cytokine research.

The discovery of MIF activity constituted a landmark (Bloom and Bennett, 1966; David, 1966), which ideally marks the beginning of a 'historical' phase of cytokine research. Shortly after the description of MIF activity, it was found that supernatants from mixed leukocyte cultures were blastogenic for lymphocytes. Morgan *et al.* (1976) reported that supernatants of mitogen-activated mononuclear cells could sustain the long-term growth of human bone marrow-derived T cells. T cell growth factor (TCGF), an acronym subsequently abandoned together with other similar ones, is now known as IL-2, a central regulator of T cell growth and function.

Two main independent pathways led to the identification of IL-1, a cytokine mainly produced by cells of the monocyte-macrophage lineage (reviewed in Oppenheim, 1994; Dinarello, 1996). *In vivo* work on endogenous pyrogen and the *in vitro* lymphocyte activating factor (LAF) assay converged on IL-1, which was instrumental to the introduction of the 'interleukin terminology'. LAF was identified as a thymocyte mitogen produced by adherent monocytes, hence a 'monokine'.

Lymphotoxin was discovered in the supernatants of activated lymphocyte cultures soon after the description of MIF activity. The related protein, tumor necrosis factor (TNF), was originally identified as a cytotoxic molecule present in the serum of animals sensitized with Bacillus Calmette-Guérin and challenged with lipopolysacharide (LPS) (Carswell *et al.,* 1975). TNF was identified as a cytotoxic protein for certain tumor cells *in vitro*, as well as a mediator of hemorrhagic necrosis of certain mouse tumors *in vivo*.

Thus, early steps in the cytokine continent were largely the results of efforts focused on 'lymphokines' or 'monokines' as mediators of immune reactions. Interferons, in contrast, were a product of research in virology. In 1957, Isaacs and Lindenmann described it as a factor produced by virus-infected cells, capable of transferring antiviral resistance to other cells. Several years later, an antiviral protein produced by activated T cells, interferon γ (IFNγ), was described.

The confines of the cytokine and growth factor worlds are ill-defined. Hematopoietic growth factors, the colony stimulating factors (CSF), were originally shown to promote the formation of granulocyte or macrophage colonies in semi-solid medium (Pluznik and Sachs, 1965; Bradley and Metcalf, 1966). These molecules affect the proliferation and differentiation of hematopoietic precursors and the function of differentiated hematopoietic cells. Non-hematopoietic growth factors also have cytokine-like activities but, with the exception of TGFβ, their prevailing function and main cellular targets are distinct from those of cytokines. TGFβ proteins are involved in the activation of leukocytes, and have anti-inflammatory/immunosuppressive activity: their spectrum of action and functions justify their inclusion among cytokines.

1.2 Nomina sunt consequentia rerum (usually)

The term 'lymphokine' was coined by Dumonde *et al.* in 1969 to identify the antigen-nonspecific polypeptide mediators produced by lymphocytes exposed to antigen. The observation that LAF/IL-1 was produced by mononuclear phagocytes pointed to the existence of non-lymphocytic derived mediators and led to the introduction of the term 'monokine' to refer to them. This observation, and the finding that cells of diverse origin produced lymphokines/monokines, led Stanley Cohen to introduce the term 'cytokine' (Cohen *et al.,* 1974). In 1978, at the Second International Lymphokine Workshop held in Interlaken, Switzerland, the term 'interleukin' was proposed as a basis for 'a system of nomenclature for proteins with the ability to act as communication signals between different populations of leukocytes'. The terms 'IL-1' and 'IL-2', coined there, were used to identify activities for which a variety of acronyms had been used. Already at that time, it was recognized that the spectrum of action of interleukins produced by hematopoietic and non-hematopoietic cells need not be confined to leukocytes. The success of the interleukin terminology is justified by their growth: at the time of writing there are 18. Although the interleukin nomenclature has been undoubtedly successful, it does not apply to a number of cytokines that retain the old names (e.g. TNF, IFNγ, etc.).

Among cytokines, members of the superfamily of chemotactic proteins, whose prototype is IL-8, have several distinguishing features in common. They are a group of about 50 (in humans) distinct small proteins, usually with the capacity of attracting leukocytes, which interact with seven-transmembrane domain, serpentine receptors. For these cytokines, the term 'chemokine', short for chemotactic cytokines, was coined at the Third International Symposium on Chemotactic Cytokines held in Baden by Vienna in 1992. Though at present there is no agreement on the naming of chemokines, it was decided at a Gordon Conference in 1996 that receptors should be named CXCR1 through 5 or CCR1 through 9, depending on which of the two main families of mediators (C–X–C or C–C) they interact with (see below).

The state of cytokine nomenclature is undoubtedly less than satisfactory. For instance, IL-3 is essentially a multi-CSF, yet it is the only CSF with an interleukin terminology. IL-8 is the only molecule among the 50 or so chemokines to have an interleukin name. Also, IL-14 is a 'phantom' molecule, as yet undefined. The nomenclature of cytokines, useful but not yet completely satisfactory, reflects the different layers of research, as well as the conflicts of personalities intrinsic to human endeavours. A historical perspective may help readers orient themselves and come to terms with the irrational components of cytokine nomenclature.

1.3 Cytokines versus hormones and growth factors

Cytokines, growth factors, and polypeptide hormones are a group of regulatory proteins involved in extracellular signalling. They have some similarities and overlaps. The similarities are profound and include structural features. The receptors for certain cytokines (e.g. IL-2, IL-3/GM-CSF/IL-5, IL-6) have structural characteristics similar to those for the hematopoietic growth factors erythropoietin and granulocyte-CSF (G-CSF) and those for the polypeptide hormones prolactin and growth hormone. The macrophage-CSF (M-CSF) and platelet-derived growth factor (PDGF) receptors have structural features in common. However, some general properties distinguish cytokines from growth factors and hormones.

Non-hematopoietic growth factors, unlike cytokines, tend to be produced constitutively and their major targets are non-hematopoietic cells. Endocrine growth hormones are generally produced by specialized tissues or cells. In contrast, cytokines are usually produced by a variety of cell types or, when their production is restricted to lymphoid cells as for IL-2 or IFN-γ, it is one of the many functions of the producing cells. Hormones are released in the circulation and act at distant sites. Cytokine production, on the other hand, is transient; they act over short distances and are not found in substantial amounts in the circulation. Polypeptide hormones are frequently restricted in their action to a limited set of cellular targets, with the notable exception of insulin. In contrast, many cytokines are pleiotropic, affecting a variety of cells and tissues. Also, unlike hormones, structurally different cytokines have overlapping actions, as illustrated by IL-1 and TNF.

None of these distinguishing features is absolute. For instance, TGFβ and M-CSF are present in substantial amounts in the circulation under normal conditions; IL-6 is produced in response to local inflammatory signals and acts distantly on the liver, contributing to the acute-phase response.

Table 1.1   Structural classification of cytokines

Group	Structure	Cytokines
1	4-α-helical bundles: short chain	IL-2, IL-3, IL-4, IL-5, IL-7, IL-9 IL-13, IL-15, IFNγ, M-CSF, GM-CSF
	4-α-helical bundles: long chain	IL-6, LIF, oncostatin M, cyliary neurotrophic factor, IL-11, IL-10
2	Long chain β-sheet structures	TNF and related molecules: IL-1 and IL-1 receptor antagonist; TGFβ
3	Short chain α/β	Chemokines
4	Mosaic structures	IL-12

1.4 Classification of cytokines

The properties of individual cytokines cannot be analyzed in detail in one chapter. This and the following section, however, will provide the reader with a general framework in which individual mediators can be put, and an overview of recurrent themes in the cytokine mode of action.

Cytokines can be classified according to various criteria. These include structural features of cytokines, their capacity to interact with classes of receptors, and their function.

Structurally, cytokines have been classified according to their overall three-dimensional structure, as this usually better reflects their evolutionary origin than amino-acid sequence similarity (Nicola, 1994) (Table 1.1). Receptor usage can serve as an additional or complementary criterion for structural classification. Many cytokines in group 1 (4-α-helical, Table 1.1) interact with receptors of the hematopoietin family. These receptors have a 200 amino-acid motif, the hematopoietin domain, and do not have tyrosine kinase activity. Notable exceptions include M-CSF, interferons and IL-10.

1.5 A functional classification of cytokines

Cytokines can be classified in functional groups on the basis of their main actions. As perhaps for any classification, functional grouping, however, is an oversimplification and should be viewed more as a tool for orientation than as an accurate reflection of reality. We find it more useful to try and look at the cytokine continent from the perspective of physiology and pathology than of structure. As diagrammatically illustrated in Fig. 1.1, functional groups of cytokines include: (1) hematopoietic cytokines; (2) cytokines involved in specific immunity; (3) primary inflammatory and secondary inflammatory cytokines of innate immunity; (4) anti-inflammatory/immunosuppressive cytokines.

1.5.1 Hematopoietic cytokines

CSFs regulate the proliferation and differentiation of hematopoietic precursors. In addition to G, GM and M-CSF, erythropoietin and thrombopoietin, some more molecules not labelled as CSF also belong to this functional group. These include IL-3 (a multi-CSF), IL-5 (an eosinophil-CSF), IL-7 (a lymphoid CSF), and stem cell factor (SCF). The primary pro-inflammatory cytokine IL-1 was also called hemopoietin-1 and acts on prim-

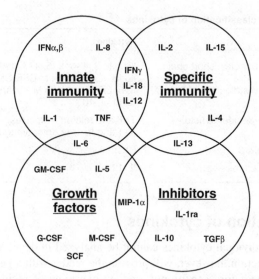

Fig. 1.1 A functional view of the cytokine world. Only selected molecules are shown. For instance, among chemokines only IL-8 is shown.

itive progenitor cells. IL-6 also has CSF activity, particularly on thrombopoiesis. Certain cytokines act as negative regulators of hematopoiesis, and these include TNF and TGFβ. The chemokine MIP-α inhibits early precursors. Besides affecting hematopoietic precursors, molecules with CSF activity regulate the function of mature differentiated cells. For instance, GM-CSF and IL-5 stimulate the survival, migration and function of mature neutrophils and eosinophils, respectively.

1.5.2 Cytokines of specific immunity

The proliferation and differentiation of T and B cells is regulated by cytokines. Various cytokines are involved in specific immunity, including IL-12, interferon-γ (IFN-γ), IL-15, IL-4, and IL-2. IL-2 has provided a paradigm for the autocrine and paracrine regulation of the proliferation and differentiation of lymphocytes and of hematopoietic cells in general. It is regulated both on the cytokine itself and on the components of the receptor. The receptor consists of an α, a β and a γ chain (γc), common to other cytokine receptors. From a pharmacological standpoint, the IL-2 system is a major target for the immunosuppressive activity of cyclosporin A, and related compounds (FK406 and rapamycin).

The T helper 1 (Th1)-Th2 paradigm has proved invaluable for understanding the role of cytokines in specific immunity (Romagnani, 1997). The CD4$^+$ lymphocytes can be classified in subsets depending on their ability to produce cytokines. The classification based on the cytokine profile extends to CD8$^+$ cells too, which produce cytokines. Thus it may be more appropriate to talk about type I and type II responses. Th1 cells produce IFNγ, IL-2 and TNF and promote the production of opsonizing and complement-fixing antibodies; these cells stimulate macrophage activation, antibody-dependent cytotoxicity and delayed-type hypersensitivity (Fig. 1.2). Therefore, Th1 cells activate phagocyte-dependent mechanisms of host resistance.

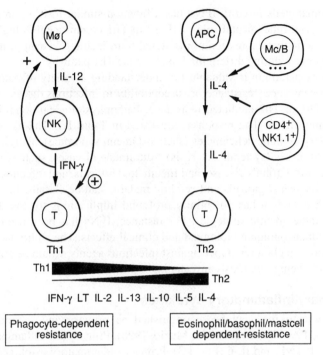

Fig. 1.2   The Th1/Th2 paradigm.

Th2 cells produce IL-4, IL-5, IL-6, IL-9, IL-10 and IL-13, and promote the humoral immune response, including the isotype switch to IgE and IgG1 (or IgG4 in humans), as well as mucosal immunity through the production of growth and differentiation factors for mast cells/basophils and eosinophils, and the promotion of IgA synthesis. Some cytokines produced by Th2 cells, such as IL-4, IL-10 and IL-13, inhibit a variety of macrophage functions. Therefore these cells activate responses independent of phagocytes and dependent on eosinophils/mast cells/basophils.

Th1 and Th2 cells are the polarized versions of a continuum of T cells that show a less distinct repertoire of cytokine production. In the absence of strong polarizing signals, T cells have a less distinct cytokine profile; these cells are usually called Th0 and are responsible for effector functions with intermediate characteristics. The heading Th0 groups a heterogeneous population of effector cells, which can either retain these intermediate properties or differentiate into polarized Th1 or Th2 populations. It is now common to use the term Th1 or Th2-like to indicate cells that produce IFNγ but not IL-4 or vice versa, without taking into consideration the whole spectrum of the cytokine repertoire.

As illustrated in Fig. 1.2, not only do cytokines provide a fingerprint for Th1 rather than Th2 cells, but they also play a central role in the differentiation of precursor cells to one or the other population. IL-12 and IFNγ, the former produced by macrophages, the latter by T cells or NK cells, promote differentiation to Th1 cells and inhibit the Th2 pathway. A similar role is played by IL-4 in commitment and promotion of Th2 differentiation. The primary source of IL-4 in starting up a Th2 response has not been clearly defined. At least with human cells *in vitro*, IFNα has a function similar to IFNγ in promoting Th1 development. The fundamental role of IL-12 in Th1 commitment is highlighted by the recent observation that expression of the signal-transducing β2 chain of the IL-12 receptor is an early event during differentiation along the Th1 pathway.

The Th1/Th2 paradigm is valuable for understanding a variety of pathophysiological processes. For instance, resistance or susceptibility to infectious diseases can be read in the light of Th1 or Th2 mediated resistance. Pathophysiological conditions associated with prevailing Th1 or Th2 responses are listed in Table 1.2. Th2-associated diseases include primary immune deficiencies (such as Omenn syndrome), allergic disorders, and autoimmune diseases (systemic sclerosis). Autoimmune diseases, such as type I diabetes, multiple sclerosis, Crohn's disease, and rheumatoid arthritis, and infectious diseases such as *Helicobacter pylori* gastritis and cerebral malaria, can be classified as Th1 disorders. The Th1/Th2 paradigm has potentially profound implications for the development of novel immunotherapeutic strategies. For instance, IFNγ has been tried in the Omenn syndrome with encouraging biological and clinical effects. The ability to redirect immunity, for instance to elicit resistance against infectious agents, would be a formidable goal and is currently being vigorously investigated.

1.5.3 Primary inflammatory cytokines

Inflammatory cytokines can be distinguished as primary and secondary mediators (Colotta *et al.*, 1994; Dinarello, 1996; Muzio, 1998). Primary pro-inflammatory cytokines are a trio: IL-1, TNF, and IL-6 (Fig. 1.3). Primary inflammatory cytokines are extremely pleiotropic, their spectrum of action encompassing different cells and tissues. In spite of the fact that they interact with structurally different receptors, their activities overlap substantially. IL-1 and TNF are unequivocally primary inflammatory cytokines, in that they set in motion the whole cascade of mediators (Figs 1.4–1.7). IL-6 tends to be more of a secondary mediator, fundamental for the acute-phase response in the liver, and has a regulatory function (Fig. 1.7). As illustrated in Fig. 1.3, the primary inflammatory cytokines, IL-1 and TNF, amplify leukocyte recruitment and survival of white cells in tissues,

Table 1.2 Pathophysiological conditions associated with a prevailing Th1 or Th2 responses

	Th1	Th2
Autoimmune	Hashimoto thyroiditis Graves ophthalmopathy Type I diabetes Multiple sclerosis Rheumatoid arthritis	Systemic sclerosis
Infectious or post-infectious	*Helicobacter pylori* gastritis Cerebral malaria Lyme disease Chronic type C virus hepatitis	Measles
Primary immunodeficiency	–	Omenn syndrome
Miscellaneous	Allograft rejection (acute) GVH disease (acute) Sarcoidosis Aplastic anemia Recurrent abortions	Atopic diseases Vernal conjuntivitis Allograft tolerance GVH disease (chronic) Normal pregnancy

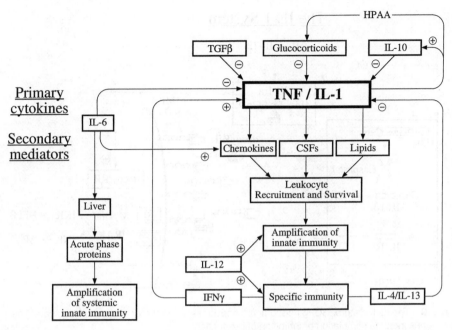

Fig. 1.3   The cascade of inflammatory cytokines. HPAA, hypothalamus-pituitary-adrenal axis.

TNFα and its receptors

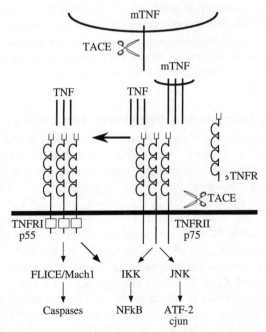

Fig. 1.4   TNF and its receptors (TNFR). m, membrane; s, soluble; R, receptor; TACE, TNFα converting enzyme.

The IL-1 System

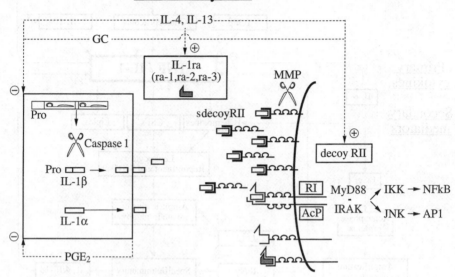

Fig. 1.5 The IL-1 system. GC, glucocorticoid hormones; ra, receptor antagonists, soluble. The + and − signs indicate stimulation or inhibition of production

through secondary mediators produced or acting on the vessel wall. Therefore, they amplify local mechanisms of innate resistance and set the stage for the activation of specific immunity. Systemically, production of IL-6 causes the production of acute-phase proteins in the liver, such as the pentraxins serum amyloid P-component and C-reactive protein, which opsonize microorganisms and debris, and activate complement, thus amplifying systemic innate immunity. As discussed below, these mediators are more than just individual agonists interacting with a receptor, and act as complex systems as illustrated in Fig. 1.5 for IL-1.

1.5.4 Secondary inflammatory cytokines: chemokines

Chemokines are a superfamily of small proteins vital to immune and inflammatory reactions and viral infection (Hedrick and Zlotnik, 1996; Baggiolini *et al.*, 1997; Rollins, 1997; Mantovani, 1999). Most chemokines cause chemotactic migration of leukocytes but they also affect angiogenesis, collagen production, and the proliferation of hematopoietic precursors. Based on a cysteine motif, a CXC, CC, C and CX3C family have been identified (Fig. 1.8). The chemokine scaffold consists of an N-terminal loop connected by Cys bonds to the more structured core of the molecule (3 β sheets) with a C terminal α helix. About 50 human chemokines have been identified.

Chemokines interact with seven transmembrane domain, G protein-coupled receptors. Ten CC (CCR1–8), five CXC (CXCR1–5) and one CX3C (CX3CR1) receptors have been identified. Receptor expression is crucial to the spectrum of action of chemokines. For instance, polarized Th1 and Th2 populations show different receptor expression and responsiveness to chemokines (Sallusto *et al.*, 1997; Bonecchi *et al.*, 1998; Loetscher *et al.*, 1998). Regulation of receptor expression during activation or deactivation of mono-

IL-1 AND TOLL RECEPTOR SIGNALING

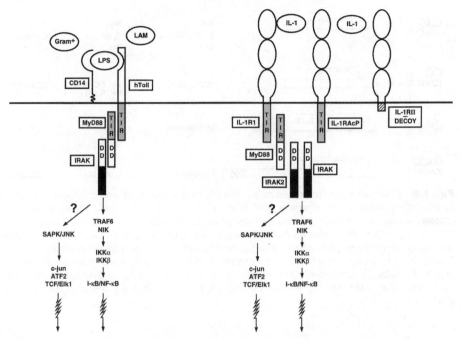

Fig. 1.6 The IL-1 receptor/Toll signaling cascade. The IL-1 receptor I (RI), in concert with the IL-1 accessory protein (AcP) and with a cytoplasmic adapter (MyD88), activates two kinases (IRAK). These, thourgh an adapter (TRAF6), activate the NIK kinase which in turn activates phosphorylation of the inhibitor of NF-kB (I-kB) through a kinase (IKKα), leading to NFkB activation. The same cascade is activated by Toll-like receptors (hToll) upon interaction with LPS, lipoarabinomannan (LAM) or Gram+ bacteria. TIR, Toll-IL-1R domain; DD, death domain.

IL-6 and its receptor

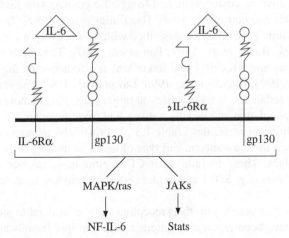

Fig. 1.7 IL-6 and its receptors. The soluble IL-6 Rα chain, present in biological fluids, forms a signal transducing complex with the agonist and with gp130 (transignaling).

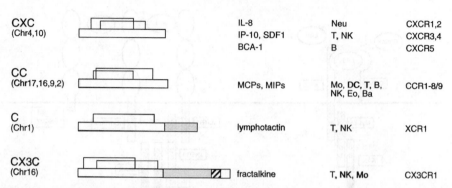

Fig. 1.8 Chemokine families: a schematic, simplified view. Acronyms and chromosomes refer to humans. Only prototypic molecules or families of molecules and main cellular targets are shown. Clusters of related molecules are identified as monocyte chemotactic proteins (MCP 1–4), macrophage inflammatory proteins (MIP), molecules with a 6 Cys motif (6 CCK). Certain molecules are bigger (lymphotactin, fractalkine), with a C terminal, mucin-like domain (dotted part). Fractalkine is expressed as a membrane molecule, with a transmembrane domain, on activated endothelial cells. The chromosomal localization is shown in parentheses and receptors are in the right-hand column. Mo, monocytes; Neu, neutrophils; Eo, eosinophils; Ba, basophils; DC, dendritic cells.

cytes is as important as regulation of chemokine production for tuning the chemokine system (Sica *et al.,* 1997; Sozzani *et al.,* 1998).

The chemokines' main function is chemotaxis for leukocytes. Schematically (Fig. 1.8), CXC (or) chemokines are mainly active on neutrophils (PMN) and T and B lymphocytes, while CC (or β) chemokines act on multiple leukocyte subtypes, including monocytes, basophils, eosinophils, T lymphocytes, dendritic cells and NK cells, but are generally not active on PMN. Eotaxins (CC) have the most restricted spectrum of action, being selectively active on eosinophilic and basophilic granulocytes (Schall, 1994; Ben-Baruch *et al.,* 1995; Sozzani *et al.,* 1996; Baggiolini *et al.,* 1997). Lymphotactin and fractalkine are the only proteins so far described with, respectively, a C and CX3C motif, (Kelner *et al.,* 1994; Bazan *et al.,* 1997; Pan *et al.,* 1997). They both act on lymphoid cells (T lymphocytes and NK cells), and fractalkine is also active on monocytes and NK cells (Kelner *et al.,* 1994; Bianchi *et al.,* 1996; Bazan *et al.,* 1997; Pan *et al.,* 1997).

Chemokines are redundant in their action on target cells. No chemokine is active only on one leukocyte population and usually a given leukocyte population has receptors for, and responds to, different molecules (Table 1.3). Interestingly, mononuclear phagocytes, in evolutionary terms the most ancient cell type of innate immunity, respond to the widest range of chemokines. These include most CC chemokines, fractalkine (CX3C) and certain CXC molecules (e.g. SDF1 and, under certain conditions, IL-8, for abbreviations, see Table 1.3).

The chemokines' interaction with their receptors show considerable promiscuity. Most known receptors have been reported to interact with multiple ligands and most ligands interact with more than one receptor. For instance, all four monocytic chemotactic pro-

Table 1.3   Expression of chemokine receptors in leukocyte populations: a simplified view

Receptor[a]	Main ligands[b]	Main cells[c]
CCR1	MCP-3, RANTES, MIP-1α	Mo, T, NK, iDC, Neu
CCR2 B/A	MCP-s (1–4)	Mo, T (act.) NK (act.)
CCR3	Eotaxin (1–3), MCP-3, RANTES	Eo, Ba, T (Th2)
CCR4	TARC, MDC	T (Th2, Tc2), NK, iDC
CCR5	MIP-1ß, MIP-1α, RANTES	Mo, T (Th1, Tc1), iDC
CCR6	MIP-3α/LARC/Exodus	T, iDC (CD34)
CCR7	ELC/MIP-3ß	T, Mo, mDC
CCR8	I309, TARC	T, (Th2/Tc2), Mo
CCR9	TECK	T, Mo, DC
CXCR1	IL-8, GCP-2	Neu
CXCR2	IL-8, GROs, NAP-2	Neu
CXCR3	IP10, MIG, ITAC	T (Th1, Tc1)
CXCR4	SDF-1	Widely expressed receptor
CXCR5	BCA-1	B
CX3CR1	Fractalkine	Mo, NK, T

[a] For certain chemokines the receptor(s) has (have) not been found yet.
[b] Only selected acronyms are presented. Abbreviations for chemokines: BCA-1, B cell-attracting chemokine 1; ELC, EBI (EBV-induced gene) 1-ligand chemokine (=MIP-3ß/CKß-11); GCP-2, granulocyte chemoattractant protein 2; IP-10, interferon γ inducible protein 10; GRO, growth-related oncogene; ITAC, interferon inducible T-cell α chemoattractant; LARC, liver and activation-regulated chemokine (MIP-3α/Exodus); MCP, monocyte chemotactic protein; MDC, macrophage-derived chemokine; MIG, monokine induced by interferon γ; MIP, macrophage inflammatory protein; RANTES, regulated on activation normal T cell expressed and secreted; SDF-1, stromal cell-derived factor; SLC, secondary lymphoid tissue chemokine; TARC, thymus and activation-regulated chemokine; TECK, thymus-expressed chemokine.
[c] (act), activated; Ba, basophils; DC, dendritic cells; iDC and mDC, immature and mature dendritic cells; DC(CD34), DC derived from CD34 cells *in vitro*; Eo, eosinophils; Mo, monocytes; Neu, neutrophils; Th, T helper; Tc, T cytotoxic.

teins (MCPs) interact with CCR2, and at least MCP-2, MCP-3, and MCP-4, also recognize other receptors (CCR1 and CCR3).

Probably all cell types can produce chemokines under appropriate conditions. Two general modes of chemokine production can be defined (Fig. 1.9). Molecules such as SDF1 or MDC (see Table 1.3. for abbreviations) are produced constitutively either by specialized cells and organs (macrophages, dendritic cells; thymus, and lymphoid organs for MDC) or in a more diffuse way as for SDF1. Most chemokines, however, are produced on cell activation. Interestingly, chemokines are also produced in a redundant way (polyspeirism, polus, many, speiro, make). Usually the same cell produces many chemokines concomitantly in response to the same stimulus. Polyspeirism is particularly striking for mononuclear phagocytes and endothelial cells exposed to bacterial products or primary inflammatory cytokines. In these cells, bacterial lipopolysaccharide, IL-1, and TNF elicit production of MCPs, MIPs, RANTES (CC), fractalkine (CCX3C), and various CXC molecules (Baggiolini *et al.*, 1994; Schall, 1994; Ben-Baruch *et al.*, 1995; Sozzani *et al.*, 1996; Mantovani *et al.*, 1997).

G protein-coupled receptors are a classic target in pharmacology. Given the role of chemokines in various human diseases, ranging from HIV infection to allergy, their pharmacology is a prime target for research. Although redundancy is a formidable stumbling block, interfering with one agonist or one receptor may be beneficial in certain disease models, as demonstrated for MCP-1 and its receptor CCR2 for monocytes, and for

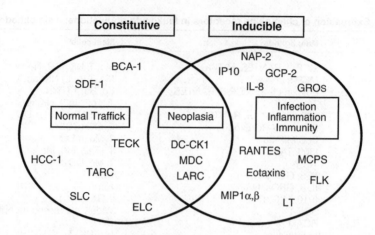

Fig. 1.9 A classification of chemokines based on the mode of production (for abbreviations, see Table 1.3). Certain chemokines are made constitutively in lymphoid organs (e.g. TARC, SLC) or by stromal cells (SDF1), whereas others are made 'on demand', in response to immune or inflammatory signals. The former are likely to play a role in basal leukocytes traffick, while the latter are responsible for recruitment in inflammatory and immune reactions. Tumors that produce inducible chemokines in a constitutive way, belong to both realms.

eotaxins and their receptor CCR3 for eosinophils and basophils. Therefore, simple chemicals with chemokine antagonistic properties or with selective inhibitory activity on chemokine production are a holy grail in present-day cytokine pharmacology.

1.5.5 Anti-inflammatory, immunosuppressive cytokines

Anti-inflammatory, immunosuppressive cytokines act as endogenous brakes for inflammation and immunity (Fig. 1.3). Suppression of inflammatory and immune responses is a property of various mediators, including IL-6, IL-13, IL-4. For these molecules, the ability to suppress the production, for instance, of IL-1 and TNF by macrophages, is one biological activity among a variety. In contrast, suppression of cytokine production is a major property of IL-10 and TGFβ. IL-10 is produced mainly by mononuclear phagocytes with kinetics somewhat delayed compared to the primary inflammatory cytokines IL-1 and TNF; its production serves as a negative feedback pathway for the inflammatory responses of these cells. In general, cytokines with anti-inflammatory activity, such as IL-4, IL-13, IL-10, TGFβ, inhibit production of IL-1 but do not interfere with, or stimulate, production of the receptor antagonist, and at least some of them increase the release of the IL-1 decoy receptor (Fig. 1.5).

1.6 Recurrent themes in the cytokine world

The mode of action of cytokines shows recurrent patterns that have profound implications for the design and implementation of therapeutic strategies. Some of these 'cytokine keywords' will be briefly discussed here.

1.6.1 Redundancy

Redundancy is a recurrent motif among cytokines. For instance, IL-1 and TNF elicit similar cellular responses *in vitro* and show remarkably similar spectra of action *in vitro* and *in vivo*. In spite of the fact that they interact with structurally different receptors, cellular responses are similar and in certain respects virtually superimposable. Notable exceptions are bone marrow hematopoietic precursors, which are stimulated by IL-1 and inhibited by TNF.

The chemokines are a second impressive example of redundancy. In this superfamily many of at least fifty molecules share the ability to elicit directional migration of leukocytes. As illustrated in Fig. 1.8, chemokines of the C–X–C family, with an ELR motif, can all elicit directional migration of neutrophils and many, if not all, molecules belonging to the C–C family induce migration of monocytes and have a broader spectrum of action. A notable feature of the chemokine system is the promiscuous usage of the receptor molecules, as illustrated in Table 1.3.

Redundancy of cytokines, illustrated here by IL-1 and TNF and chemokines, poses obvious problems for the design of therapeutic strategies. Which is the dominant mediator for a given human pathology? In the case of IL-1 and TNF, will one eventually need to block both mediators, which are usually synergistic, to obtain an appreciable therapeutic result? In the case of chemokines, which molecule(s) play(s) a dominant role in recruitment in a given disease? Will blocking one molecule/one receptor system give worthwhile therapeutic results? Is there a hierarchy?

1.6.2 Cascades and networks

Cytokines typically act as cascades or networks (Fig. 1.3). For instance, after administration of bacterial endotoxin to mimic septic shock, one can measure production first of TNF then of IL-1, IL-6, IL-10 and chemokines. In human rheumatoid arthritis, it has been suggested that TNF is produced as a consequence of an as yet undefined autoimmune reaction, setting in motion the whole cytokine cascade (see Chapter 5). TNF was, therefore, selected as a primary target for therapeutic intervention, using first blocking monoclonal antibodies and then soluble receptors. Under conditions in which a primary causative agent elicits concomitant production of different cytokines resulting more in a network than a cascade, given the possible synergistic interactions such as those between IL-1 and TNF, blocking one mediator may be sufficient to obtain a pharmacological effect.

1.6.3 Molecules and systems

Certain cytokines are complex systems with peculiar intrinsic regulatory pathways. The most dramatic illustration of a complex system is IL-1 (Fig. 1.5). The IL-1 system includes two agonists, α and β, a specific converting enzyme, IL-1 converting enzyme (ICE), now called caspase-1, a receptor antagonist, of which three isoforms have been cloned, and three IL-1 'receptors'; the type I receptor and the accessory protein (type III) are signal transducing molecules essential for IL-1 activity. The type II receptor represents a unique pathway of negative regulation acting as a decoy for IL-1; it is expressed on the cell surface and released in medium and biological fluids. Thus, the IL-1 system includes two unique negative pathways of regulation, the receptor antagonists and the decoy receptor, which have no counterparts for other cytokines or growth factors. The presence of these negative pathways of regulation highlights the need for tight control of the action of IL-1.

From a pharmacological point of view, it is of interest that certain endogenous anti-inflammatory agents coordinatedly regulate different elements in the system. For instance, anti-inflammatory cytokines such as IL-4 and IL-13 inhibit IL-1 production, increasing at the same time production of the receptor antagonist and the expression and release of the type II decoy receptor.

References

Atkins, E. and Wood, W. B. J. (1955). Studies on the pathogenesis of fever. II. Identification of an endogenous pyrogen in the bloodstream following the injection of typhoid vaccine. *J. Exp. Med.*, **102**, 499–516.

Atkins, E., Allison, F. J., Smith, M. R., and Wood, W. B. J. (1955). Studies on the antipyretic action of cortisone in pyrogen-induced fever. *J. Exp. Med.*, **101**, 353–66.

Auron, P. E., Webb, A. C., Rosenwasser, L. J., Mucci, S. F., Rich, A., Wolff, S. M., *et al.* (1984). Nucleotide sequence of human monocyte interleukin 1 precursor cDNA. *Proc. Natl. Acad. Sci. USA.*, **81**, 7907–11.

Baggiolini, M., Dewald, B., and Moser, B. (1994). Interleukin-8 and related chemotactic cytokines—CXC and CC chemokines. *Adv. Immunol.*, **55**, 99–179.

Baggiolini, M., Dewald, B., and Moser, B. (1997). Human chemokines: An update. *Annu. Rev. Immunol.*, **15**, 675–705.

Bazan, J. F., Bacon, K. B., Hardiman, G., Wang, W., Soo, K., Rossi, D., *et al.* (1997). A new class of membrane-bound chemokine with a CX3C motif. *Nature*, **385**, 640–4.

Ben-Baruch, A., Michiel, D. F., and Oppenheim, J. J. (1995). Signals and receptors involved in recruitment of inflammatory cells. *J. Biol. Chem.*, **270**, 11703–6.

Bianchi, G., Sozzani, S., Zlotnik, A., Mantovani, A., and Allavena, P. (1996). Migratory response of human NK cells to lymphotactin. *Eur. J. Immunol.*, **26**, 3238–41.

Bloom, B. R. and Bennett, B. (1966). Mechanism of a reaction *in vitro* associated with delayed-type hypersensitivity. *Science*, **153**, 80–2.

Bonecchi, R., Bianchi, G., Bordignon, P. P., D'Ambrosio, D., Lang, R., Borsatti, A., *et al.* (1998). Differential expression of chemokine receptors and chemotactic responsiveness of type 1 T helper cells (Th1) and Th2. *J. Exp. Med.*, **187**, 129–34.

Bradley, T. R. and Metcalf, D. (1966). The growth of mouse bone marrow cells *in vitro*. *Aust. J. Exptl. Biol. Med. Sci.*, **44**, 287–99.

Carswell, E. A., Old, L. J., Kassel, R. L., Green, S., and Fiore, N. (1975). An endotoxin-induced serum factor that causes necrosis of tumors. *Proc. Natl. Acad. Sci. USA.*, **72**, 3666–70.

Centanni, E. (1931). *Trattato di Immunologia*. Milano, Casa Editrice Ambrosiana.

Cohen, S., Bigazzi, P. E., and Yoshida, T. (1974). Similarities of T cell function in cell-mediated immunity and antibody production. *Cell Immunol.*, **12**, 150–9.

Colotta, F., Dower, S. K., Sims, J. E., and Mantovani, A. (1994). The type II 'decoy' receptor: novel regulatory pathway for interleukin-1. *Immunol. Today.*, **15**, 562–6.

David, J. R. (1966). Delayed hypersensitivity *in vitro*: its mediation by cell-free substances formed by lymphoid cell-antigen interaction. *Proc. Natl. Acad. Sci. USA.*, **56**, 72–7.

Dinarello, C. A. (1996). Biological basis for IL-1 in disease. *Blood*, **87**, 2095–147.

Dinarello, C. A. and Wolff, S. M. (1982). Molecular basis of fever in humans. *Am. J. Med.*, **72**, 799–819.

Dinarello, C. A., Renfer, L., and Wolff, S. M. (1977). Human leukocytic pyrogen: purification and development of a radioimmunoassay. *Proc. Natl. Acad. Sci. USA*, **74**, 4624–7.

Dumonde, D. C., Wolstencroft, R. A., Panayi, G. S., Matthew, M., and Howson, W. T. (1969). 'Lymphokines': non-antibody mediators of cellular immunity generated by lymphocyte activation. *Nature*, **224**, 38–42.

Fessler, J. H., Cooper, K. E., Cranston, W. I., and Vollum, R. L. (1961). Observations on the production of pyrogenic substances by rabbit and human leukocytes. *J. Exp. Med.*, **113**, 1127.

George, M. and Vaughan, J. H. (1962). *In vitro* cell migration as a model for delayed hypersensitivity. *Proc. Soc. Exp. Biol. Med.*, **111**, 514–21.

Hedrick, J. A. and Zlotnik, A. (1996). Chemokines and lymphocyte biology. *Curr. Opin. Immunol.*, **8**, 343–7.

Isaacs, A. and Lindenmann, J. (1957). Virus interference. I. The interferon. *Proc. Roy. Soc. Series B*, **147**, 258–67.

Kelner, G. S., Kennedy, J., Bacon, K. B., Kleyensteuber, S., Largaespada, D. A., Jenkins, N. A., *et al.* (1994). Lymphotactin: A cytokine that represents a new class of chemokine. *Science*, **266**, 1395–9.

Loetscher, P., Uguccioni, M., Bordoli, L., Baggiolini, M., Moser, B., Chizzolini, C., *et al.* (1998). CCR5 is characteristic of Th1 lymphocytes. *Nature*, **391**, 344–5.

Mantovani, A. (1999). The chemokine system: redundancy for robust outputs. *Immunol. Today.*, **20**, 254–7.

Mantovani, A., Bussolino, F., and Introna, M. (1997). Cytokine regulation of endothelial cell function: from molecular level to the bed side. *Immunol. Today.*, **18**, 231–9.

Morgan, D. A., Ruscetti, F. W., and Gallo, R. (1976). Selective *in vitro* growth of T lymphocytes from normal human bone marrows. *Science*, **193**, 1007–8.

Muzio, M. (1998). Signaling by proteolysis: death receptors induce apoptosis. *Int. J. Clin. Lab. Res.*, **28**, 141–7.

Nicola, N. A. (1994). *Guidebook to cytokines and their receptors* Sambrook and Tooze, Oxford

Oppenheim, J. J. (1994) Foreword. In *The cytokine handbook* (ed. A. W. Thomson), pp. xvii–xx, Academic Press, London

Pan, Y., Lloyd, C., Zhou, H., Dolich, S., Deeds, J., Gonzalo, J. A., *et al.* (1997). Neurotactin, a membrane-anchored chemokine upregulated in brain inflammation. *Nature*, **387**, 611–7.

Pluznik, D. H. and Sachs, L. (1965). The cloning of normal 'mast' cells in tissue culture. *J. Cell Physiol.*, **66**, 319–4.

Rich, A. R. and Lewis, M. R. (1932). The nature of allergy in tuberculosis as revealed by tissue culture studies. *Bull. Johns Hopkins Hosp.*, **50**, 115–31.

Rollins, B. J. (1997). Chemokines. *Blood*, **90**, 909–28.

Romagnani, S. (1997). The Th1/Th2 paradigm. *Immunol. Today.*, **18**, 263–6.

Sallusto, F., Mackay, C. R., and Lanzavecchia, A. (1997). Selective expression of the eotaxin receptor CCR3 by human T helper 2 cells. *Science*, **277**, 2005–7.

Schall, T. J. (1994). The Chemokines. In *The cytokine handbook* (ed. A. Thomson), pp. 419–60. Academic Press, London

Sica, A., Saccani, A., Borsatti, A., Power, C. A., Wells, T. N. C., Luini, W., *et al.* (1997). Bacterial lipopolysaccharide rapidly inhibits expression of C-C chemokine receptors in human monocytes. *J. Exp. Med.*, **185**, 969–74.

Sozzani, S., Locati, M., Allavena, P., Van Damme, J., and Mantovani, A. (1996). Chemokines: a superfamily of chemotactic cytokines. *Int. J. Clin. Lab. Res.*, **26**, 69–82.

Sozzani, S., Ghezzi, S., Iannolo, G., Luini, W., Borsatti, A., Polentarutti, N., *et al.* (1998). Interleukin-10 increases CCR5 expression and HIV infection in human monocytes. *J. Exp. Med.*, **187**, 439–44.

Waksman, B. H. and Matoltsy, M. (1958). The effect of tuberculin on peritoneal exudate cells of sensitized guinea pigs in surviving cell culture. *J. Immunol.*, **81**, 220–34.

Zinsser, H. and Tamiya, T. (1926). An experimental analysis of bacterial allergy. *J. Exp. Med.*, **44**, 753–78.

Part I

Pharmacology

2 *Inhibitors of cytokine production and action*

Since the first reports of protective effects of anti-cytokine antibodies in disease, industrial research has actively attempted to identify synthetic, simple chemicals to inhibit cytokine production or action. In particular, efforts have been aimed at developing receptor antagonists, an approach that has been successful in other areas of pharmacology. However, while the interest was obviously in identifying synthetic, orally active compounds, the really significant finding in this direction was the cloning of IL-1ra in 1990. More recently, screening of recombinant peptide display libraries has led to the identification of smaller peptides. With the advent of molecular modeling, the development of non-peptide inhibitors is forseeable in the future. For now, the general lack of success in the search for receptor antagonists has directed research towards inhibitors of cytokine synthesis or action by acting on specific signal transduction pathways implicated in the pro-inflammatory activities of cytokines. Table 2.1 gives a map of this chapter, and indicates the major classes of chemicals discussed.

Finally, in order to critically evaluate these pages, as well as future papers reporting on inhibitory or protective effect of drugs acting on cytokines, it is necessary to be familiar with the experimental models used to identify such drugs. In fact, while new classes of chemicals and pharmacological targets are likely to be discovered, the experimental models used for their identification and characterization have not changed much over the last ten years. We have, therefore, included a 'methodology' section on the experimental models used for the identification of cytokine inhibitors, which it is hoped will help in interpreting the actual meaning of the term 'cytokine inhibitor'.

2.1 Inhibitors of cytokine production

2.1.1 Glucocorticoids (GC)

This chapter will deal with the effects of exogenously administered GC on cytokine production and action. The physiological role of endogenous GC, as well as the elevation of their levels, will be dealt with in a separate chapter (Chapter 8) on hormonal regulation of cytokines. The effect of GC on chemokine production and receptor expression will be discussed later (Chapter 7).

Table 2.1 Classes of cytokine inhibitors and their main activities

Drugs	Major effects (cytokine production versus action)	Notes
Glucocorticoids	Production; induction of inhibitors	
Other steroids	Same as glucocorticoids	
Retinoids	Production	
Phosphodiesterase inhibitors	Production	Acts by elevating cAMP
Nitric oxide synthase inhibitors	Action (in small part also production)	
Prostaglandins	Production	Mostly by elevating cAMP; include PPARγ agonists
	action	
Cyclo-oxygenase inhibitors (NSAIDs)	Production/action	Include inhibitors of cytochromes P-450
Lipoxygenase inhibitors	Production/action	
Phospholipase A2 inhibitors	Production	
Protein kinase inhibitors	Production/action	Include p38 MAPK inhibitors and tyrphostins
Antioxidants	Production	Also see lazaroids (other steroids); include NF-κB inhibitors
Anti-endotoxin molecules	Mainly production	Peptides and proteins that bind LPS
Miscellaneous compounds	Mainly production	Thalidomide, CNI-1493, Benzydamine
Neurotransmitter receptors agonists and antagonist	Production	See Chapter 8
Psychotropic drugs	Action, production	See Chapter 8
MSH	Action	See Chapter 8
Tryptophan metabolism inhibitors		

Inhibition of cytokine production

Synthetic GC have been widely used as anti-inflammatory agents. They were the first drugs described that inhibit the synthesis of pro-inflammatory cytokines, because inhibition of IL-1 production (Snyder and Unanue, 1982) was reported in the early 1980s. A list of cytokines whose production was reported to be inhibited by GC is given in Table 2.2 (for review, see Almawi *et al.*, 1996). This includes cytokine production induced by bacteria or bacterial products, such as lipopolysaccharide (LPS), as well as that induced by other cytokines in a cascade fashion. *In vivo*, GC inhibit the production of circulating tumor necrosis factor (TNF), IL-1, IL-6 and IFN-γ in mice and rats treated with LPS or anti-CD3 antibodies (Staruch and Wood, 1985; Waage, 1987; Ferran *et al.*, 1990; Ulich *et al.*, 1990). Studies with LPS-treated human volunteers have also shown inhibition of circulating TNF and IL-6 levels (Rock *et al.*, 1992; Barber *et al.*, 1993).

GC reduce IL-1 production at both the transcriptional (Nishida *et al.*, 1988) and post-transcriptional level (Knudsen *et al.*, 1987; Lee S.W. *et al.*, 1988). GC block expression of the IL-1β transcript in IL-1-stimulated astrocytoma cells (Nishida *et al.*, 1989) and in LPS-activated monocytes (Lew *et al.*, 1988) and U937 cells (Knudsen *et al.*, 1987). Although one study failed to report GC-induced suppression of IL-1 transcription, the high LPS concentration used in that study (10 μg/ml) could have overcome GC activity (Kern *et al.*, 1988). The molecular mechanism for inhibition of IL-1 production seems also to involve a decrease in mRNA stability (Lee S.W. *et al.*, 1988). It should be noted that GC are not inhibitory when PMA, rather than LPS, is used as an inducer, probably because PMA stabilizes IL-1 mRNA (Hurme *et al.*, 1991). Also, TNF and IL-8 production are not inhibited by GC when PMA is used as stimulus (Debets *et al.*, 1989; Anttila *et al.*, 1992). The susceptibility of the various cytokines to the inhibitory effect of GC *in vivo* is not the same and TNF is generally more sensitive to GC (Zuckerman *et al.*, 1991; Sironi *et al.*, 1992).

The inhibitory effect of GC is mediated primarily through the type II GC receptor, as inhibition of TNF production in human and murine monocytic cells is antagonized by

Table 2.2 Cytokines whose synthesis is inhibited by GC

Cytokine	Selected references
Pro-inflammatory cytokines	
IL-1β	(Arend and Massoni, 1986; Knudsen *et al.*, 1987; Ghezzi and Dinarello, 1988)
IL-2	(Tracey *et al.*, 1988)
IL-6	(Waage *et al.*, 1990; Tobler *et al.*, 1992)
IL-8	(Brown *et al.*, 1991; Anttila *et al.*, 1992; Tobler *et al.*, 1992)
IL-12	(Kubin *et al.*, 1994)
IFNγ	(Gessani *et al.*, 1988; Kunicka *et al.*, 1993)
MCP-1	(Villiger *et al.*, 1992)
TNF	(Beutler *et al.*, 1986; Debets *et al.*, 1989)
Hemopoietic cytokines	
GM-CSF	(Hamilton *et al.*, 1992; Tobler *et al.*, 1992)
G-CSF	(Hamilton *et al.*, 1992; Kerner *et al.*, 1992)
M-CSF	(Campbell *et al.*, 1993)
IL-3	(Culpepper and Lee, 1985)
Others	
IL-4	(Byron *et al.*, 1992; Kunicka *et al.*, 1993)
IL-5	(Volterra *et al.*, 1992)

the type II GC receptor antagonist RU38486 (Fantuzzi *et al.*, 1995*a*; Di Santo *et al.*, 1996*b*).

Two models have been proposed for the inhibition of cytokine production by GC, as reviewed by Almawi *et al*, (Almawi *et al.*, 1996). In one model, the activated GC receptor would bind to GC response elements present in cytokine genes, thus resulting in transcriptional repression. In a second model, the GC receptor acts by inhibiting transcription factors implicated in cytokine gene transcription, including AP-1, NF-AT and NF-κB. Recent results have shown that GC decrease NF-κB activation by inducing its cytoplasmic inhibitor, IκB (Auphan *et al.*, 1995; Scheinman *et al.*, 1995) or through the interaction between the p65 subunit of transcription factor NF-κB and the GC receptor (Ray and Prefontaine, 1994), thus stressing the opposing role of GC and NF-κB in inflammation.

GC inhibition of NF-κB might well contribute to the inhibition of synthesis of several cytokines as the promoter sequences of many of them have NF-κB sites (Baeuerle and Henkel, 1994; Baldwin Jr., 1996).

Inhibition of IL-1 gene expression by GC is reversed by inhibition of protein synthesis (Lee S.W. *et al.*, 1988). This is reminiscent of the fact that some of the anti-inflammatory activities of GC require protein synthesis because they are mediated by lipocortins (Hiralta *et al.*, 1980; Flower, 1988). In fact, one study has shown that a lipocortin-1 N-terminal fragment (amino acids 1–188) inhibits TNF production in human peripheral blood mononuclear cells and, more importantly, that dexamethasone suppression of LPS-stimulated TNF production was reversed by a polyclonal antibody to lipocortin-1 N-terminal fragment (Sudlow *et al.*, 1996). The effect of GC on the production of IL-1 or TNF can be modulated by other cytokines in a complex fashion. The anti-inflammatory cytokine IL-4 potentiates the inhibitory action of GC on IL-1, TNF and PGE2 production by human monocytes (Hart *et al.*, 1990). Also, ciliary neurotrophic factor (CNTF) potentiates the inhibitory effect of dexamethasone (decreasing its inhibitory concentration, IC_{50}) on TNF production in mouse splenocytes (Benigni *et al.*, 1995).

On the contrary, inhibition of TNF production by GC in mouse peritoneal macrophages is partially reversed by IFN-γ (Luedke and Cerami, 1990), which acts by increasing TNF mRNA levels in LPS-treated macrophages. This GC-antagonizing effect of IFN-γ is particularly important as IFN-γ is often increased in infectious and inflammatory diseases.

Another interesting observation emerges from recent studies on macrophage migration inhibitory factor (MIF). This cytokine, originally discovered as an inhibitor of macrophage migration, has been shown to be a toxic mediator of endotoxic shock, as demonstrated by the protective effect of anti-MIF antibodies in animal models (Bernhagen *et al.*, 1993). Calandra *et al.*, have shown (1995) that very low concentrations of GC (10^{-10}–10^{-14} M) induce, rather than inhibit, MIF production by macrophages. MIF produced in this way is then able to overcome inhibition of TNF secretion mediated by GCs and thus could antagonize GC protection against endotoxemia. The bottom line of this observation is that GC may, at very low concentrations, amplify the cytokine-mediated inflammatory response rather than inhibit it.

Another example of cytokines overriding an inhibitory effect of GC is the report that IFN-γ and IL-4 can antagonize the inhibition of IL-1ra production by GC (Kovalovsky *et al.*, 1998).

Interestingly, the LPS-induced production of the anti-inflammatory cytokine IL-10 (which inhibits IL-1 and TNF production) is increased, both *in vivo* in mice and in mouse peritoneal macrophages *in vitro*, by the synthetic GC dexamethasone (Mengozzi *et al.*, 1994) and methylprednisolone (Marchant *et al.*, 1996). It should be mentioned that one study (Kunicka *et al.*, 1993) reported that in lymphocytes stimulated with anti-CD3 monoclonal antibodies, the *in vitro* production of all cytokines, including IL-2, IFNγ, TNF, IL-4, IL-6, and IL-10, is inhibited by an *in vivo* pretreatment with dexamethasone.

While most of the attention has been focused on the direct, acute inhibitory effect of GC on cytokine production, GC may change the balance between Th1 and Th2 production pattern. In fact, 3–4 day incubation of CD4+ T cells with dexamethasone promotes a Th2 response, increasing the production of IL-4, IL-10 and IL-13 (Ramirez *et al.*, 1996). Furthermore, a recent review suggested that physiological concentrations of GC down-regulate Th1 cytokines and up-regulate Th2 cytokines (Rook *et al.*, 1994).

The effect of GC on cytokine production by different stimuli, relevant to specific pathologies different from bacterial infection, was also studied. GC inhibit the production of TNF in a murine model of partial hepatectomy (Satoh *et al.*, 1991), that of IL-6 in a rat model of adjuvant arthritis (Theisen-Popp *et al.*, 1992) and that of IL-1 in a rat model of zymosan-induced pleurisy (Perretti *et al.*, 1992).

Ex vivo studies on cells from patients with sarcoidosis (Zabel *et al.*, 1990), Crohn's disease (Andus *et al.*, 1991) or rheumatoid arthritis (Seitz *et al.*, 1991) found decreased IL-1, IL-6 and IL-8 production after GC treatment.

GC are still the most potent inhibitors of cytokine production and are often used both as reference compounds in the identification of novel inhibitors of cytokines and as reference inhibitors of cytokine production in order to verify the role of cytokines in pathogenic models. Thus, it is difficult to understand that GC may not be beneficial in animal models of IL-1- or TNF-mediated diseases. It should be noted, however, that when GC act by inhibiting TNF or IL-1 production, they have to be given before (or shortly after) endotoxin or bacteria. This may be an important point in considering the lack of efficacy of GC in septic shock reported in some clinical trials (Bone *et al.*, 1987; Veterans Administration Systemic Sepsis Cooperative Study Group, 1987). One exception to this might be in the case of bacterial meningitis where, in some cases, the peak of cytokine release due to the LPS release induced by treatment with antibiotics can be predicted (see Chapter 8)

The effect of GC on IL-1ra is controversial. While some reports show an inhibition of IL-1ra production by GC (Arzt *et al.*, 1994; Sauer *et al.*, 1996; Kovalovsky *et al.*, 1998), others report no effect, even in the presence of an inhibited IL-1 production (Santos *et al.*, 1993; Sousa *et al.*, 1997). While the reports of an inhibition of IL-1ra production by GC used *in vitro* models, those reporting a lack of effect were *in vivo* studies. Thus, a possible explanation for the discrepancy is that IL-1ra is less sensitive to GC inhibition than IL-1. One report indicated that the mRNA for an intracellular form of IL-1ra is induced by GC (Levine *et al.*, 1996). *In vitro*, induction of IL-1ra synthesis by the two anti-inflammatory cytokines, IL-4 and IL-10, is also inhibited by GC (Joyce *et al.*, 1996)

Another anti-inflammatory effect of GC on the IL-1 system is the induction of type II IL-1 receptor (Colotta and Mantovani, 1994; Re *et al.*, 1994), which acts as a decoy receptor (see Chapter 1). This effect is part of a general up-regulation of cytokine receptors by GC, which was reported for other cytokines, including IL-2, IL-6, IFNγ, CSF-1 and GM-CSF (Almawi *et al.*, 1996; Wiegers and Reul, 1998). More recently, GC were reported to up-regulate the chemokine receptor CXCR4 and CCR2 (Wang *et al.*, 1998; Penton-Rol *et al.*, 1999).

Up-regulation of cytokine production

As discussed above, GC tend to augment or, at least, spare the production of anti-inflammatory cytokines, including IL-10, IL-1ra and the IL-1 decoy receptor. The inhibitory effect of GC on pro-inflammatory cytokine production is clear when they are given as a pretreatment or a co-treatment, normally from 0 to 60 min before administration of LPS. When the pretreatment time is longer than 12 h, a paradoxical increase in TNF production has been observed. This was observed in mice when GC (dexamethasone) was given as a single dose 24–48 h before LPS or chronically for 4 days, followed by a 2-day washout period (Fantuzzi *et al.*, 1994). Also, in healthy human volunteers given a bolus of LPS, GC (hydrocortisone) had an inhibitory effect (almost 100% inhibition) on serum TNF and IL-6 levels when LPS was given within 6 h of GC administration. Conversely, an increased TNF and IL-6 production (5–10-fold) was observed when the interval between GC pretreatment and LPS was 12 h or 6 days (Barber *et al.*, 1993). This paradoxical increase in cytokine production induced by early GC pretreatment might be regarded as a classical pharmacological rebound effect, well known for GC. One possible explanation is that GC pretreatment desensitizes the hypothalamus-pituitary-adrenal axis (as observed after chronic stress), thus blocking the feedback response mediated by endogenous GC. This effect would be evident only when the exogenously administered GC is washed out, thus explaining the need for a 12-h interval. In fact, this desensitization (the lack of corticosterone elevation in response to LPS) was observed in GC pretreated mice (Fantuzzi *et al.*, 1994). However, some dissociation between the ability of GC pretreatment to up-regulate TNF production and to inhibit the hypothalamus-pituitary-adrenal axis response was observed. In fact, a 48-h dexamethasone pretreatment in mice still potentiated TNF production without affecting neither basal nor LPS-induced CS levels (Fantuzzi *et al.*, 1994). Furthermore, the same effect was observed in humans in which a 6-day hydrocortisone pretreatment before LPS increased TNF levels without any change in circulating cortisol (Barber *et al.*, 1993). Thus other mechanisms might be responsible for the observed effect. One possibility is that this is due to GC induction of cytochrome P-450 3A, which is known to produce nitric oxide (NO). In fact, the up-regulating effect of dexamethasone on TNF production is associated with increased NO production and both the up-regulation of NO and of TNF production by dexamethasone are inhibited by co-administration of the P-450 3A inhibitor troleandomycin. These data suggest that P-450 3A-generated NO might be involved in TNF induction. Thus, this paradoxical increase in TNF production by early GC pretreatment might suggest the existence of other pharmacological targets to inhibit TNF production (Fantuzzi *et al.*, 1995).

2.1.2 Other steroids

In addition to GC, other steroids that do not act through the GC receptor affect cytokine production.

Androgens and estrogens

Lack of gonadal hormones induced by orchiectomy in mice elevates serum IL-6 and this effect can be reversed by administration of testosterone (Bellido *et al.*, 1995). *In vitro*, dihydrotestosterone inhibits IL-6 transcription through activation of the androgen receptor, in part but not exclusively, by inhibition of NF-κB (Keller *et al.*, 1996). It was hypothesized that as IL-6 levels increase with age, this might be related to age-associated decrease of androgen levels (Keller *et al.*, 1996). Inhibition of IL-6 production by 17-β-estradiol, androstenedione, androstenediol and progesterone was also reported (Pottratz *et al.*, 1994; Bellido *et al.*, 1995). This matter will be discussed again when dealing with bone resorption.

Estrogens also modulate cytokine production. Reports on the effects of estrogens, such as estradiol, on TNF production, ranged from increased TNF production to a decrease in TNF production, depending on the experimental models. On the other hand, most reports show that estrogens inhibit IL-6 production. Most of these reports investigate IL-6 production in relation to bone resorption.

The fact that trasngenic mice overexpressing sTNFR (Amman *et al.*, 1997) or IL-6-deficient mice (Poli *et al.*, 1994) are resistant to bone loss induced by estrogen deficiency, strenghten the importance of these observations. Estrogens also inhibit osteoclast expression of IL-1RI, while increasing IL-1RII expression and sIL-1RII release, suggesting they may thus counteract also IL-1 action (Sunyer *et al.*, 1999)

Neurosteroids

This term indicates a series of steroids including progesterone and dehydroepiandrosterone (DHEA) that are intermediates in the synthesis of sex hormones. Neurosteroids are synthesized in the adrenals and the gonads but can be produced in the brain, where they have a role as endogenous modulators of the gamma-aminobutyric acid receptor. They were reported to inhibit LPS-induced TNF production, and to be protective in a murine model of LPS toxicity (Danenberg *et al.*, 1992; Di Santo *et al.*, 1996*b*). They do not activate the GC receptor and their inhibitory effect on TNF production is not reversed by RU38486, indicating that their mechanism of action is different from that of GC (Di Santo *et al.*, 1996*b*). A recent report suggested that DHEA might inhibit cytokine production by acting on the peroxisome proliferator-activated receptor-α (Poynter and Daynes, 1998).

The inhibition of TNF production could be ascribed either to an antioxidant activity of DHEA sulfate (DHEAS) or to its interaction with the γ-aminobutyric acid (GABA) receptor, as suggested by the reversal of its inhibitory effect by GABA (Di Santo *et al.*, 1996*a*). DHEAS declines by 80–90% with aging and its administration to old mice decreases age-associated IL-6 production (Daynes *et al.*, 1993). In mice infected with a murine leukemia retrovirus, DHEAS administration partially reversed the infection-associated decrease in the production of two Th1 cytokines, IL-2 and IFN-γ, and inhibited the increase of IL-6 and TNF production (Araghi-Niknam *et al.*, 1997).

Lazaroids (21-aminosteroids)

21-aminosteroids (also termed lazaroids) are methylprednisolone derivatives, which are devoid of GC or mineralcorticoid activity. They were originally developed for neuroprotection based on the concept that the efficacy of high doses of methylprednisolone in spinal cord injury, stroke, and subarachnoid hemorrhage (for which lazaroids are currently in phase III trials) is not mediated by the GC receptor (Hall *et al.*, 1994). Although the mechanism of action is far from being established, it was suggested that lazaroids act as antioxidants (Hall *et al.*, 1994).

The data on their effects on cytokine production are contrasting. One study on human peripheral blood mononuclear cells stimulated with LPS and phytoemagglutinin (PHA), reported no inhibition of TNF or IL-6 production by lazaroids U-74389G (16-desmethyl tirilazad) and U-74500A. This data was used to confirm that 21-aminosteroids do not act through the GC receptor (Buttgereit *et al.*, 1995). On the other hand, *in vivo* administration of U74389F to mice inhibits pulmonary expression of IL-1 beta, IL-6, IL-10, TNF-alpha and IFNγ induced by hemorrhage (Shenkar and Abraham, 1995), while U74500A reduced production of IL-1β by monocytes exposed to myelin (Fisher *et al.*, 1993).

2.1.3 Retinoids

Vitamin A and its analogues are important regulators of cell growth and differentiation. Retinoids are ligands for nuclear receptors (retinoic acid receptors, RAR) that belong to the superfamily of GC/thyroid hormone nuclear receptors, and also have antioxidant activity. Retinoic acid is an inhibitor of IL-1-induced IL-6 production in human lung fibroblasts (Zitnik *et al.*, 1994). Furthermore, one study with several synthetic retinoids has shown a correlation between their ability to inhibit IL-1-induced IL-6 production in the MC3T3-E1 mouse osteogenic fibroblast cell line with their affinity to the nuclear retinoic acid receptor (Kagechika *et al.*, 1997). However, this inhibition was dependent on the stimulus used (it inhibited IL-1-induced, not TNF-induced, IL-6 production) and cell specific (it did not inhibit IL-1-induced IL-6 production in other cell types) suggesting that the effect is not specific for the IL-6 promoter (Zitnik *et al.*, 1994).

Vitamin D also has important immunosuppressive effects and inhibits EAE (Lemire and Archer, 1991). Peripheral blood monocytes from healthy volunteers treated with vitamin D produce less TNF and IL-1 (Muller *et al.*, 1991), and similar effects were reported *in vitro* (Muller *et al.*, 1992). Vitamin D3 inhibits IL-12 production by activated macrophages and dendritic cells, possibly by down-regulation of NF-κB (D'Ambrosio *et al.*, 1998). Also the up-regulation by vitamin D of TGF-beta and IL-4 might contribute to its protective effect in EAE (Cantorna *et al.*, 1998). Vitamin D compound also inhibit the synthesis of RANTES and IL-8 (Harant *et al.*, 1997; Fukuoka *et al.*, 1998).

2.1.4 Drugs acting by increasing cAMP levels

The most important effect of cAMP on cytokine production is its inhibition of TNF production (Renz *et al.*, 1988; Spengler *et al.*, 1989; Bailly *et al.*, 1990). The efficiency of cAMP as a TNF inhibitor has also been exploited by leukemia viruses. In fact, the CSK-17 envelope protein of leukemia viruses augments cAMP levels and suppresses TNF production (Haraguchi *et al.*, 1997). Chemokine (MIP-1 alpha, MIP-1 beta and MCP-1) mRNA expression in macrophage cell lines is also inhibited by cAMP-elevating agents (Martin and Dorf, 1991). This effect, however, seems specific for TNF and the synthesis of other cytokines is increased by cAMP. cAMP induces the following cytokines: IL-5 in the D10A Th2 cell line (Muñoz *et al.*, 1992); IL-6 in fibroblasts (Zhang *et al.*, 1988), mouse BMS2 cells (Gimble *et al.*, 1991), and anterior pituitary cells (Spangelo *et al.*, 1990); IL-8 in human monocytes (Anttila *et al.*, 1992); and IL-10 in monocytes/macrophages and *in vivo* (Strassmann *et al.*, 1994; Platzer *et al.*, 1995; Kambayashi *et al.*, 1995; Meisel *et al.*, 1996).

Induction of IL-1 by cAMP was also reported in human monocytes or myelomonocytic cell lines (Kaissis *et al.*, 1989; Sung and Walters, 1991; Serkkola *et al.*, 1992) and mouse P388D1 cells (Okamoto *et al.*, 1990) or macrophages (Ohmori *et al.*, 1990). In some cases, cAMP (or PGE2 or forskolin) did not induce IL-1 expression alone but potentiated that induced by phorbol myristate acetate (PMA) (Hurme *et al.*, 1990). This cAMP-potentiated IL-1 induction was insensitive to the protein kinase A inhibitor HA1004 (Hurme *et al.*, 1990). It should be noted, however, that other studies on the effect of cAMP on IL-1 synthesis reported no effect (Endres *et al.*, 1991) or even inhibition (Knudsen *et al.*, 1986; Tannenbaum and Hamilton, 1989; Hurme, 1990).

The studies of the effect of cAMP on cytokine production were prompted by initial observations that phosphodiesterase inhibitors inhibited TNF production by macrophages (Strieter *et al.*, 1988). The inhibitory effect of cAMP was then demonstrated using cell permeable cAMP analogues (e.g. dibutyril cAMP). Raising cAMP formation with agents that stimulate adenylate cyclase, such as PGE_2, forskolin, or cholera toxin, also inhibit production of TNF (Spengler *et al.*, 1989, Tannenbaum and Hamilton, 1989), IL-1 (Sung and Walters, 1991) and IL-2 (Anastassiou *et al.*, 1992). The latter study showed that the inhibitory effect of cAMP (and cAMP-elevating agents PGE2 and cholera toxin) on IL-2 expression was both at the transcriptional and post-transcriptional levels and was reversed by the protein kinase A inhibitor, N-[2-(Methylamino)ethyl]-5-isoquinolinesulfonamide (H8) (Anastassiou *et al.*, 1992).

cAMP has also been suggested to be responsible for the inhibition of TNF production observed *in vitro* with human immunoglobulin preparations for intravenous use (Shimozato *et al.*, 1991). cAMP-mediated inhibition of TNF production was inhibited by H-8, an inhibitor of cyclic nucleotide-dependent protein kinases, suggesting they are involved in this effect of cAMP (Shimozato *et al.*, 1991).

This pharmacological target might be particularly important in consideration of the fact that LPS inhibits the response to PGE_2 and epinephrine in terms of cAMP elevation, possibly by activating a phosphodiesterase (Hazechi *et al.*, 1986; Okonogi *et al.*, 1991). This suggests that inflammatory stimuli may deactivate the mechanism leading to augmented cAMP levels.

From the pharmacological point of view, phosphodiesterase inhibitors are actively studied as inhibitors of TNF production. In fact, some inhibitors are selective for various phosphodiesterase isozyme families. The phosphodiesterases include: (I) Ca++/calmodulin-dependent, (II) cGMP-stimulated, (III) cGMP-inhibited, (IV) cAMP-specific, and (V) cGMP specific (Beavo and Reifsnyder, 1990) (Table 2.3). There is a particular interest toward phosphodiesterase (PDE) IV inhibitors, which would specifically increase cAMP.

Table 2.3 Nomenclature of major PDE gene families

PDE family	Designation	Specific inhibitors
I	Ca++-calmodulin-dependent PDE	Phenothiazines, vinpocetine
II	cGMP-stimulated PDE	–
III	cGMP-inhibited PDE	Cilostamide, milrinone, enoximone, imadozan, SKF94120, trequinsin, quazinone, indolidan, carbazeran, anagrelide
IV	cAMP-specific PDE	Rolipram, RO201724
V	cGMP-specific PDE	Dipyridamole, zaprinast

Reviewed in (Beavo and Reifsnyder, 1990; Beavo *et al.*, 1994).

Among the PDE inhibitors, pentoxifylline has been the subject of most efforts. This drug is currently used to treat peripheral vascular diseases (Serafin, 1996). Its inhibition of TNF production and protective effect on LPS toxicity (Strieter *et al.*, 1988; Noel *et al.*, 1990) has prompted several studies that show its efficacy in animal models of various diseases where TNF is implicated. These diseases include EAE, meningitis, and acute respiratory distress syndrome (ARDS) (Saez-Llorens *et al.*, 1990; Nataf *et al.*, 1993; van Leenen *et al.*, 1993) and will be discussed in specific chapters. In guinea-pigs, pentoxifylline inhibits the second peak of LPS-induced fever (which is probably TNF-mediated), leaving intact the early peak (Goldbach *et al.*, 1997). Studies in LPS-treated human volunteers have confirmed its inhibition of TNF production (Zabel *et al.*, 1989). A double-blind, placebo-controlled study has shown that pentoxifylline is able to decrease serum TNF (but not IL-6 or IL-8) levels in patients with septic shock, although no improvement in the hemodynamics was observed (Zeni *et al.*, 1996). As an expected consequence of its inhibitory effect on cytokine production, pentoxifylline, like dexamethasone, impairs macrophage defense against *Mycobacterium avium* complex, suggesting a potentially harmful effect of inhibitors of TNF synthesis in AIDS patients (Sathe *et al.*, 1995). Pentoxifylline was also documented to up-regulate the production of IL-10 by monocytes (Platzer *et al.*, 1995).

Non-specific PDE inhibitors, such as theophylline, pentoxifylline, and 3-isobutyl-1-methylxanthine, selectively decrease TNF production (and its mRNA levels) in monocyte/macrophages (Renz *et al.*, 1988; Strieter *et al.*, 1988; Endres *et al.*, 1991; Molnar-Kimber *et al.*, 1992). One study that compared different PDE inhibitors for their effect on TNFα and IL-1β production by human monocytes *in vitro* (Molnar-Kimber *et al.*, 1992) reported that PDE I inhibitors (vinpocetine) did not affect TNF or IL-1 production, while PDE III inhibitors (CI 930 and milrinone) only slightly inhibited TNF production and did not affect that of IL-1. PDE IV inhibitors (rolipram, nitraquazone) markedly inhibited TNF production ($IC_{50} = 0.2–0.3$ μM) and, to a lesser extent, IL-1 production. In contrast, zaprinast, a PDE V inhibitor that should raise cGMP levels, slightly increased TNF production in agreement with other reports of a stimulatory, rather than inhibitory, role of cGMP on TNF production (Renz *et al.*, 1988; Sprenger *et al.*, 1991).

There is a particular interest towards PDE IV inhibitors, which would specifically increase cAMP. One of these, rolipram, also inhibits TNF production, protects mice from experimental autoimmune encephalomyelitis (EAE) (Sinha *et al.*, 1995; Sommer *et al.*, 1995; Greten *et al.*, 1996) and has anti-inflammatory activity in a murine model of zymosan-induced inflammation (Klemm *et al.*, 1996).

The inhibitory effect of cAMP on TNF production takes place at the transcriptional level (Tannenbaum and Hamilton, 1989; Taffet *et al.*, 1989). However, part of it seems to be mediated by the cAMP-induced up-regulation of IL-10 production. As anti-IL-10, antibodies partially reverse the TNF inhibitory effect of PGE2, both in murine peritoneal macrophages *in vitro* and in LPS-treated mice *in vivo* (Strassmann *et al.*, 1994). The same authors have shown that cAMP elevation attained with the PDE IV inhibitors rolipram and RO-20–1724, up-regulate IL-10 and inhibit TNF production *in vivo* and *in vitro*, while non-PDE IV specific inhibitors OPC 13013, 8-methoxymethyl-isobutyl methylxanthine and quinazone (which do not increase macrophage cAMP) did not (Kambayashi *et al.*, 1995). Interestingly, *in vivo* rolipram increases spleen IL-10 mRNA levels but does not inhibit TNF mRNA (Kambayashi *et al.*, 1995), which would suggest a post-transcriptional inhibition of TNF production.

Adrenergic receptor agonists

Beta-adrenergic agonists have long been known to inhibit TNF production (Hetier *et al.*, 1991), and this probably contributes to the increased TNF production observed in adrenalectomized (Zuckerman *et al.*, 1989) or sympathectomized animals (Chelmicka-Schorr *et al.*, 1992). More recently, β2-agonists have been shown to inhibit IL-12 production in human monocytes and dendritic cells, possibly by elevating cAMP levels. Furthermore, one of these drugs, solbutamol, inhibited IL-12 production *in vivo* in mice (Panina-Bordignon *et al.*, 1997). The effect of adrenaline and β-adrenergic agonists, such as isoproterenol, are likely mediated by an elevation of intracellular cAMP (Severn *et al.*, 1992).

This inhibitory pathway can be defective in infectious and inflammatory diseases; in fact, TNF, IL-1 and the HIV coat protein gp120, inhibit the adrenergic responsiveness in terms of elevation of cAMP (Gulick *et al.*, 1989; Levi *et al.*, 1993). TNF was also reported to decrease the expression of β-adrenergic receptors in adipose tissue (Berkowitz *et al.*, 1998).

2.1.5 Drugs acting on the nitric oxide (NO) pathway

Nitric oxide (NO) is one of the most studied mediators of cytokine action and will be discussed in detail below. A number of studies have shown that, on the contrary, NO can regulate cytokine production. This has an immediate pharmacological relevance because several inhibitors of NO production have been developed. The pathologies in which inhibition of NO production can be tested are often the same pathologies where TNF is produced, hence it is important to know the effect of endogenous NO on TNF production.

Most authors report that NO donors stimulate the release of TNF (Lander *et al.*, 1993; Wang *et al.*, 1997) and of IL-8 (Remick and Villarete, 1996) and activate NF-κB (Lander *et al.*, 1993), although one report indicated an inhibitory effect of NO donors (Eigler *et al.*, 1995).

The main biological activities of NO (including vasorelaxation) are mediated by activation of guanylate cyclase and, in this respect, NO can be regarded as a cGMP-elevating agent. As mentioned above, there are reports that cGMP, either exogenously added or increased by cGMP-elevating agents, up-regulates TNF production *in vitro* (Renz *et al.*, 1988; Sprenger *et al.*, 1991). Others have shown a dissociation between elevation of cGMP, and induction of TNF and activation of NF-κB by NO donors, suggesting that these might act by decreasing cAMP (Lander *et al.*, 1993; Wang *et al.*, 1997).

The fact that some NO donors used *in vitro* also release cyanide makes these data difficult to interpret. It is also possible that low concentrations of NO potentiate TNF production, while high concentrations inhibit it.

A second aspect is the role of endogenously produced NO. NO can be studied using inhibitors of NO synthase (NOS), and the results are suggestive of a stimulatory role of endogenous NO. In fact, inhibitors of NOS, such as L-N-monomethylarginine (L-NMMA) or N-iminoethyl-L-ornithine, attenuated TNF production by LPS-stimulated mouse J774 cells (Deakin *et al.*, 1995) or human THP-1 cells (Zinetti *et al.*, 1995). Similarly, L-NMMA reduced serum TNF release *in vivo* in LPS-treated mice (Rojas *et al.*, 1993). Along this line, it was shown that human U937 cells transfected with NOS cDNA produced more TNF than control transfectant, and this difference was inhibited by L-NMMA (Yan *et al.*, 1997).

2.1.6 Drugs acting on arachidonic acid metabolism and other lipid mediators

Inhibitors of arachidonic acid metabolism

Classical anti-inflammatory agents, normally used as reference controls in the testing of new drugs, include inhibitors of arachidonic acid metabolism. In fact, arachidonic acid oxygenation products, particularly prostaglandins (Fig. 2.1) are inflammatory mediators strictly related to pro-inflammatory cytokines, and both the synthesis and the action of these two classes of mediators are largely interdependent.

Earlier studies on pharmacomodulation of IL-1, IL-6 and TNF production, investigating the effect of non-steroidal anti-inflammatory drugs (NSAID) that act by inhibiting cyclooxygenase (COX), described an apparently paradoxical effect. In fact, NSAID, particularly indomethacin, increased rather than inhibited, LPS-induced cytokine (TNF and IL-1) production, thus leading to the discovery that prostaglandins, particularly PGE2, are potent inhibitors of TNF and IL-1 production (Brandwein, 1986; Knudsen *et al.*, 1986; Kunkel *et al.*, 1986, 1988). This was known since 1980, when IL-1 was still termed lymphocyte-activating factor (LAF) (Oppenheim *et al.*, 1980). The mechanism for this inhibition is, at least in part, mediated by cAMP (whose levels are increased by PGE2) (Knudsen *et al.*, 1986; Spengler *et al.*, 1989), but other mechanisms are possible. For instance, reactive cyclopentenone prostaglandins, such as PGA1, inhibit NF-κB and this might result in inhibition of synthesis of several cytokines (Rossi *et al.*, 1997). In human peripheral blood mononuclear cells (PBMC), indomethacin increases production of TNF, IFNγ, and IL-2, while inhibiting that of IL-6 (Tsuboi *et al.*, 1995). Up-regulated TNF and IL-6 production by indomethacin and ibuprofen was also reported *in vivo* in LPS-treated mice (Sironi *et al.*, 1992), while in human volunteers receiving LPS, ibuprofen up-regulated serum TNF, IL-6, and IL-8 levels (Martich *et al.*, 1991; Spinas *et al.*, 1991). This phenomenon is probably at the basis of the toxic effects of indomethacin and ibuprofen in gram-negative sepsis or endotoxic shock in mice (Pettipher and Wimberly, 1994; Campanile *et al.*, 1996). Also *in vitro*, ibuprofen potentiates IL-1 production, although to a lesser extent than indomethacin (Kunkel *et al.*, 1986). In agreement with these reports,

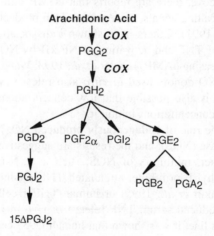

Fig. 2.1 The cyclooxygenase pathway.

we observed that ibuprofen increases TNF production in mice undergoing sepsis induced by cecal legation and puncture (Villa *et al.*, 1995). By contrast, others reported that ibuprofen lowers TNF levels in pigs infused with live *Pseudomonas aeruginosa* (Lepper-Wooford *et al.*, 1991) and does not inhibit IL-1 production by human PBMC (Okamoto *et al.*, 1991). It is not clear whether this discrepancy is due to the difference in the models used but, in any case, these results suggest a lower potency of ibuprofen compared to indomethacin.

Although most studies were carried out with indomethacin, other NSAIDs were reported to potentiate IL-1 production, including ibuprofen, piroxicam, and sodium meclofenate (Kunkel *et al.*, 1986; Bahl *et al.*, 1994).

It should be noted, however, that some papers reported an inhibitory effect of NSAIDs on cytokine production. The effect of aspirin is controversial: *in vitro* no up-regulation of IL-1 production was observed (Kunkel *et al.*, 1986; Bahl *et al.*, 1994), while another report indicates that in healthy humans oral aspirin, like ibuprofen, increases cytokine-induced synthesis of IL-1β and of TNF *ex vivo* (Endres *et al.*, 1996). Another report shows that aspirin and sodium salicylate inhibit TNF production *in vitro* in human monocytes (Osnes *et al.*, 1996). In fact, one paper has suggested, on the basis of dose–response studies of various NSAIDs for their ability to inhibit PGE2 production and to increase that of IL-1, that NSAIDs may have additional, unknown mechanisms that explain their effect on IL-1 synthesis (Bahl *et al.*, 1994). This might also be true for their effect on TNF and other cytokines. In human monocytic THP-1 cells, several NSAIDs inhibited the expression of cytokines, and this was suggested to be mediated by activation of stress genes (Housby *et al.*, 1999).

One possibility is that COX inhibition might divert arachidonic acid metabolism towards lipooxygenases. Also, not all prostaglandins have the same effect on cytokines. For instance, PGE1 and PGE2, but not PGD2, inhibit the production of TNF and increase that of IL-6 in mast cells (Leal-Berumen *et al.*, 1995). PGE2 also induces IL-6 production in macrophages (Hinson *et al.*, 1996), probably via cAMP (Zhang *et al.*, 1988). The ability of PGE2 to induce IL-6 might explain why, in inflammatory conditions, where PGE2 synthesis is induced, NSAIDs inhibit IL-6 production (Shacter *et al.*, 1992; Theisen-Popp *et al.*, 1992; Anderson *et al.*, 1996; Romano *et al.*, 1997a). The importance of this pathway is supported by the reduction of IL-6 production by neutralizing anti-PGE2 antibodies in a rat model of carrageenan-induced paw edema (Portanova *et al.*, 1996). Not only PGE2, but also addition of arachidonic acid, inhibits expression of TNFα and IL-1α induced by LPS or PMA in porcine aortic endothelial cells (Stuhlmeier *et al.*, 1996).

On the other hand, the fact that NSAID up-regulate IL-6 production in some cases might be secondary to their effect on TNF production. In fact, *in vivo*, LPS-induced IL-6 production is largely mediated by TNF, as shown by the IL-6-lowering effect of anti-TNF antibodies in sepsis (Jansen *et al.*, 1996). This might explain the fact that controversial results were obtained for the effect of NSAID on its production, in some cases. In fact, IL-6 is produced later than TNF, both *in vivo* and *in vitro*, and its production could well be influenced by TNF. It should be noted, however, that, when tested at high concentrations (2–5 mM), aspirin and salicylate inhibit NF-κB (Kopp and Ghosh, 1994) and this may result in inhibition of synthesis of several cytokines, as already mentioned for GC. In fact, aspirin and salicylate inhibit NF-κB and TNF production in human monocytes (Osnes *et al.*, 1996).

More recently, two different forms of COX were identified, one constitutive, COX-1, and one inducible, COX-2 (Cromlish and Kennedy, 1996), and it is likely that future studies with selective inhibitors will give a clear idea of the action of NSAIDs on cytokine production. For instance, selective inhibition of COX-2 with SC-58125 reduces IL-6 levels in arthritic rats (Anderson *et al.*, 1996).

Finally, tenidap, naproxen, and meloxicam (but not ibuprofen, indomethacin, piroxicam nor diclofenac) inhibited IL-1-induced IL-6 production in human astrocytes. This finding may have some relevance for the therapy of inflammatory component of Alzheimer's disease (Fiebich *et al.*, 1996).

Anti-inflammatory activities of prostaglandins (PGs)

As mentioned above, PGs are potent inhibitors of TNF production. While we have discussed this aspect only to explain why NSAIDs up-regulate TNF production, one cannot overlook the pharmacological implications for the development of inhibitors of TNF production.

Several PGs were in fact reported to have anti-inflammatory or protective activities. These include not only the inhibition of TNF production discussed at length in the previous chapters, but also anti-inflammatory activities. In particular, iloprost, a stable prostacyclin derivative, inhibits TNF production by macrophages (Grundmann *et al.*, 1992; Jörres *et al.*, 1997) and has protective effects against endotoxic shock (Grundmann *et al.*, 1992). PGE1 was also reported to have inhibitory effects on animal models of autoimmunity (Zurier *et al.*, 1977) or adjuvant arthritis (Zurier and Quagliata, 1971).

As mentioned above, cAMP was suggested as mediating the inhibitory activities of prostaglandins on TNF production. However, the picture is more complex. In fact, three types of PGE receptors have been defined pharmacologically: EP1, EP2, and EP3 (Sugimoto *et al.*, 1992; Honda *et al.*, 1993; Watabe *et al.*, 1993). Of the three receptor subtypes, only EP2 is linked to activation of adenyl cyclase (Honda *et al.*, 1993), while EP3 is an inhibitor of adenyl cyclase (Sugimoto *et al.*, 1992) and EP1 act on the mobilization of Ca^{2+} (Watabe *et al.*, 1993). Interestingly, only EP3 was significantly expressed (at the mRNA level) in the mouse brain (Sugimoto *et al.*, 1992, 1994), while no mRNA for EP1 or EP2 were found (Honda *et al.*, 1993; Watabe *et al.*, 1993). Thus, binding of PGE_2 to brain PGE receptor subtype EP3 would not cause an elevation, but might even produce a decrease, of cAMP. This difference between the central nervous system (CNS) and peripheral tissues was already noted in a review by Schaad *et al.* (1991), who observed that, in contrast to activation of adenylate cyclase observed in all studies using tissues other than the CNS, PGI2 and 6-keto-PGE1 paradoxically reduced the stimulation of cAMP formation in mouse neurocortical slices.

Thus, EP2-specific agonists might inhibit TNF production, but EP3-specific antagonists might have the same effect, particularly in the CNS. This might explain why NSAIDs, while up-regulating TNF production in peripheral tissues induced by LPS or inflammatory diseases (e.g. animal models of rheumatoid arthritis), inhibit TNF levels in the CNS induced by LPS injection, by cerebral ischemia or experimental autoimmune encephalomyelitis (Sacco *et al.*, 1998).

Agonists of the peroxisome proliferator-activated receptors (PPAR)

It was recently discovered that some prostaglandins, particularly PGJ2 and its derivatives, are ligands for the, until then, orphan nuclear receptor PPARγ (peroxisome proliferator-activated receptor γ) (Forman *et al.*, 1996; Kliewer *et al.*, 1997). Agonists of this receptor, including PGJ2 and high concentrations of some anti-inflammatory drugs, were found to inhibit production of TNF, IL-1, and IL-6 at the mRNA level (Jiang *et al.*, 1998). It is important to note that the inhibitory effect of PPARγ agonists was restricted to phorbol ester-induced cytokine production and did not affect that induced by LPS. As several agonists of this receptor were developed, this clearly indicates that PPARγ represents a valuable pharmacological target to modulate cytokine production.

More recently, *in vivo* administration of PPARα agonists were reported to inhibit the synthesis of IL-6 and IL-12, possibly by inhibiting NF-κB (Poynter and Daynes, 1998).

Lipoxins

Lipoxins are trihydroxytetraene-containing eicosanoids synthesized during a neutrophil (PMN)–platelet interaction, involving both the 5-lipoxygenase (5-LO) and 12-LO, or an interactions between the 5-LO and 15-LO (Serhan *et al.*, 1996). 15-epi-lipoxin A4 is a potent anti-inflammatory agent and inhibits several PMN functions, including adhesion, transmigration, and chemotaxis (Takano *et al.*, 1997; Gronert *et al.*, 1998).

Recently a human enterocyte Lipoxin A4 (LXA4) receptor was cloned, and interaction of LXA4 or its stable analogues with this receptor resulted in inhibition of TNF and IL-8 production (Gronert *et al.*, 1998).

Interestingly, IL-4 and IL-13 activate the LXA4 synthetic pathway (Nassar *et al.*, 1994). More interestingly, one pathway of LXA4 synthesis is triggered by aspirin through acetylation of prostaglandin H synthase-II (PGHS-II) in endothelial cells and by its interaction with 5-LO in leukocytes that generate novel 15-epi-lipoxins (Claria and Serhan, 1995), suggesting a role for LXA4 in the anti-inflammatory action of aspirin.

Thus, as outlined in Fig. 2.2, different prostaglandins may have inhibitory or stimulatory effects on TNF

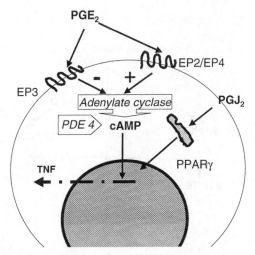

Fig. 2.2 Differential effects of PG on cAMP and TNF production. PGE2 receptors EP2/EP4 activate adenyl cyclase, while EP3 inhibits adenyl cyclase. The levels of cAMP are also decreased by phosphodiesterase (PDE) IV. cAMP then inhibits TNF production. In addition, PGJ2, and other ligands, bind the nuclear receptor PPARγ, which also causes inhibition of TNF production.

Other arachidonic acid metabolites

Two lipoxygenase products,15(s)-hydroxy-5,8,11,13-eicosatetraenoic acid (15-HETE) and 15(s)-hydroperoxy-5,8,11,13-eicosatetraenoic acid (15-HPETE) were also reported to inhibit TNF production by LPS-stimulated monocytes or by leukocytes stimulated with mitogens, possibly by inhibiting translocation of protein kinase C (Ferrante *et al.*, 1997).

Inhibitors of lipoxygenases (LO) and phospholipase A2 (PLA2)

In addition to the COX pathway, which produces prostaglandins and thromboxanes, arachidonic acid can be metabolized via the LO pathway to various metabolites, including monohydroxy fatty acids and leukotrienes. (Fig. 2.3), and several LO inhibitors have been described. Early studies reported that LO inhibitors block LPS-induced IL-1 and TNF production *in vitro* and/or *in vivo* (Dinarello *et al.*, 1984; Schade *et al.*, 1989), as well as IL-2 production *in vitro* (Dornand *et al.*, 1987; Dornand and Gerber, 1991). Inhibition of IL-1 production was also reported by anti-inflammatory agents acting as dual COX/LO inhibitors, such as SK&F 86002 (Lee *et al.*, 1988) and tenidap (Sipe *et al.*, 1992).

In this respect, PLA2 represent another pharmacological target. In fact, this enzyme releases arachidonic acid from membrane lipids thus providing the substrate for both LO and COX. In fact, PLA2 activity is increased by LPS (Mohri *et al.*, 1990) and the PLA2 inhibitors quinacrine (mepacrine) and bromophenacyl bromide potently inhibit LPS-induced production of TNF *in vitro* and *in vivo* (Mohri *et al.*, 1990; Spriggs *et al.*, 1990; Bertini *et al.*, 1993), thus suggesting that the requirement for LO metabolites is predominant over the inhibitory effects of COX metabolites. A further support to the concept that eicosanoids (at least some of them) may participate in the cascade of events leading to cytokine production, comes from the finding that PLA2-activating protein (PLAP) and melittin, a bee venom peptide that activates PLA2 and thus stimulates production of LO products (Salari *et al.*, 1985), induce TNF and IL-1 synthesis in human monocytes (Bomalaski *et al.*, 1995).

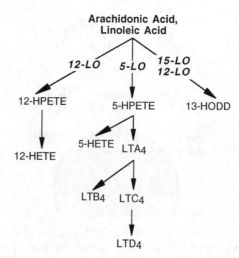

Fig. 2.3 The lipoxygenase pathway.

The fact that exogenously-added LTB4 induces production of IL-1 and TNF *in vitro*, initially indicated a role for these metabolites (Rola-Pleszczynski and Lemaire, 1985; Rola-Pleszczynski *et al.*, 1988). However, two studies using site-specific inhibitors of LO found that selective 5-LO inhibitors did not inhibit TNF production *in vivo* and *in vitro* (Schade *et al.*, 1991; Fantuzzi *et al.*, 1993). Also, a dual COX/5-LO inhibitor, tebufelone, increased, rather than inhibited, TNF and IL-1 production at concentrations that blocked formation of LTB4 (Sirko *et al.*, 1991).

The studies by Schade *et al.*, (1991) led to the identification of a 15-LO metabolite, 13-hydroxyoctadecadienoic acid (13-HODD), which is probably important in the signaling pathway leading to TNF production.

It was also reported that two inhibitors of thromboxane (TX) synthase, UK38485 (dezmegrel) and OKY046, inhibit TNF production by human alveolar macrophages (Kuhn *et al.*, 1993) and that carboxyheptyl imidazole inhibited zymosan-induced TNF and IL-1 production in PBMC (Caughey *et al.*, 1997). Addition of a TXA2 mimetic (carbocyclic TXA2) reverted the inhibition of TNF and IL-1 production by carboxyheptyl imidazole, while two TXA2 receptor antagonists, pinane and SQ29548, inhibited TNF and IL-1 production. These data also suggest that TXA2, which would act as a paracrine or autocrine facilitator of TNF and IL-1 production, could represent a pharmacological target for inhibiting cytokine production.

Inhibitors of cytochrome P-450

Cytochrome P-450 is the key electron transport cytochrome involved in the oxidative metabolism of several xenobiotics, including drugs. However, cytochromes of this family are also implicated in the metabolism of endogenous compounds (e.g. leukotrienes and other arachidonate metabolites, vitamin D).

It was reported that two inhibitors of cytochrome P-450, metyrapone and SKF252A, blocked TNF production *in vivo* and *in vitro* (Fantuzzi *et al.*, 1993). This might be explained by postulating that: (1) a TNF-inducing metabolite of an endogenous substrate is formed by a cytochrome P-450-like enzyme upon LPS treatment; or (2) the constitutive presence of such a metabolite is required for a normal TNF production.

It is of interest to note that *in vivo* administration of most cytokines, including interferons, IL-1 and TNF, depresses the levels of cytochrome P-450 (Ghezzi *et al.*, 1986a, 1986b, 1986c). It is tempting to hypothesize that this effect represents a mechanism by which inflammatory cytokines down-regulate TNF production. However, it is not known whether the isoforms of cytochrome P-450 involved in TNF induction, are among those which are depleted *in vivo* by cytokines.

2.1.7 Inhibitors of protein kinases

Fig. 2.4 shows some of the pathways of cytokine induction involving protein kinases and the effect on their inhibitors. As protein kinase inhibitors are typically small molecules, there has been considerable interest in this area and some of the kinases involved will be described in more detail below.

Inhibitors of protein kinase C (PKC)

The fact that the synthesis of most LPS-inducible cytokines can also be induced by PMA (Nishida *et al.*, 1988), a PKC activator, is suggestive of a role of PKC in the signaling

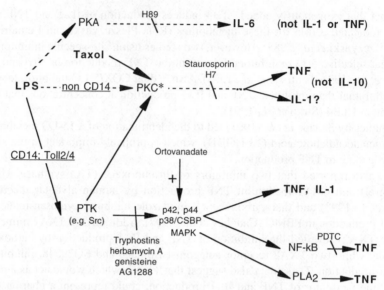

Fig. 2.4   Role of protein kinases in LPS-induced signaling, involved in the production of pro-inflammatory cytokines. Compiled from information obtained from: Barnes *et al.*, 1990; Mengozzi *et al.*, 1991; Chung *et al.*, 1992; Geng *et al.*, 1993; Sironi *et al.*, 1993; Stefanova *et al.*, 1993; Weinstein *et al.*, 1993; Beaty *et al.*, 1994; Lee J.C. *et al.*, 1994; Liu *et al.*, 1994; Novogrodsky *et al.*, 1994; Shapira *et al.* 1994; Jun *et al.*, 1995; Lang *et al.*, 1995; Meisel *et al.*, 1996.

* Activation of PKC alone is not sufficient for inducing TNF (Chung *et al.*, 1992)

pathway leading to cytokine production. This hypothesis was probed by Kovacs *et al.* (1988) using two inhibitors of PKC, 1-(5)-isoquinolinesulfonyl)-2-methylpiperazine hydrochloride (H7) and retinal in mouse peritoneal macrophages. The results indicated that the induction of mRNA for both TNF and IL-1α or β was inhibited by PKC inhibitors. On the other hand, inhibitors of calmodulin-dependent kinase (calmidazolum, trifluoperazine, and W7, N-(6-aminobutyl)-5-chloro-2-naphtalene sulfonamide) inhibited only IL-1 mRNA expression, not TNF (Kovacs *et al.*, 1988).

Another activator of PKC, bryostatin-1, currently tested in phase I trials as an anti-cancer agent, induced TNF-alpha mRNA and secretion of TNF in the human cell line MONO-MAC-6 (Steube and Drexler, 1995).

The effect of PKC inhibitors on chemokine production is more complex. In human keratinocytes, staurosporine and auranofin (another inhibitor of PKC, (Jordan *et al.*, 1996)) inhibit PMA-stimulated IL-8 production but potentiate TNF- and IL-1-induced IL-8 protein and mRNA production (Chabot Fletcher *et al.*, 1994). Also, the more specific PKC inhibitor chelerythrine (staurosporine also inhibits PKA and phosphorylase kinase (Bradshaw *et al.*, 1993)), up-regulates IL-1-induced IL-8 mRNA in human synovial fibroblasts (Jordan *et al.*, 1996). Interestingly, two specific PKC inhibitors of the substi-tuted bisindolylmaleimide family, Ro 31–8220 and GF109203X, have a concentration-dependent biphasic effect on IL-1α- or TNF-induced expression of IL-8, MCP-1 and RANTES. At low concentrations, Ro 31–8220 and GF109203X up-regulate chemokine production, while at higher concentrations (IC$_{50}$ in the 1–10 μM range) they inhibit chemokine production (both at the protein and mRNA levels) (Jordan *et al.*, 1996). The authors speculate that, as the higher concentrations of these bisindolylmaleimides are required to inhibit an isoform of PKC (PCK epsilon, or zeta), the latter is important in chemokine expression induced by IL-1 or TNF.

Inhibitors of p38 mitogen-activated kinase (MAPK)

Another protein kinase implicated in the synthesis of pro-inflammatory cytokines is p38-MAPK (mitogen-activated protein kinase). Its role in cytokine synthesis, as well as its relevance as a pharmacological target, became particularly evident by a study carried out by Young and Lee (Lee J.C. *et al.*, 1988, 1993). They developed a class of pyridinyl imidazole anti-inflammatory agents, the prototype of which was SK&F86002, that proved to be a potent inhibitor of IL-1 synthesis, but actually was a dual cyclo-oxygenase/lipo-oxygenase inhibitor. Various derivatives of it were developed, including SB203580, and based on the hypothesis that they had a novel mechanism of action, biochemical studies were performed to identify their molecular targets. The molecular targets of SB203580 were found to be a pair of mitogen-activated protein kinase homologues termed by Lee *et al.* (Lee *et al.*, 1988, 1993), 'cytokine suppressive binding protein' (CSBP); SB203580 and its analogues were named 'cytokine suppressive anti-inflammatory drug' (CSAID, a registered trademark). CSBP was actually identical to p38 or reactivating-kinase (RK) (Han *et al.*, 1994; Rouse *et al.*, 1994). SB203580 showed an activity in several models of inflammation, including some relatively resistant to COX/LO inhibitors (Badger *et al.*, 1996). It should be noted that SB203580 might still retain an inhibitory activity on COX (Kramer *et al.*, 1996).

Finally, it should be pointed out that although much emphasis was put on the inhibitory effect of SB203580 on cytokine synthesis, other actions of this molecule might be important in its pharmacological activity. In fact, p38 is also important in cytokine signaling and p38 inhibitors inhibit several actions of cytokines (Kramer *et al.*, 1996; Pouliot *et al.*, 1997; Read *et al.*, 1997; Ridley *et al.*, 1997).

Inhibitors of tyrosine kinases

Tyrphostins are derivatives of benzylidene malononitrile that inhibit tyrosine kinases. Some tyrphostins (AG556 and AG126), which inhibit tyrosine phosphorylation of a p42MAPK, inhibit TNF production and protect against septic or endotoxic shock (Novogrodsky *et al.*, 1994; Sevransky *et al.*, 1997).

While inhibitors of TNF production usually need to be administered prior to LPS treatment in order to be protective, AG126 is also active when given 2 h later, when peak TNF levels have already been attained (Vanichkin *et al.*, 1996). This suggests that AG126 can have effects downstream of the TNF signaling pathway. Recent reports indicate that tyrphostins also inhibit ICAM-1 and E-selectin up-regulation and neutrophil adhesion (Kelly *et al.*, 1998).

2.1.8 Antioxidants

Inhibitors of cytokine production

In biological aerobic organisms, molecular oxygen (O_2) participates in a variety of metabolic processes. The most important of these processes is mitochondrial respiration, where O_2 is reduced to H_2O. This process requires four electrons and some oxygen intermediates are generated by one-step electron processes (Fig. 2.5).

In addition, O_2^- participates as a cofactor for various *oxidases*, a class of enzymes that oxidize their substrate and can use O_2 as an electron acceptor, thus generating a reduced oxygen molecule, such as superoxides or H_2O_2 (two such examples are NAD(P)H oxidases and xanthine oxidase). O_2 is also a substrate for various *oxygenases*, that insert one or two (if they are mono- or di- oxygenases) oxygen atoms into their substrate. In this latter case, oxygen, in order to be inserted into the substrate has to be *activated* to a reactive form.

No matter how these intermediates originate, their main feature is a high instability and consequently, reactivity, hence the term reactive oxygen intermediates, ROI. These molecules avidly tend to react with other molecules and go down to the reduced (H_2O) state. In biological systems, reactivity inevitably results in toxicity. Thus, aerobic organisms have developed an armamentarium of antioxidants. These include enzymes that detoxify ROI: superoxide dismutase (SOD), which catalyzes the reduction (disproportionation or dismutation) of O_2^- to H_2O_2 and O_2; catalase, decomposing H_2O_2 to O_2 and H_2O; and glutathione (GSH) peroxidase (GSH-PX) that detoxifies various hydroperoxides using GSH and generating oxidized GSH (GSSG). Part of the antioxidant defense is also the so-called free radical scavengers, which act as traps for ROI such as GSH and vitamin E.

ROI have been considered, among other things, inflammatory mediators, particularly those produced by phagocytes upon stimulation. In fact, antioxidants have some anti-inflammatory actions. The fields of GSH and TNF lit up in 1990 when some papers reported that N-acetylcysteine (NAC, an antioxidant itself and a precursor of GSH synthesis) inhibited TNF-induced HIV replication and activation of NF-κB (Roederer *et al.*, 1990; Staal *et al.*, 1990; Kalebic *et al.*, 1991). These works stemmed from the original observation that HIV patients have low levels of plasma thiols and intracellular GSH (Eck *et al.*, 1989). In the same years, two works have indicated that NAC and GSH inhibit the release of TNF *in vivo* and *in vitro* (Chaudri and Clark, 1989; Peristeris *et al.*, 1992). This is probably mediated through the inhibitory effects of antioxidants on NF-κB. The antioxidant and metal chelator pyrrolidine dithiocarboxylic acid (PDTC), widely used as an inhibitor of NF-κB (Schreck *et al.*, 1992), inhibits not only the production of TNF but the production of a variety of cytokines (Table 2.4) (Meisel *et al.*, 1996; Munoz *et al.*, 1996; Baeuerle and Baichwal, 1997). One of these studies reported no effect of PDTC on TNF production by human monocytes but this was associated with inhibition of IL-10 production, so that the inhibitory effect on TNF production might be masked by the removal of its inhibitory cytokine (Meisel *et al.*, 1996). PDTC inhibited IL-10 production even if the human IL-10 promoter, unlike the murine promoter, does not contain classical NF-κB consensus binding sites (Meisel *et al.*, 1996). *In vivo*, at a dose of 200 mg/kg, PDTC inhibits mRNA expression of IL-1β and MCP-1 in a rat model of nephrotoxic

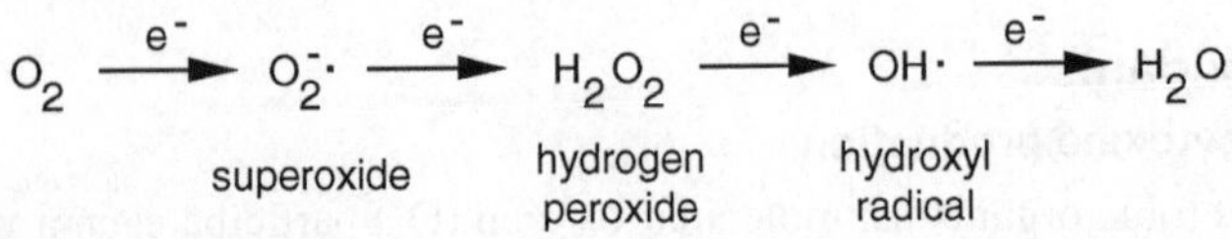

$$O_2 \xrightarrow{e^-} O_2^-\cdot \xrightarrow{e^-} H_2O_2 \xrightarrow{e^-} OH\cdot \xrightarrow{e^-} H_2O$$

superoxide   hydrogen peroxide   hydroxyl radical

Fig. 2.5 Reactive intermediates in the reduction of molecular oxygen.

Table 2.4 Cytokine genes with NF-κB sites

Pro-inflammatory cytokines
IL-1β
IL-2
IL-6
IL-8
IL-12
Chemokines
IP-10
KC, IL-8
M-CSF
MCP-1
MIP-1a
Hemopoietic cytokines
G-CSF
GM-CSF
IL-3

glomerulonephritis (Sakurai *et al.*, 1996). Along the same line, antisense phosphorothioate oligonucleotides to the p65 subunit of NF-κB have a protective effect in a murine model of colitis (Neurath *et al.*, 1996).

In a paper where several antioxidants were studied on human peripheral blood mononuclear cells stimulated with LPS, staphylococci, silica or zymosan, it was reported that buthylated hydroxyanisole, tetrahydropapaveroline, nordihydroguaiaretic acid, and 10,11-dihydroxyaporphine were potent inhibitors (IC_{50} in the low micromolar range) of the production of TNFα, IL-1β, and IL-6 (Eugui *et al.*, 1994). Other antioxidants (ascorbic acid, trolox, alpha-tocopherol, butylated hydroxytoluene) were not inhibitory and it was not clarified whether this reflected a different antioxidant potency of the molecules tested in terms of the reactive species scavenged or in the subcellular distribution or in the half-life of the antioxidant.

The organoselenium compound [2-(N-phenyl-carboxamido)]phenyl diselenide, 2-phenyl-1,2-benzisoselenazol-3(2H)-one (Ebselen), which acts as an antioxidant by mimicking the selenium-dependent antioxidant enzyme GSH-peroxidase, induces, rather than inhibits, TNF and IFNγ production by human peripheral blood leukocytes (Inglot *et al.*, 1990).

Administration of the antioxidant enzymes catalase or superoxide dismutase also inhibits serum TNF levels in galactosamine-sensitized mice injected with LPS (Neihörster *et al.*, 1992).

Administration of the antiatherogenic drug probucol inhibits production of IL-1 *ex vivo* by peritoneal macrophages (Ku *et al.*, 1990). This action is suggested to be due to the antioxidant action of probucol. However, probucol did not affect TNF production in the same system, neither did it affect IL-1 production when added *in vitro* to macrophages, which is different from what one might expect for an antioxidant.

The cyclic nitrone antioxidant MDL101002 was reported to reduce organ dysfunction and cytokine secretion (strong inhibition of TNF levels; slight effect on IL-1) induced by LPS administration in rats (Downs *et al.*, 1995).

Another molecule that inhibits TNF production, probably via its antioxidant activity, is melatonin (N-acetyl-5-methoxytryptamine). This molecule inhibits LPS-induced production of TNF *in vivo* and *in vitro*. By studying other, structurally related indolamines

(N-acetyl-5-hydroxytryptamine, 5-methoxytryptamine, and 5-hydroxytryptamine) it was found that only those that maintain the antioxidant action of melatonin, which is due to its 5-methoxy group, inhibit TNF production (Sacco *et al.*, 1998*b*).

Two sources of free radicals are particularly important in cytokine-mediated pathologies. Phagocytes (particularly neutrophils) represent one source, where reactive oxygen intermediates are secreted as part of their bactericidal weapons (the so-called oxidative burst). The other source is the intracellular enzyme, xanthine oxidase (XO) (Fig. 2.6), which is an interferon-inducible enzyme (Ghezzi *et al.*, 1984; Falciani *et al.*, 1992) and is elevated in mice after LPS administration (Faggioni *et al.*, 1994; Ghezzi *et al.*, 1984) or viral infection (Akaike *et al.*, 1990), as well as in patients with sepsis syndrome and acute respiratory distress syndrome (ARDS) (Grum *et al.*, 1987; Galley *et al.*, 1996). The XO inhibitor, allopurinol, was reported to inhibit the induction of lung IL-1 and TNF following hemorrhagic shock and the induction of TNF following LPS/galactosamine administration (Neihörster *et al.*, 1992), suggesting that XO-generated ROI might be implicated in cytokine induction (Schwartz *et al.*, 1995). Allopurinol also inhibits TNF production by human peripheral blood mononuclear cells *in vitro* (Olah *et al.*, 1994). However, caution should be used in interpreting these data as a demonstration of the role of XO since, normally, allopurinol must be used at high doses to inhibit XO, and at this concentration it could act as an antioxidant itself (i.e. scavenge all ROI, whether or not produced by XO).

IL-8 is also regulated by oxidant/antioxidant balance. Both the pro-oxidant herbicide paraquat (Bianchi *et al.*, 1993) and H_2O_2 (DeForge *et al.*, 1993) stimulate IL-8 production and IL-8 mRNA in human peripheral blood mononuclear cells, fibroblasts, whole blood or the pulmonary epithelial cell line A549. Antioxidants, such as dimethylsulfoxide, inhibited LPS-induced IL-8 production (DeForge *et al.*, 1993), similarly to what was observed for TNF. H_2O_2 also induces the synthesis of IL-10 and TNF in human monocytes (Le Moine *et al.*, 1996).

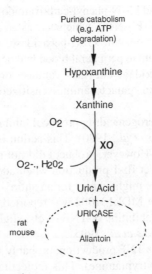

Purine catabolism
(e.g. ATP
degradation)

Hypoxanthine

Xanthine

O_2

XO

O_2-., H_2O_2

Uric Acid

URICASE

rat
mouse

Allantoin

Fig. 2.6 The xanthine oxidase pathway.

One cautionary note, which is not only semantic, should be stated at the end of this section on the inhibition of cytokine production by antioxidants. The two terms, 'antioxidant' and 'free radical scavengers', are often used interchangeably. To be precise, a free radical scavenger will only react with (i.e. eliminate or deactivate) free radicals. Free radicals are molecules with an unpaired electron (e.g. O_2^- and $OH\cdot$). H_2O_2 is reactive but is not a radical; however, the term 'free radical scavenger' is often extended to include molecules that will inactivate (or degrade) H_2O_2.

The term 'antioxidant' has a more general meaning and denotes a molecule that inhibits an oxidation process. Thus, many antioxidants will also inhibit a biological oxidation carried out by an enzyme.

This brings us to the cautionary note we want to leave the reader with: in many cases there is no clear distinction between an antioxidant and a lipo-oxygenase inhibitor. Thus, when dealing with inhibitors of TNF production that supposedly act through one of the two mechanisms (antioxidant activity or inhibition of lipo-oxygenase), one should confirm which of the mechanisms is at work.

Immunopotentiating effects of thiol antioxidants

In the case of thiol antioxidants, the use of immunostimulants has also been envisaged. In particular, addition of 2-mercaptoethanol (2-ME) to culture medium has long been known to stimulate several lymphocyte functions (Heber-Katz and Click, 1972). Other thiols were reported to have lymphocyte-stimulatory properties. The first molecule of this kind was diethyldithiocarbamate, a metal chelator used to treat metal poisoning, which was proposed as an immunostimulatory drug under the name of imuthiol, or its disulfide precursor, disulfiram. Imuthiol was studied in AIDS patients with controversial results (Lang *et al.*, 1988; Group, 1993). However, the molecule is far from being specific. Although it is an antioxidant, it is also a metal chelator. Encouraging results have recently been obtained with NAC (Herzenberg *et al.*, 1997), a drug used as a mucolytic agent and to cure acetaminophen poisoning.

In fact, some antioxidants were actually reported to potentiate the production or action of cytokines, particularly IL-2, and this effect was studied in relation to AIDS. 2-mercaptoethanol and the GSH precursor, NAC, were reported to enhance T cell colony formation in AIDS patients or healthy individuals. Augmenting intracellular GSH levels using L-2-oxothiazolidine-4-carboxylate (OTC) or 2-ME potentiates T-cell proliferation (Fidelus and Tsan, 1986).

2-ME was reported to augment IL-2 production *in vitro* (Lyte, 1988), and enhanced concanavalin A- or anti-CD3-induced T cell mitogenesis by NAC is also associated with an augmentation of IL-2 production (Eylar *et al.*, 1993; Chen *et al.*, 1994; Eylar *et al.*, 1995).

Thiol antioxidants also potentiate IL-2 action. 2-ME is essential for IL-2-dependent proliferation of a mouse lymphocyte cell line (Sugama *et al.*, 1987) and for the induction of lymphokine-activated killer cells (LAK) activity by IL-2 in rat splenocytes (Kuppen *et al.*, 1991). Also, GSH stimulates IL-2-induced LAK activity and NK cell proliferation (Yamauchi and Bloom, 1993). The molecular mechanisms for the potentiated IL-2 action, and lymphocyte function in general, are far from being completely understood, and the inhibitory effect of thiol antioxidants on NF-κB may act as a confounding factor, particularly when very high drug concentrations are used *in vitro* (for instance, IL-2 has a NF-κB site). However, some studies have suggested possible mechanisms for the stimulating effect of GSH. In particular, it was reported that GSH depletion in human T lymphocytes or cell lines decreases anti-CD3-stimulated calcium flux (Staal *et al.*, 1994) and that 2-ME increases PKC translocation in concanavalin A-stimulated murine T cells (Fong and Makinodan, 1989).

While dithiocarbamates are inhibitors of the production of several cytokines, through inhibition of NF-κB, it was also reported that diethyldithiocarbamate induces production of GM-CSF, G-CSF, IL-6, IL-1 beta, and TNF-alpha in human bone marrow cells (East *et al.*, 1992).

2.1.9 Anti-endotoxin molecules

Cytokine synthesis can be triggered by a variety of agents, as shown in Table 2.5. However, the one most extensively studied is LPS. Clearly, inhibition of the stimulation pathways activated by LPS is of major importance in the pharmacology of cytokines and it might conceptually be achieved by inhibiting binding of LPS to its receptors, as well as by the post-receptor signaling mechanisms.

Not only is LPS the most popular inducer of cytokine production used in research laboratories but it is, obviously, the main trigger of the cytokine cascade in gram-negative sepsis. Endotoxin is present in the blood of patients with gram-negative sepsis and in febrile patients, and endotoxemia is associated with a high risk of developing septic shock (Levin *et al.*, 1970; van Deventer *et al.*, 1988). Thus, detoxification/neutralization of LPS has been attempted using various strategies.

It is clear that the various biological activities of LPS, including those that are toxic and inflammatory, are induced through its lipid A moiety (Morrison and Ryan, 1987; Raetz *et al.*, 1991), which is the actual target for neutralization. According to the currently accepted picture on which there is substantial agreement, the most important LPS binding molecule is CD14 (Wright *et al.*, 1990; Raetz *et al.*, 1991). At low LPS concentrations, LPS requires a carrier protein (LPS-binding protein, LBP) present in serum, to optimally bind and activate CD14. However, other LPS receptors may exist. In fact, blockade of CD14 with antibodies does not completely inhibit LPS responsiveness, including induction of cytokines. Recently, a Toll-like receptors (TLR) 2 and 4 (Toll is a receptor that participates to immunity and development of *Drosophila*) have been implicated as components of the LPS receptor signaling complex. Mutation of TLR4 leads to LPS resistance in mice (Muzio *et al.*, 1998; Kirschning *et al.*, 1998; Poltorak *et al.*, 1998; Yang *et al.*, 1998; Zhang *et al.*, 1999).

While anti-CD14 inhibits TNF production in the presence of low (10–100 ng/ml) concentrations of LPS, it does not affect TNF induced by high (> 1 μg) LPS concentrations. Mice over-expressing CD14 are more sensitive to LPS, while CD14 knockouts are more resistant (Haziot *et al.*, 1996). However, it should be mentioned that LBP-deficient mice have normal susceptibility to LPS *in vivo* (Wurfel *et al.*, 1997).

Detoxification of LPS *in vivo* in mice by polymyxin B, a peptide antibiotic, was described in the 1960s (Rifkind, 1967), and is due to stoichiometric binding of polymyxin B to lipid A (Morrison and Jacobs, 1976). However, although polymyxin B is widely used *in vitro* to neutralize LPS, its human use has always been hampered by high toxicity.

Another approach has consisted of the search for LPS-binding proteins. Some of them were isolated by the horseshoe crab *Limulus polyphemus*. In fact, the lysate of *Limulus*

Table 2.5   Non-microbial inducers of IL-1

Stress factors
Hyperosmolarity
Hypoxia/hyperoxia; ischemia/reperfusion
UV light
Radiation
Thermal injury

Neuroactive substances
Substance P
Excititoxins (kainic acid)
Melatonin

Inflammatory substances
C5a; C5b
Urate crystals
Advanced glycation end-products
Phtalates; dioxin; silica; asbestos

Cell matrix
Collagen; fibronectin

Clotting factors
Fibrin degradation products; plasmin; thombin

Lipids
Platelet-activating factor

Cytokines and growth factors
IL-1; TNF; IL-3; IL-12; GM-CSF; M-CSF; SCF; PDGF

Miscellaneous
Phorbol esters
Bleomycin; colchicine; taxol
Phytoemagglutinin; concanavalin A
Anti-CD3

Reproduced with kind permission from Dinarello (1996).

amoebocytes gels in the presence of LPS. The occurrence of this reaction, which is at the basis of the most used assay for LPS, the 'LAL test', indicates that the *Limulus* must contain a factor that can bind LPS. This protein has been identified as a 15-kDa protein (LALF, for LAL factor) and is an inhibitor of LPS action. Another LPS-binding protein was originally described as an antibacterial protein secreted by neutrophils, bactericidal/permeability-increasing protein (BPI) (Weiss *et al.*, 1978). Later on, this 55-kDa human protein was studied for its ability to neutralize LPS, thus inhibiting LPS-induced cytokine production and toxicity (Marra *et al.*, 1992; Jin *et al.*, 1995). In human volunteers receiving an LPS injection, BPI inhibited release of circulating cytokines, indicating that it effectively neutralizes LPS *in vivo* (von der Möhlen *et al.*, 1995). Other LPS-binding proteins include CAP-18, also present in neutrophils (Larrik *et al.*, 1991) and the LPS receptor CD14.

A study in which the amino acid sequence of the lipid A binding site of polymyxin B was mapped (Rustici *et al.*, 1993), has led to the identification of the minimal and optimal sequence requirements of peptides for binding and detoxifying lipid A. This allowed for the design of various synthetic anti-endotoxin peptides (SAEP) mimicking the primary and secondary structure of polymyxin B (Rustici *et al.*, 1993). These SAEP have shown anti-LPS activity *in vitro* and *in vivo* in endotoxemic mice and rabbits (Rustici *et al.*, 1993; Velucchi *et al.*, 1994; Demitri *et al.*, 1996). The mechanism by which SAEP do this lies in their ability to diffuse into tissues and inhibit systemic and local LPS-induced TNF production, as well as LPS-induced local Schwartzman reaction in rabbits (Rustici *et al.*, 1993; Velucchi *et al.*, 1994; Demitri *et al.*, 1996). The characterization of the structural basis for recognition by natural polypeptides has led to the identification of SAEP-related sequences in various natural polypeptides that bind LPS, including CD14, LBP, LALF, BPI, magainin, melittin, tubulin, and CAP-18, all of which were in one way or another known to bind LPS or possess antibacterial properties (Porro, 1994; Porro *et al.*, 1998). This model seems to be predictive of lipid A binding and neutralization by natural polypeptides. In fact, a sequence search led to the identification of a SAEP-like sequence in nociceptin, a dynorphin-related peptide involved in the sensation of pain (Porro *et al.*, 1998). When tested to determine the hypothesis, nociceptin was found to inhibit, as predicted, the LAL assay, LPS-induced cytokine production *in vitro* and *in vivo*, and local Schwartzman reaction (Porro *et al.*, 1998).

A second strategy to neutralize LPS is the development of non-toxic lipid A analogueues that might act as lipid A antagonists. Inhibition of LPS activity was reported with lipid X, a biosynthetic precursor of lipid A isolated from a variant of E. coli and some derivatives (Danner *et al.*, 1987), or non-toxic lipid A molecules derived from *Rhodobacter spheroides* and *R. capsulatum* (Christ *et al.*, 1995).

Last but not least, several monoclonal antibodies (e.g. E5, HA-1A) directed against LPS have been tested in clinical trials in septic shock. Some of these are still under investigation, however the first studies encountered the same problems that were met by the various septic shock trials (IL-1ra, anti-TNF antibodies, etc.), i.e. the difficulty of improving the 28-day survival endpoint, possible efficacy in subpopulations (see Chapter 14). It should be mentioned, however, that the preclinical studies (published) with these antibodies have been scarce, and there were no clear-cut published works showing that these antibodies could effectively neutralize LPS activity, at least *in vitro* (for a critical review of this, see Warren *et al.*, 1991).

Other inhibitors of cytokine production

Various compounds, which do not fit in the previous sections, have been reported to inhibit cytokine production with different mechanisms of action. Some of them have been the subject of several studies (e.g. CNI 1493) or have already been tested in clinical trials (e.g. thalidomide) or are in clinical use (e.g. benzidamine). Other agents have been put in a 'miscellaneous' section. We decided not to list all the compounds reported to inhibit cytokine production, but only those for which we felt that the original report had some follow-up, or when we thought the compound was important, either because it is already a registered drug or the mechanism of action was novel or somehow interesting.

Thalidomide

Thalidomide, which caused an unprecedented medical tragedy in the early 1960s due to its teratogenic properties, is now reconsidered for the therapy of a series of autoimmune diseases (rheumatoid arthritis, systemic lupus erythematosus, multiple sclerosis, inflammatory bowel diseases), for leprosy, tubercolosis, AIDS-associated aphtous ulcers, graft-versus-host disease, as well as for cancer- and AIDS-associated cachexia (reviewed in Stirling *et al.*, 1997). The US Food and Drug Administration has approved the drug for one form of leprosy (Nightingale, 1998), and clinical trials for some of the diseases mentioned above are under way.

The finding that it is an inhibitor of TNF production, as indicated by several reports, renewed the interest in thalidomide as a cytokine inhibitor. Thalidomide inhibits LPS-induced TNF production *in vivo* (Schmidt *et al.*, 1996) and *in vitro* in mononuclear cells stimulated with LPS (Corral *et al.*, 1996; Tavares *et al.*, 1997), possibly by enhancing mRNA degradation (Moreira *et al.*, 1993). This was associated with protection against LPS lethality (Schmidt *et al.*, 1996) and reduction of the brain inflammatory response in experimental meningitis in rabbit (Burroughs *et al.*, 1995). It was shown to have an efficacy in leprosy and tuberculosis (Sampaio *et al.*, 1993; Tramontana *et al.*, 1995) and against aphtous ulcers in AIDS patients (although the latter effect may not have been due to inhibition of TNF production (Jacobson *et al.*, 1997)). On the other hand, a clinical trial of a combination of thalidomide with pentoxifylline in rheumatoid arthritis, although reducing TNF levels, did not show a significant effect (Huizinga *et al.*, 1996).

It should also be noted that the inhibitory effect of thalidomide on TNF production is cell type- and inducer-specific. While inhibition of LPS-induced TNF production was reported in most studies, some papers have shown that thalidomide enhances phorbol ester-induced TNF production (Nishimura *et al.*, 1994; Miyachi *et al.*, 1996a, 1996b) or even LPS-induced TNF production in some monocyte populations (Shannon and Sandoval, 1996).

Using analogues of thalidomide or separating its enantiomers, some studies have indicated the possibility of dissociating its inhibitory effect on TNF production from its side-effects (Corral *et al.*, 1996; Wnendt *et al.*, 1996; Marriott *et al.*, 1998; Corral *et al.*, 1999).

Guanylhydrazones (CNI-1493)

CNI-1493 is a bulky aromatic compound possessing 4 guanidinium groups (N,N'-bis [3,5-diacetyl phenyl]decanediamide tetrakis [amino hydrazone] tetrahydro chloride). This tetravalent guanylhydrazone was originally described for its ability to inhibit arginine transport and NO production (Bianchi *et al.*, 1995).

It was later found to be effective in preventing other responses induced by activated macrophages, including production of pro-inflammatory cytokines. In LPS-stimulated human mononuclear cells, CNI-1493 inhibits the production of TNF, IL-1β, MIP-1α, MIP-1β, IL-6 (Bianchi *et al.*, 1996) with an estimated IC_{50} of 30–70 nM for IL-1 and TNF inhibition, and 125–175 nM for the inhibition of IL-6 and MIP-1. This inhibitory effect is not restricted to LPS-induced activation of macrophages, since it also suppresses TNF production by macrophages stimulated with toxic shock syndrome toxin (TSST)-1. The specificity of the effect of CNI-1493 was evaluated by assay of the production of TGFβ and the expression of MHC class II antigens, which were not inhibited, even by a high concentration of CNI-1493 (Bianchi *et al.*, 1996). In contrast to the macrophage suppressive action of dexamethasone, which is overridden in the presence of IFNγ (Leudke and Cerami, 1990), CNI-1493 retains its suppressive effect even in the presence of IFNγ. This is particularly important to the anti-inflammatory strategies *in vivo*, where IFNγ is ubiquitously induced in acute and chronic inflammation and may limit the usefulness of GCs.

CNI-1493 inhibits macrophage TNF synthesis through suppression of TNF translation efficiency (Cohen *et al.*, 1996). CNI-1493 blocked neither the LPS-induced increases in the expression of TNF mRNA nor the translocation of NF-κB to the nucleus in LPS-treated macrophages, indicating that CNI-1493 does not interfere with early NF-κB-mediated transcriptional regulation of TNF. The synthesis if the 26-kDa membrane form of TNF was also effectively blocked by CNI-1493, indicating a translational suppressive effect. Previous work suggests that after macrophage activation, discrete signaling pathways regulate the p38 MAP kinase-dependent increases of TNF translation and the NF-κB-dependent enhancement of TNF transcription. It is possible that these signaling pathways diverge upstream of MEKK, the raf-1 homologue implicated in activation of JNK/p38 MAP kinase family. Although the molecular target of CNI-1493 is still unknown, it was shown that fetuin is necessary for macrophages to respond to it (Wang, *et al.*, 1998). More recently, CNI-1493 was reported to block the activation of p54 and p38 MAP kinases by IL-2 (Hunt *et al.*, 1999).

CNI-1493 has been studied in animal models of cytokine-mediated diseases, such as cancer-induced wasting (cachexia), experimental autoimmune encephalomyelitis, stroke, rheumatoid arthritis, allograft rejection, and cecal legation and puncture-induced peritoneal sepsis. *In vivo* studies have shown that CNI-1493 is protective against endotoxic shock or sepsis induced by cecal legation and puncture (Bianchi *et al.*, 1996; Cohen *et al.*, 1996) and collagen-induced arthritis (Kerlund *et al.*, 1999). It inhibits brain TNF production and is protective in a rat model of stroke (Meistrell III *et al.*, 1997).

Miscellaneous compounds

Benzidamine is a compound with anti-inflammatory properties currently in clinical use for the topical treatment of mucosal infections or inflammatory conditions. This agent, which does not affect arachidonate metabolism, was recently shown to inhibit the production of IL-1, TNF, and MCP-1 *in vitro* and *in vivo* (Sironi *et al.*, 1996). In contrast, it does not affect the anti-inflammatory cytokines IL-10 and IL-1ra.

Tenidap, an anion transport inhibitor with anti-inflammatory properties, inhibits production of IL-1, IL-6, and TNF (Sipe *et al.*, 1992; Laliberte *et al.*, 1994). Decrease in plasma IL-6 was also demonstrated in clinical trials with rheumatoid arthritis (RA) patients, where the drug proved effective (Littman *et al.*, 1995; Wylie *et al.*, 1995). Tenidap, however, did not decrease serum IL-6 levels in AIDS patients (Dezube *et al.*, 1997), suggesting a sort of specificity for RA. Fenspiride, an anti-inflammatory drug used in the treatment of inflammatory diseases of the upper respiratory tract, also inhibits TNF production *in vivo* (De Castro *et al.*, 1995).

Okamoto *et al.* (1991) investigated the effect of anti-inflammatory agents on IL-1β production in human peripheral blood mononuclear cells. They found that auranofin and sulphasalazine suppress IL-1 production (whereas bucillamine, lobenzarit and penicillamine did not). It should be noted, however, that auranofin also inhibits PKC (Chabot Fletcher *et al.*, 1994).

The macrolide antibiotics erythromycin and roxithromycin were reported to inhibit TNF, IL-1, and IL-8 (Iino *et al.*, 1992; Oishi *et al.*, 1994; Yoshimura *et al.*, 1995). Erythromycin also ameliorates bleomycin-induced pulmonary fibrosis by inhibiting TNF production (Chen *et al.*, 1997).

Suramin, an anticancer agent that inhibits protein-protein interactions, has been shown to dissociate the TNF trimer into inactive oligomers, thus inhibiting its receptor binding and biological activity (Grazioli *et al.*, 1992; Alzani *et al.*, 1993, 1995). It should be noted that dimethylsulfoxide also deoligomerizes TNF (Corti *et al.*, 1992; De Groote *et al.*, 1993) and there have been reports of an antiarthritic effect of dimethylsulfoxide (Watson *et al.*, 1985; Santos and Tipping, 1994).

Ferulic acid, an active component of *Cimifuga*, a plant used as an anti-inflammatory drug in Japanese traditional medicine, inhibits production of TNF-alpha and MIP-2 in the murine macrophage cell line, RAW264.7 (Sakai *et al.*, 1997).

Linomide (LS-2626) is an immunomodulator known to ameliorate autoimmune diseases and has been clinically tested for the treatment of multiple sclerosis (Karussis *et al.*, 1996) and inhibits the production of TNF and IL-1 by activated macrophages (Hortelano *et al.*, 1997).

Adenosine and adenosine receptor agonists inhibit TNF production in various experimental models (Hetier *et al.*, 1991; Prabhakar *et al.*, 1995; Brodie *et al.*, 1998; Wagner *et al.*, 1998). This has been reported for agonists of both adenosine A3 receptor (Bowlin *et al.*, 1997) and A2 receptor (Brodie *et al.*, 1998), but the mechanism has not been identified. While adenosine receptor agonist also block the induction of nitric oxide production (Brodie *et al.*, 1998), they up-regulate that of IL-6 (Ritchie *et al.*, 1997) and IL-10 (Hasko *et al.*, 1996).

Carnitine inhibits the synthesis of TNF, IL-1 and IL-6 in LPS-treated or tumor-bearing rats (Winter *et al.*, 1995) and administration of high-dose L-carnitine to AIDS patients lowers circulating TNF levels (De Simone *et al.*, 1993). This might be at least in part related to the antioxidant properties of carnitine (Arduini, 1992).

Other molecules have been reported to inhibit TNF production, including pentamidine, chloroquine, fusidic acid, angiotensin-converting enzyme. Some of these miscellaneous inhibitors have been mentioned by Newton and Decicco in their excellent review on TNF inhibitors (Newton and Decicco, 1999).

2.2 Inhibitors of cytokine action

2.2.1 Inhibitors of eicosanoids synthesis

Probably the inhibitor of cytokine action that has been used for the longest time is aspirin. However, the drug was used to inhibit fever before knowing that the endogenous mediators of fever are prostaglandins, and aspirin's mechanism of action was elucidated in the 1960s (Vane, 1971), before finding that prostaglandins are actually induced by pyrogenic cytokines (Dinarello and Wolff, 1982; Dinarello *et al.*, 1988). If aspirin and other NSAIDs were identified by screening IL-1-induced PGE2 production, we would probably classify them as specific inhibitors of cytokine action. That is, some of the pathways activated by cytokines that mediate inflammation were identified when cytokines were still not known. In this case, the knowledge of the existence of pro-inflammatory cytokines did not bring any real new strategy for the identification of drugs inhibiting critical steps of these pathways, such as cyclo-oxygenases or lipo-oxygenases.

2.2.2 Antioxidants and inhibitors of ROI generation

Another example is that of antioxidant molecules. It is now established that cytokines exert some of their activities by activation of NF-κB and this transcription factor is inhibited by various antioxidants. This, therefore, represents a strategy to inhibit this cytokine-activated pathway. Antioxidants like N-acetyl-cysteine, which inhibit NF-κB activation, also inhibit cytokine-stimulated HIV replication (Roederer *et al.*, 1990; Staal *et al.*, 1990).

It should be noted that inhibition of cytokine-activated NF-κB by antioxidants does not necessarily demonstrate that cytokines increase reactive oxygen intermediate production. It is more likely that some redox-sensitive step is implicated in NF-κB activation (Schreck *et al.*, 1991).

Cytokines can also exert some activities through an increased production of reactive oxygen intermediates by several mechanisms. One of these is the increased generation of ROI by IFNγ, TNF, G- and GM-CSF observed in PMN or macrophages. This is probably the first experimental model where the effect of cytokines on ROI production was studied and is important both in the microbicidal activity of phagocytes, as well as in their inflammatory, tissue damaging actions. Actually, experimental models of IFNγ- and/or PMA-stimulated PMN have been widely used to screen for 'antioxidant' agents. It should be noted that in this case the term 'antioxidant' is used incorrectly, as it refers to any compound that might block PMN activation.

Several studies have also pointed out a role of ROI in TNF-mediated cytotoxicity *in vitro*. Various groups have reported a protective effect of antioxidants against the *in vivo* and *in vitro* toxicity of recombinant TNF (Zimmerman *et al.*, 1989) and it was proposed that this toxicity was due to overproduction of ROI in mitochondria, more precisely at the level of the mitochondrial respiratory chain (Schulze-Osthoff *et al.*, 1992).

It was also reported that various IFNs (α, β and γ) (Ghezzi *et al.*, 1984, 1986; Falciani *et al.*, 1992) and IL-12 (Villa *et al.*, unpublished) induce xanthine oxidase, a well-known superoxide- and hydrogen peroxide-generating enzyme (McCord and Fridovich, 1968). However, while xanthine oxidase generates ROI, its product, uric acid, is an antioxidant and thus the induction of this enzyme might be regarded both as pro-oxidant and antioxidant. It was reported that xanthine oxidase is elevated in arthritis (Miesel and Zuber, 1993) and administration of its inhibitor, allopurinol, suppresses arthritis in mice (Miesel *et al.*, 1994). In murine models of influenza infection, xanthine oxidase is elevated, probably through IFNs, and its inhibition has protective effects (Akaike *et al.*, 1990; Maeda, 1997).

This enzyme is also induced in EAE (Agnello *et al.*, unpublished), but in this case it was associated with increased levels of uric acid in the spinal cord (Langemann *et al.*, 1992), and its inhibition with allopurinol has no protective effects. As administration of uric acid, which has antioxidant properties, is protective against EAE (Hooper *et al.*, 1997), a protective role of xanthine could be envisaged.

As in the case of ROI generation by phagocytes, induction of xanthine oxidase might have anti-infective actions. For instance, it was shown that high serum xanthine oxidase levels are protective against trypanosomal infection (Muranjan *et al.*, 1997).

2.2.3 Inhibitors of tryptophan metabolism

Another redox enzyme that is induced by IFNs is indoleamine dioxygenase. This flavin-dependent enzyme was discovered because it was found that D-tryptophan could be metabolized to kynurenine, and the known enzyme present in the liver that catalyzes such reaction, tryptophan dioxygenase, is specific for L-tryptophan. Indoleamine dioxygenase, however, can metabolize both D- and L-tryptophan and several other indoleamines (Shimizu *et al.*, 1978). This enzyme requires superoxides as cofactors and is markedly induced in mice infected with influenza virus or injected with IFN (Yoshida *et al.*, 1979; Hayaishi *et al.*, 1994).

The earlier studies focused on the role of indoleamine dioxygenase in the antiproliferative and antimicrobial effects of IFN, where a role for the depletion of tryptophan due to increased indoleamine dioxygenase was demonstrated (Hayaishi *et al.*, 1994). More recently, however, it was pointed out that this metabolic pathway leads to formation, among other metabolites, of quinolinic acid (see Fig. 2.7 and Kerr *et al.*, 1997). Quinolinic acid is a neurotoxin, acting through the N-methyl-D-aspartate (NMDA) receptor (Kerr *et al.*, 1997; Heyes *et al.*, 1991). Its concentrations are increased in the cerebrospinal fluid of patients with AIDS dementia and were suggested to be associated with production of cytokines (Griffin, 1997; Kerr *et al.*, 1997). Some inhibitors of indoleamine dioxygenase have been reported to inhibit quinolinic acid formation by interferon-gamma-stimulated monocytes: norharmane, 4-chloro-3-hydroxyanthranilate and 6-chloro-D-tryptophan (Saito *et al.*, 1993). Furthermore, the latter was shown to reduce the neurotoxicity of supernatants from HIV-infected macrophages (Kerr *et al.*, 1997). A recent study, using 6-chloro-D-tryptophan to inhibit indoleamine dioxygenase, has suggested that tryptophan catabolism associated with induction of this enzyme, might play a role in the prevention of allogeneic fetal rejection (Munn *et al.*, 1998), thus indicating a possible immunosuppressive role of this enzyme.

2.2.4 Inhibitors of nitric oxide synthesis

Among the so-called autacoids, the role of NO in biological systems was discovered only recently, and almost concomitantly with the identification of IL-1 and TNF as pathogenic mediators. The role of endogenous NO as a hypotensive agent (endothelium-derived relaxing factor) was defined in 1987, although a 1985 paper reported the production of inorganic nitrites by LPS-stimulated macrophages (Stuehr and Marletta, 1985). Shortly after that, it was found that the inducible form of NO synthase (iNOS) is inducible by LPS and several cytokines, alone or in combination, including TNF, IL-1 and IFNγ (reviewed in: Nathan and Xie, 1994; Moncada and Higgs, 1995).

As nitric oxide uses arginine as a substrate, inhibitors were rapidly developed and tested in animal models of septic shock of cytokine toxicity. The NOS inhibitor L-N-monomethyl-L-arginine (L-NMMA) prevents TNF-induced hypotension in dogs (Kilbourn *et al.*, 1990). As early as 1991 a preliminary report was published showing that L-NMMA and L-N-nitro-L-arginine methyl ester (L-NAME, another NOS inhibitor) had improved blood pressure in two patients with septic shock (Petros *et al.*, 1991). It should be noted, however, that NO is probably important in the LPS-induced hypotension but is not necessarily a critical mediator of LPS-induced mortality, as knock-out mice lacking iNOS are not protected for LPS toxicity (Laubach *et al.*, 1995).

While inhibition of NOS can be achieved with arginine analogues, another approach is to block its induction by endotoxin or pro-inflammatory cytokines. For instance, dexamethasone inhibits the expression of iNOS (Knowles *et al.*, 1990; Radomski *et al.*, 1990; Rees *et al.*, 1990).

2.2.5 Phosphodiesterase inhibitors

Although agents that increase cAMP are studied mainly as inhibitors of cytokine production, there is much evidence that they can also block the pro-inflammatory activity of

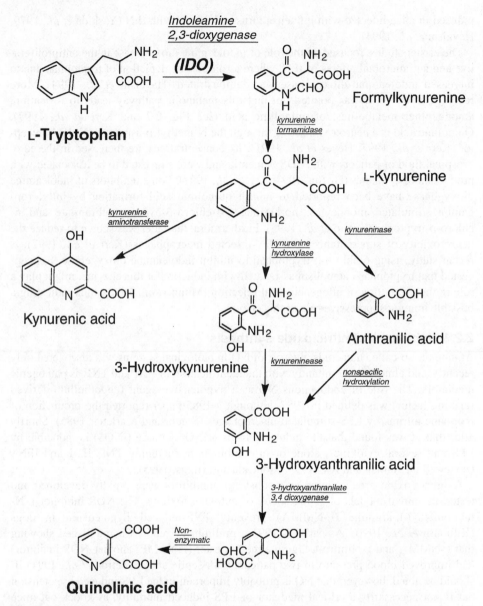

Fig. 2.7 Tryptophan metabolism through the indoleamine 2,3-dioxygenase pathway. (Reproduced with kind permission from Kerr *et al.*, 1997.)

cytokines *in vivo* and *in vitro*, although the mechanism for this action is unspecific as cAMP protects endothelial cells from a variety of insults. For instance, pentoxifylline inhibits TNF-induced endothelial cell cytotoxicity and neutrophil respiratory burst (Zheng *et al.*, 1990) or IL-1 activation of PMN (Sullivan *et al.*, 1988). Also, in a model of cecal legation and puncture, pentoxifylline was protective even using a treatment schedule that did not result in inhibition of TNF production. In this case, its protective action was explained on the basis of its effect on neutrophil trafficking, by augmenting PMN infiltration at the site of infection, while decreasing it in the lung (Hadjiminas *et al.*, 1994). More recently, it was reported that cyclic AMP inhibits NF-κB-mediated transcription in human monocytic cells and endothelial cells (Ollivier *et al.*, 1996).

2.3 Experimental models used for the identification of inhibitors of cytokine synthesis

Most of the published papers reporting the identification of inhibitors of cytokine production deal with TNF or IL-1, as these are probably the most extensively studied, as well as the most toxic cytokines. When various compounds are tested *in vitro* for inhibition of cytokine production, other cytokines, including those discovered more recently, are often measured.

On the other hand, in examining *in vivo* models, TNF is often the only cytokine for which inhibition is described. This is due to two reasons: TNF is more easily induced *in vivo* (IL-1 can hardly be detected in the circulation of endotoxemic animals or patients) and is probably the most important mediator of death by a lethal dose of endotoxin, an *in vivo* model that is widely used.

2.3.1 In vitro models for the study of inhibitors of cytokine synthesis

IL-1 was originally described as a product from endotoxin-stimulated macrophages that activated lymphocyte proliferation termed lymphocyte-activating factor (LAF). Thus, the model in which the production of this cytokine is studied is based on LPS-stimulated monocytes or macrophages. In this case, cells are cultured with endotoxin (or other stimuli such as phorbol esters) and IL-1 is measured in the supernatants after a period of, in most cases, 24 h. In the case of TNF, the kinetics of production is more rapid with a culture period of 4 h. This time period is known for the model of LPS-stimulated monocyte-macrophages.

When reading papers that describe inhibitors of cytokine production some aspects of the experimental models should be considered.

The first point is the method used to measure cytokines, for example, bioassay, ELISA or mRNA. In earlier studies, IL-1 was measured by means of a bioassay based on its LAF activity (i.e. induction of proliferation of thymocytes). In this case, a non-specific inhibition by the test compounds, carried over into the assay system, could give false-positive results. More recently, ELISAs for IL-1 have been made available and the old bioassay abandoned. Thus, this problem is to be kept in mind when revisiting 'old' reports on IL-1 synthesis inhibitors.

An example of such an artifact is given by the study of the effect of cAMP-inducing agents on IL-1 synthesis. While earlier reports measuring IL-1 using a bioassay showed a strong inhibition of synthesis by various phosphodiesterase inhibitors (up to 90%), subsequent data generated by using specific immunoassays did not confirm such an effect (Endres *et al.*, 1991). Furthermore, measurement of IL-1 mRNA will avoid this kind of artifact.

Similar problems arise with TNF. This cytokine is still measured largely by a bioassay based on the cytotoxic activity of TNF on some tumor cell lines (such as LM and L929 cells or WEHI164). In many cases, a description of a novel inhibitor of TNF synthesis reported using this bioassay should be confirmed using an ELISA. In fact, a compound that protects the cellular target from TNF cytotoxicity could be wrongly considered an inhibitor of TNF production. Another critical factor is whether cytokines are measured in the supernatant or in the cell lysate. In fact, as discussed below, both IL-1 and TNF require processing in order to be secreted. For these, as for any cytokine that is not immediately secreted (as happens with cytokines that have a signal peptide), secretion may not be an indicator of production or synthesis. When culture supernatants are harvested, and therefore only secreted protein is measured, an inhibitor of processing will give an apparent blocking effect. On the other hand, if overall synthesis is evaluated, for instance by measuring cytokines in both supernatant and cell lysate or by measuring cytokine mRNA, no effect of the inhibitor may be observed.

Cell system

Various experimental models have been used to identify inhibitors of TNF or IL-1 production. All of these are based on cells of the monocyte-macrophage lineage, the major producers of IL-1 and TNF.

Various cell preparations of monocytes, macrophages or peripheral blood mononuclear cells are used, including murine peritoneal macrophages, human monocytes or monocyte-derived macrophages, or total human peripheral blood mononuclear cells. Mouse cells have the obvious limitation of the animal species, but data obtained using this system are often better related to *in vivo* animal experiments. Attention should be paid to the use of peritoneal macrophages. These can be resident or elicited and, in the latter case, the number and activity of peritoneal macrophages is increased by injection of inflammatory agents, such as thioglycollate, peptone or casein.

Human cells, on the other hand, are subject to intra-donor variability. Data from more than one donor, possibly at least three, are often reported to support the reproducibility of the observations.

Recently, many studies have used whole blood as a cytokine-producing system. This model is very close to the use of peripheral blood mononuclear cells. The latter system is potentially suitable for the study of peptide inhibitors because these can be unstable in whole blood.

Various cytokines (e.g. IL-6, IL-8, MCP-1) are produced by endothelial cells stimulated with other cytokines, particularly IL-1 (Sironi *et al.*, 1989; Romano *et al.*, 1997*b*).

Cytokine-inducing agents

In most studies, LPS is used as a stimulus for the production of IL-1 and TNF. The inhibitors identified are generally active on IL-1 and TNF produced upon stimulation with other agents as well. However, in some cases specific stimuli are used for studies targeted to specific diseases. Anti-CD3 antibodies may be used to study TNF synthesis inhibitors in autoimmunity, myelin basic protein for multiple sclerosis, and others. Furthermore, some drugs may inhibit cytokine production only when this is induced by specific stimuli. For instance, PPAR-γ agonists were originally reported to inhibit only phorbol ester-induced, but not LPS-induced, cytokine production (Jiang *et al.*, 1998).

A typical experiment will consist of incubating cells (for instance, monocytes) with LPS in both the presence and the absence of the test drug. When a compound turns out to be an inhibitor of cytokine production some obvious controls will be required, such as the viability of the cells (a toxic compound will inevitably give false-positive results), as well as total protein synthesis (non-specific inhibitor of protein synthesis will also be a false-positive). Particular attention should be paid to the vehicle in which the test compound is dissolved. Dimethyl sulfoxide (DMSO) and ethanol are the most used solvents for water insoluble compounds. In these cases, one should be careful since these compounds have non-specific effects and are potent inhibitors of cytokine production in several experimental models. DMSO is an antioxidant and dissociates protein–protein interactions including the trimeric structure of TNF (Corti *et al.*, 1992) and ethanol is a phospholipase D inhibitor (Bauldry *et al.*, 1991).

Mechanisms of action: specific versus non-specific inhibition

The specificity of an inhibitor of cytokine synthesis should be investigated at various levels. If a compound has proven effective in inhibiting the synthesis of one or more cytokines *in vitro*, one should affirm that this is not due to a toxic effect on the cells. It could be possible that the test compound inhibits overall protein synthesis. This can be checked with a standard approach by measuring protein synthesis by incorporation of labeled amino acid. Furthermore, one should consider that cytokine production by monocyte/macrophages (and thus inhibition) is always studied in the presence of a stimulus. Thus, one should check that the activation pathway is not down-regulated in a generalized way. Measuring other cytokines or effects of macrophage activation can accomplish this task. For instance, induction of MHC class II antigens, or of TGF-β, have been successfully used to rule out such non-specific effects of an agent that inhibits production of pro-inflammatory cytokines (Bianchi *et al.*, 1996).

Obviously, if other cytokines induced in the same cells with the same stimulus (e.g. LPS-stimulated macrophages) are not inhibited, this would represent one of the best controls for the specificity. However, one must take into account differences in the time course of cytokine induction. For instance, TNF production generally peaks at 4 h, while other cytokines (e.g. IL-1, IL-6) often require longer (up to 24 h) incubations. Hence, it is conceivable that an inhibitor may be present in active concentrations for a short time and then be degraded, which would result in an inhibitory effect on TNF rather than IL-1 or IL-6.

Mechanism of inhibition: effects on the cytokine network or on the pathway of stimulation

Another aspect to consider is that cytokines constitute a network with positive and negative effects on one another synthesis (Chapter 1). For instance, TNF and IL-10 are both induced by LPS, and IL-10 is an inhibitor of TNF production. This means that any drug that up-regulates IL-10 synthesis will be picked up as an inhibitor of TNF production, if the endpoint is measurement of TNF produced. The existence of such a negative loop can be demonstrated by using anti-IL-10 antibodies and also measuring IL-10. For instance, PGE2 inhibits TNF production in part via IL-10, as anti-IL-10 antibodies partially reverse its inhibitory effect on TNF (Strassmann *et al.*, 1994).

However, one should test the possibility that other inhibitory cytokines are up-regulated. This can only be ruled out by determining whether the inhibitory effect on TNF production depends on protein synthesis. This can be done measuring TNF mRNA, instead of the protein, induced in the presence of an inhibitor of protein synthesis, such as cycloheximide.

In addition, the stimulatory loops among cytokines should be considered. For instance, TNF and IL-1 induce IL-6, IL-8, and other cytokines. TNF represents an important inducer of IL-6 and, in fact, anti-TNF antibodies inhibit IL-6 levels induced by LPS (Jansen *et al.*, 1996), so that any compound that inhibits TNF production, will also inevitably inhibit IL-6 production. Thus, in screening for an IL-6 synthesis inhibitor, this possibility has to be considered. For instance, one could use TNF as the inducer or measure IL-6 mRNA as discussed above.

2.3.2 In vivo models to study inhibitors of cytokine synthesis

In selecting the animal model, one should obviously keep in mind the pathology for which inhibitors of cytokines are developed. LPS is the most obvious inducer when the pathology is gram-negative sepsis. However, LPS is also used as a generic stimulus to cytokine production for the screening of inhibitors of cytokine production.

The model consists in injecting animals (normally mice or rats) with LPS. An intraperitoneal or intravenous injection of LPS will induce circulating levels of TNF and IL-6, with a peak between 1 and 2 h. Unfortunately, usually no IL-1 can be detected in the circulation in this model. In most cases, IL-1 can be measured in tissue homogenates (e.g. spleen, liver) of these animals (Gnocchi *et al.*, 1992).

The test compound is administered before or after LPS. Schedules may vary. However, since cytokines are detected in the circulation 1–2 h after LPS administration, the compound to be tested cannot be given too late: TNF gene expression in monocytes was reported to be activated as early as 5–10 min after LPS addition (Gallay *et al.*, 1993).

When serum TNF or IL-6 are measured, one must check, as in the case of *in vitro* experiments, for the possible interference of the compound in the assay (bioassay or ELISA).

While 'generic' inhibitors of cytokine synthesis can be identified using the LPS model, some more 'pathology-oriented' models may be necessary (e.g. live bacteria for sepsis; models of inflammation for arthritis; cerebral TNF production in meningitis, etc.). These will be discussed in specific chapters.

As in the case of *in vitro* models, toxicity of the test drug might result in false-positive results. In most cases, this is less of a problem *in vivo* as toxicity will be evident as lethality or sick appearance of the animal. Furthermore, *in vivo* one should make sure that a drug that inhibits cytokine production, does not act simply by elevating serum corticosteroid levels (see Chapter 8)—an effect that may also result from non-specific toxicity of the drug.

In a few cases, studies were done using human volunteers or monkeys. In such cases, the experiments have taken advantage of the availability of ELISA for almost all human cytokines. For instance, in LPS-treated humans, IL-8 can also be measured (there is no clear mouse homologue of human IL-8) in addition to IL-6 and TNF. Also, in the case of human volunteers, little or no IL-1 can be found in the circulation after LPS (Michie *et al.*, 1988).

2.3.3 Positive controls

As in most tests for the identification of novel compounds, reference inhibitors are normally included in the studies. Synthetic glucocorticoids are probably the most active inhibitors of cytokine synthesis *in vivo* and *in vitro*. More specific agents should be included for testing inhibitors of specific cytokines or their processing. It should be noted, as one of the main areas of research of cytokine inhibitors is inflammation, that non-steroidal anti-inflammatory drugs acting as cyclo-oxygenase inhibitors may inhibit or increase LPS-induced cytokine production, depending on the experimental model used. While the biochemical basis for this 'paradoxical' effect will be given below, it is important to remember that these do not represent good reference compounds for inhibition of cytokine production (although they can be used as reference inhibitors of cytokine-mediated inflammation).

References

Akaike, T., Ando, M., Oda, T., Doi, T., Ijiri, S., Araki, S. *et al.* (1990). Dependence on O_2^- generation by xanthine oxidase of pathogenesis of influenza virus infection in mice. *J. Clin. Invest.*, **85**, 739–45.

Almawi, W. Y., Beyhum, H. N., Rahme, A. A. and Rieder, M. J. (1996). Regulation of cytokines and cytokine receptor expression by glucocorticoids. *J. Leukoc. Biol.*, **60**, 563–72.

Alzani, R., Corti, A., Grazioli, L., Cozzi, E., Ghezzi, P. and Marcucci, F. (1993). Suramin induces deoligomerization of human tumor necrosis factor alpha. *J. Biol. Chem.*, **268**, 12526–9.

Alzani, R., Cozzi, E., Corti, A., Temponi, M., Trizio, D., Gigli, M. *et al.* (1995). Mechanism of suramin-induced deoligomerization of tumor necrosis factor alpha. *Biochemistry*, **34**, 6344–50.

Amman, P., Rizzoli, R., Bonjour, J.-P., Bourrin, S., Meyer, J.-M. and Vassalli, P. (1997). Transgenic mice expressing soluble tumor necrosis factor-receptor are protected against bone loss caused by estrogen deficiency. *J. Clin. Invest.*, **99**, 1699–703.

Anastassiou, E. D., Paliogianni, F., Balow, J. P., Yamada, H. and Boumpas, D. T. (1992). Prostaglandin E2 and other cyclic AMP-elevating agents modulate IL-2 and IL-2Rα gene expression at multiple levels. *J. Immunol.*, **148**, 2845–52.

Anderson, G. D., Hauser, S. D., McGarity, K. L., Isakson, P. C. and Gregory, S. A. (1996). Selective inhibition of cylooxygenase (COX)-2 reverses inflammation and expression of COX-2 and interleukin 6 in rat adjuvant arthritis. *J. Clin. Invest.*, **97**, 2672–9.

Andus, T., Gross, V., Casar, I., Krumm, D., Hosp, J., David, M. *et al.* (1991). Activation of monocytes during inflammatory bowel disease. *Pathobiology*, **59**, 166–70.

Anttila, H. S. I., Reitamo, S., Ceska, M. and Hurme, M. (1992). Signal trasduction pathways leading to the production of IL-8 by human monocytes are differentially regulated dy dexamethasone. *Clin. Exp. Immunol.*, **89**, 509–12.

Araghi-Niknam, M., Liang, B., Zhang, Z., Ardestani, S. K. and Watson, R. R. (1997). Modulation of immune disfunction during murine leukemia retrovirus infection of old mice by dehydroepiandrosterone sulphate (DHEAS). *Immunology*, **90**, 344–9.

Arduini, A. (1992). Carnitine and its acyl esters as secondary antioxidants? [letter]. *Am. Heart J.*, **123**, 1726–7.

Arend, W. P. and Massoni, R. J. (1986). Characteristics of bacterial lipopolysaccharide induction of interleukin 1 synthesis and secretion by human monocytes. *Clin. Exp. Immunol.*, **64**, 656–64.

Arzt, E., Sauer, J., Pollmacher, T., Labeur, M., Holsboer, F., Reul, J. M. *et al.* (1994). Glucocorticoids suppress interleukin-1 receptor antagonist synthesis following induction by endotoxin. *Endocrinology*, **134**, 672–7.

Auphan, N., DiDonato, J. A., Rosette, C., Helmberg, A. and Karin, M. (1995). Immunosuppression by glucocorticoids: inhibition of NF-kB activity through induction of IkB synthesis. *Science*, **270**, 286–90.

Badger, A. M., Bradbeer, J. N., Votta, B., Lee, J. C., Adams, J. L. and Griswold, D. E. (1996). Pharmacological profile of SB 203580, a selective inhibitor of cytokine suppressive binding protein/p38 kinase, in animal models of arthritis, bone resorption, endotoxin shock and immune function. *J. Pharmacol. Exp. Ther*, **279**, 1453–61.

Baeuerle, P. A. and Baichwal, V. R. (1997). NF-kappa B as a frequent target for immunosuppressive and anti- inflammatory molecules. *Adv Immunol*, **65**, 111–37.

Baeuerle, P. A. and Henkel, T. (1994). Function and activation of NF-kB in the immune system. *Ann. Rev. Immunol.*, **12**, 141–79.

Bahl, A. K., Dale, M. M. and Foreman, J. C. (1994). The effect of non-steroidal anti-inflammatory drugs on the accumulation and release of interleukin-1-like activity by peritoneal macrophages from the mouse. *Br. J. Pharmacol.*, **113**, 809–14.

Bailly, S., Ferrua, B., Fay, M. and Gougerot-Pocidalo, M. A. (1990). Differential regulation of IL-6, IL-1 alpha, IL-1 beta and TNF alpha production in LPS-stimulated human monocytes: role of cyclic AMP. *Cytokine*, **2**, 205–10.

Baldwin Jr., A. S. (1996). The NF-kB and IkB proteins: new discoveries and insights. *Ann. Rev. Immunol.*, **14**, 649–81.

Barber, A. E., Coyle, S. M., Marano, M. A., Fischer, E., Calvano, S. E., Fong, Y. *et al.* (1993). Glucocorticoid therapy alters hormonal and cytokine responses to endotoxin in man. *J. Immunol.*, **150**, 1999–2006.

Barnes, P. J., Belvisi, M. G. and Rogers, D. F. (1990). Modulation of neurogenic inflammation: novel approaches to inflammatory disease. *Trends Pharmacol. Sci.*, **11**, 185–9.

Bauldry, S. A., Bass, D. A., Cousart, S. L. and McCall, C. E. (1991). Tumor necrosis factor alfa priming of phospholipase D in human neutrophils. Correlation between phosphatidic acid production and superoxide generation. *J. Biol. Chem.*, **266**, 4173–9.

Beaty, C. D., Franklin, T. L., Uehara, Y. and Wilson, C. B. (1994). Lipopolysaccharide-induced cytokine production in human monocytes: role of tyrosine phosphorylation in transmembrane signal transduction. *Eur. J. Immunol.*, **24**, 1278–84.

Beavo, J. A. and Reifsnyder, D. H. (1990). Primary sequence of cyclic nucleotide phosphodiesterase isozymes and the design of selective inhibitors. *Trends Pharmacol. Sci.*, **11**, 150–5.

Beavo, J. A., Conti, M. and Heaslip, R. J. (1994). Multiple cyclic nucleotide phosphodiesterases. *Mol. Pharmacol.*, **46**, 399–405.

Bellido, T., Jilka, R. L., Boyce, B. F., Girasole, G., Broxmeyer, H., Dalrymple, S. A. *et al.* (1995). Regulation of interleukin-6 osteoclastogenesis and bone mass by androgens. The role of androgen receptor. *J. Clin. Invest.*, **95**, 2886–95.

Benigni, F., Villa, P., Demitri, M. T., Sacco, S., Sipe, J. D., Lagunowich, L. *et al.* (1995). Ciliary neurotrophic factor (CNTF) inhibits brain and peripheral TNF production and, in association with its soluble receptor, protects mice against LPS toxicity. *Molecular Medicine*, **1**, 568–75.

Berkowitz, D. E., Brown, D., Lee, K. M., Emala, C., Palmer, D., An, Y. *et al.* (1998). Endotoxin-induced alteration in the expression of leptin and beta3- adrenergic receptor in adipose tissue. *Am. J. Physiol.*, **274**, E992–7.

Bernhagen, J., Calandra, T., Mitchell, R. A., Martin, S. B., Tracey, K. J., Voelter, W. *et al.* (1993). MIF is a pituitary-derived cytokine that potentiates lethal endotoxemia. *Nature*, **365**, 756–9.

Bertini, R., Garattini, S., Delgado, R. and Ghezzi, P. (1993). Pharmacological activities of chlorpromazine involved in the inhibition of tumor necrosis factor production *in vivo* mice. *Immunology*, **79**, 217–9.

Beutler, B., Krochin, N., Milsark, I. W., Luedke, C. and Cerami, A. (1986). Control of cachectin (tumor necrosis factor) synthesis: mechanism of endotoxin resistance. *Science.*, **232**, 975–9.

Bianchi, M., Fantuzzi, G., Bertini, R., Perin, L., Salmona, M. and Ghezzi, P. (1993). The pneumotoxicant paraquat induces IL-8 mRNA in human mononuclear cells and pulmonary epithelial cells. *Cytokine*, **5**, 525–30.

Bianchi, M., Ulrich, P., Bloom, O., Meistrell III, M., Zimmerman, G. A., Schmidtmayerova, H. *et al.* (1995). An inhibitor of macrophage arginine transport and nitric oxide production (CNI-1493) prevents acute inflammation and endotoxin lethality. *Molecular Medicine*, **1**, 254–66.

Bianchi, M., Bloom, O., Raabe, T., Cohen, P. S., Chesney, J., Sherry, B. *et al.* (1996). Suppression of proinflammatory cytokines in monocytes by a tetravalent guanylhydrazone. *Journal of Experimental Medicine*, **183**, 927–36.

Bomalaski, J. S., Ford, T., Hudson, A. P. and Clark, M. A. (1995). Phospholipase A₂-activating protein induces the synthesis of IL-1 and TNF in human monocytes. *J. Immunol.*, **154**, 4027–31.

Bone, R. C., Fisher, C. J. J., Clemmer, T. P., Slotman, G. J., Metz, C. A., Balk, R. A. *et al.* (1987). A controlled clinical trial of high-dose methylprednisolone in the treatment of severe sepsis and septic shock. *New Engl. J. Med.*, **317**, 653–8.

Bowlin, T. L., Borcherding, D. R., Edwards, C. K., 3rd and McWhinney, C. D. (1997). Adenosine A3 receptor agonists inhibit murine macrophage tumor necrosis factor-alpha production *in vitro* and *in vivo*. *Cell Mol. Biol. (Noisy-le-grand)*, **43**, 345–9.

Bradshaw, D., Hill, C. H., Nixon, J. S. and Wilkinson, S. E. (1993). Therapeutic potential of protein kinase C inhibitors. *Agents Action*, **38**, 135–47.

Brandwein, S. R. (1986). Regulation of interleukin 1 production by mouse peritoneal macrophages. Effects of arachidonic acid metabolites, cyclic nucleotides and interferons. *J. Biol. Chem.*, **261**, 8624–32.

Brodie, C., Blumberg, P. M. and Jacobson, K. A. (1998). Activation of the A2A adenosine receptor inhibits nitric oxide production in glial cells. *FEBS Lett*, **429**, 139–42.

Brown, Z., Strieter, R. M., Chensue, S. W., Ceska, M., Lindley, J., Neild, G. H. *et al.* (1991). Cytokine-activated human mesangial cells generate the neutrophil chemoattractant, interleukin 8. *Kidney Int.*, **40**, 86–90.

Burroughs, M. H., Tsenova-Berkova, L., Sokol, K., Ossig, J., Tuomanen, E. and Kaplan, G. (1995). Effect of thalidomide on the inflammatory response in cerebrospinal fluid in experimental bacterial meningitis. *Microb. Pathog.*, **19**, 245–55.

Buttgereit, F., Brink, I., Thiele, B., Burmester, G. R., Hiepe, F. and Hall, E. D. (1995). Effects of methylprednisolone and 21-aminosteroids on mitogen-induced interleukin-6 and tumor necrosis factor-alpha production in human peripheral blood mononuclear cells. *J. Pharmacol. Exp. Ther.*, **275**, 850–3.

Byron, K. A., Varigos, G. and Wootton, A. (1992). Hydrocortisone inhibition of human interleukin-4. *Immunology*, **77**, 624–6.

Calandra, T., Bernhagen, J., Metz, C. N., Spiegel, L. A., Bacher, M., Donnelly, T. *et al.* (1995). MIF is a glucocorticoid-induced modulator of cytokine production. *Nature*, **377**, 68–71.

Campanile, F., Giampietri, A., Grohmann, U., Belladonna, M. L., Fioretti, M. C. and Puccetti, P. (1996). Evidence for tumor necrosis factor α as a mediator of the toxicity of a cyclo-oxygenase inhibitor in gram-negative sepsis. *Eur. J. Pharmacol.*, **307**, 191–9.

Campbell, I. K., Ianches, G. and Hamilton, J. A. (1993). Production of macrophage colony-stimulating factor (M-CSF) by human articular cartilage and condrocytes. Modulation by interleukin-1 and tumor necrosis factor. *Biochim. Biophys. Acta*, **1182**, 57–63.

Cantorna, M. T., Woodward, W. D., Hayes, C. E. and DeLuca, H. F. (1998). 1,25-dihydroxyvitamin D3 is a positive regulator for the two anti- encephalitogenic cytokines TGF-beta 1 and IL-4. *J. Immunol.*, **160**, 5314–9.

Caughey, G. E., Pouliot, M., Cleland, L. G. and James, M. J. (1997). Regulation of tumor necrosis factor-α and IL-1β synthesis by thromboxane A2 in nonadherent human monocytes. *J. Immunol.*, **158**, 351–8.

Chabot Fletcher, M., Breton, J., Lee, J., Young, P. and Griswold, D. E. (1994). Interleukin-8 production is regulated by protein kinase C in human keratinocytes. *J. Invest. Dermatol.*, **103**, 509–15.

Chaudri, G. and Clark, I. A. (1989). Reactive oxygen species facilitate the *in vitro* and *in vivo* lipopolysaccharide-induced release of tumor necrosis factor. *J. Immunol.*, **143**, 1290–4.

Chelmicka-Schorr, E., Kwasniewski, M. N. and Czlonkowska, A. (1992). Sympathetic nervous system modulates macrophage function. *Int. J. Immunopharmacol.*, **14**, 841–6.

Chen, B., Jiang, L., Zhao, W., Yu, R. and Hou, X. M. (1997). Ameliorating effect of erythromycin on bleomycin-induced pulmonary fibrosis: role of alveolar macrophage activation and cytokine release. *Respirology*, **2**, 151–5.

Chen, G., Wang, S. H. and Converse, C. A. (1994). Glutathione increases interleukin-2 production in human lymphocytes. *Int. J. Immunopharmacol.*, **16**, 755–60.

Christ, W. J., Asano, O., Robidoux, A. L. C., Perez, M., Wang, Y., Dubuc, G. R. *et al.* (1995). E5531, a pure endotoxin antagonist of high potency. *Science*, **268**, 80–3.

Chung, I. Y., Kwon, J. and Benveniste, E. N. (1992). Role of protein kinase C activity in tumor necrosis factor-α gene expression: involvement at the transcriptional level. *J. Immunol.*, **149**, 3894–902.

Claria, J. and Serhan, C. N. (1995). Aspirin triggers previously undescribed bioactive eicosanoids by human endothelial cell-leukocyte interactions. *Proc. Natl. Acad. Sci. USA*, **92**, 9475–9.

Cohen, P. S., Nakshatri, H., Dennis, J., Caragine, T., Bianchi, M., Cerami, A. *et al.* (1996). CNI-1493 inhibits monocyte/macrophage tumor necrosis factor by suppression of translation efficiency. *Proc. Natl. Acad. Sci. USA*, **93**, 3967–71.

Colotta, F. and Mantovani, A. (1994). Induction of the interleukin-1 decoy receptor by glucocorticoids. *Trends Pharmacol. Sci.*, **15**, 138–9.

Corral, L. G., Muller, G. W., Moreira, A. L., Chen, Y., Wu, M., Stirling, D. *et al.* (1996). Selection of novel analogues of thalidomide with enhanced tumor necrosis factor alpha inhibitory activity. *Mol. Med.*, **2**, 506–15.

Corral, L. G., Haslett, P. A., Muller, G. W., Chen, R., Wong, L. M., Ocampo, C. J. *et al.* (1999). Differential cytokine modulation and T cell activation by two distinct classes of thalidomide analogueues that are potent inhibitors of TNF- alpha. *J. Immunol.*, **163**, 380–6.

Corti, A., Fassina, G., Marcucci, F., Barbanti, E. and Cassani, G. (1992). Oligomeric tumor necrosis factor α slowly converts into inactive forms at bioactive levels. *Biochem. J.*, **284**, 905–10.

Cromlish, W. A. and Kennedy, B. P. (1996). Selective inhibition of cyclo-oxygenase-1 ans -2 using intact insect cell assays. *Biochem. Pharmacol.*, **52**, 1777–85.

Culpepper, J. A. and Lee, F. (1985). Regulation of IL-3 expression by glucocorticoids in cloned murine T lymphocytes. *Lymphokine*, **13**, 275–80.

D'Ambrosio, D., Cippitelli, M., Cocciolo, M. G., Mazzeo, D., Di Lucia, P., Lang, R. *et al.* (1998). Inhibition of IL-12 production by 1,25-dihydroxyvitamin D3. Involvement of NF-kappaB down-regulation in transcriptional repression of the p40 gene. *J. Clin. Invest.*, **101**, 252–62.

Danenberg, H. D., Alpert, G., Lustig, S. and Ben-Nathan, D. (1992). Dehydroepiandrosterone protects mice from endotoxin toxicity and reduces tumor necrosis factor production. *Antimicrob. Agents Chemother.*, **36**, 2275–9.

Danner, R. L., Joiner, K. A. and Parrillo, J. E. (1987). Inhibition of endotoxin-induced priming of human neutrophils by lipid X and 3-Aza-lipid X. *J. Clin. Invest.*, **80**, 605–12.

Daynes, R. A., Araneo, A. B., Ershler, W. B., Maloney, C., Li, G. Z. and Ryu, S. Y. (1993). Altered regulation of IL-6 production with normal aging. Possible linkage to the age-associated decline in DHEA and its sulfated derivatives. *J. Immunol.*, **150**, 5219–30.

Deakin, A. M., Payne, A. M., Whittle, B. J. and Moncada, S. (1995). The modulation of IL-6 and IFN-alpha release by nitric oxide following stimulation of J774 cells with LPS and IFN-gamma. *Cytokine*, **7**, 408–16.

Debets, J. M. H., Ruers, T. J. M., Van der Linden, M. P. M. H., Van der Linden, C. J. and Buurman, W. A. (1989). Inhibitory effect of corticosteroids on the secretion of tumour necrosis factor (TNF) by monocytes is dependent on the stimulus inducing TNF synthesis. *Clin. Exp. Immunol.*, **78**, 224–9.

De Castro, C. M., Nahori, M. A., Dumarey, C. H., Vargaftig, B. B. and Bachelet, M. (1995). Fenspiride: an anti-inflammatory drug with potential benefits in the treatment of endotoxemia. *Eur. J. Pharmacol.*, **294**, 669–76.

DeForge, L. E., Preston, A. M., Takeuchi, E., Kenney, J., Boxer, L. A. and Remick, D. G. (1993). Regulation of interleukin 8 gene expression by oxidant stress. *J. Biol. Chem.*, **268**, 25568–76.

De Groote, D., Grau, G. E., Dehart, I. and Franchimont, P. (1993). Stabilisation of functional tumor necrosis factor-alpha by its soluble TNF receptors. *Eur. Cytokine Netw.*, **4**, 359–62.

Demitri, M. T., Velucchi, M., Bracci, L., Rustici, A., Porro, M., Villa, P. *et al.* (1996). Inhibition of LPS-induced systemic and local TNF production by a synthetic anti-endotoxin peptide (SAEP-2). *Journal of Endotoxin Research*, **3**, 445–454.

De Simone, C., Tzantzoglou, S., Famularo, G., Moretti, S., Paoletti, F., Vullo, V. *et al.* (1993). High dose L-carnitine improves immunologic and metabolic parameters in AIDS patients. *Immunopharmacol. Immunotoxicol.*, **15**, 1–12.

Dezube, B. J., Lederman, M. M., Chapman, B., Georges, D. L., Dogon, A. L., Mudido, P. *et al.* (1997). The effect of tenidap on cytokines, acute-phase proteins, and virus load in human immunodeficiency virus (HIV)-infected patients: correlation between plasma HIV-1 RNA and proinflammatory cytokine levels. *J. Infect. Dis.*, **176**, 807–10.

Dinarello, C. A. (1996). Biologic basis for interleukin-1 in disease. *Blood*, **87**, 2095–147.

Dinarello, C. A. and Wolff, S. M. (1982). Molecular basis of fever in humans. *Am. J. Med.*, **72**, 799–819.

Dinarello, C. A., Bishai, J., Rosenwasser, L. J. and Coceani, F. (1984). The influence of lipoxygenase inhibitors on the *in vitro* production of human leukocytic pyrogen and lymphocyte activating factor (interleukin 1). *Int. J. Immunopharmacol.*, **6**, 43–50.

Dinarello, C. A., Cannon, J. G. and Wolff, S. M. (1988). New concepts in the pathogenesis of fever. *Rev. Infect. Dis.*, **10**, 168–89.

Di Santo, E., Foddi, M. C., Ricciardi-Castagnoli, P., Mennini, T. and Ghezzi, P. (1996a). DHEA inhibits TNF production in monocytic, astrocitic and microglial cells. *Neuroimmunomodulation*, **3**, 285–8.

Di Santo, E., Sironi, M., Mennini, T., Zinetti, M., Savoldi, G., Di Lorenzo, D. *et al.* (1996b). A glucocorticoid receptor-independent mechanism for neurosteroid inhibition of tumor necrosis factor production. *Eur. J. Pharmacol.*, **299**, 179–86.

Dornand, J. and Gerber, M. (1991). Mechanisms of IL-2 production impairment by lipoxygenase inhibitors in activated Jurkat cells. *Journal of Lipid Mediators*, **4**, 23–38.

Dornand, J., Sekkat, C., Mani, J. C. and Gerber, M. (1987). Lipoxygenase inhibitors suppress IL-2 synthesis: relationship with rise of [Ca++]i and the events dependent on protein kinase C activation. *Immunology Letters*, **16**, 101–6.

Downs, T. R., Dage, R. C. and French, J. F. (1995). Reduction in endotoxin-induced organ dysfunction and cytokine secretion by a cyclic nitrone antioxidant. *Int. J. Immunopharmacol.*, **17**, 571–80.

East, C. J., Abboud, C. N. and Borch, R. F. (1992). Diethyldithiocarbamate induction of cytokine release in human long-term bone marrow cultures. *Blood*, **80**, 1172–7.

Eck, H.-P., Gmunder, H., Hartmann, M., Petzoldt, D., Daniel, V. and Dröge, W. (1989). Low concentrations of acid-soluble thiol (cysteine) in the blood plasma of HIV-1-infected patients. *Hoppe*, **370**, 101–8.

Eigler, A., Moeller, J. and Endres, S. (1995). Exogenous and endogenous nitric oxide attenuates tumor necrosis factor synthesis in the murine macrophage cell line RAW 264.7. *J. Immunol.*, **154**, 4048–54.

Endres, S., Fulle, H.-J., Sinha, B., Stoll, D., Dinarello, C. A., Gerzer, R. *et al.* (1991). Cyclic nucleotides differentially reguate the synthesis of tumour necrosis factor-α and interleukin-1β by human mononuclear cells. *Immunology*, **72**, 56–60.

Endres, S., Whitaker, R. E. D., Ghorbani, R., Meydani, S. N. and Dinarello, C. A. (1996). Oral aspirin and ibuprofen increase cytokine-induced synthesis of IL-1β and of tumour necrosis factor-α ex vivo. *Immunology*, **87**, 264–70.

Eugui, E. M., DeLustro, B., Rouhafza, S., Ilnicka, M., Lee, S. W., Wilhelm, R. *et al.* (1994). Some antioxidants inhibit, in a co-ordinate fashion, the production of tumor necrosis factor-alpha, IL-beta, and IL-6 by human peripheral blood mononuclear cells. *Int. Immunol.*, **6**, 409–22.

Eylar, E., Rivera-Quinones, C., Molina, C., Baez, I., Molina, F. and Mercado, C. M. (1993). N-acetylcysteine enhances T cell functions and T cell growth in culture. *Int. Immunol.*, **5**, 97–101.

Eylar, E. H., Baez, I., Vazquez, A. and Yamamura, Y. (1995). N-acetylcysteine (NAC) enhances interleukin-2 but suppresses interleukin-4 secretion from normal and HIV+ CD4+ T-cells. *Cell Mol. Biol. (Noisy-le-grand)*, **41**, S35–40.

Faggioni, R., Gatti, S., Demitri, M. T., Delgado, R., Echtenacher, B., Gnocchi, P. *et al.* (1994). Role of xanthine oxidase and reactive oxygen intermediates in LPS- and TNF-induced pulmonary edema. *J. Lab. Clin. Med.*, **123**, 394–9.

Falciani, F., Ghezzi, P., Terao, M., Cazzaniga, G. and Garattini, E. (1992). Interferons induce xanthine dehydrogenase gene expression in L929 cells. *Biochem. J.*, **285**, 1001–8.

Fantuzzi, G., Cantoni, L., Sironi, M. and Ghezzi, P. (1993). Inhibitors of cytochrome P-450 suppress tumor necrosis factor production. *Cell. Immunol.*, **150**, 417–24.

Fantuzzi, G., Demitri, M. T. and Ghezzi, P. (1994). Differential effect of glucocorticoids on tumor necrosis factor production in mice: up-regulation by early pretreatment with dexamethasone. *Clin. Exp. Immunol.*, **96**, 166–9.

Fantuzzi, G., Di Santo, E., Sacco, S., Benigni, F. and Ghezzi, P. (1995a). Role of the hypothalamus-pituitary-adrenal axis in the regulation of tumor necrosis factor production in mice: effect of stress and inhibition of endogenous glucocorticoids. *J. Immunol.*, **155**, 3552–5.

Fantuzzi, G., Galli, G., Zinetti, M., Fratelli, M. and Ghezzi, P. (1995b). The upregulating effect of dexamethasone on tumor necrosis factor production is mediated by a nitric oxide-producing cytochrome P450. *Cell. Immunol.*, **160**, 305–8.

Ferran, C., Dy, M., Merite, S., Sheehan, K., Schreiber, R., Leboulenger, F. *et al.* (1990). Reduction of morbidity and cytokine release in anti-CD3 MoAb-treated mice by corticosteroids. *Transplantation*, **50**, 642–8.

Ferrante, J. V., Huang, Z. H., Nandoskar, M., Hii, C. S. T., Robinson, B. S., Rathjen, D. A. *et al.* (1997). Altered responses of human macrophages to lipopolysaccharide by hydroperoxy eicosatetraenoic acid, hydroxy eicosatetraenoic acid, and arachidonic acid. Inhibition of tumor necrisos factor production. *J. Clin. Invest.*, **99**, 1445–52.

Fidelus, R. K. and Tsan, M. F. (1986). Enhancement of intracellular glutathione promotes lympho-cyte activation by mitogen. *Cell Immunol.*, **97**, 155–63.

Fiebich, B. L., Lieb, K., Hüll, M., Berger, M. and Bauer, J. (1996). Effects of NSAIDs on IL-1β-induced IL-6 mRNA and protein synthesis in human astrocytoma cells. *Neuroreport*, **7**, 1209–13.

Fisher, M., Plante, G. M. and Doyle, E. M. (1993). Inhibition of inflammatory cell-mediated myelin oxidation and interleukin-1 beta generation by a 21-aminosteroid, U74500A. *J. Neurol. Sci.*, **119**, 189–94.

Flower, R. J. (1988). Lipocortin and the mechanism of action of the glucocorticoids. *Br. J. Pharmacol.*, **94**, 987–1015.

Fong, T. C. and Makinodan, T. (1989). Preferential enhancement by 2-mercaptoethanol of IL-2 responsiveness of T blast cells from old over young mice is associated with potentiated protein kinase C translocation. *Immunol. Lett*, **20**, 149–54.

Forman, B. R., Tontonoz, P., Chen, J., Brun, R. P., Spiegelman, B. M. and Evans, R. M. (1996). 15-deoxy-D^{12,14}-prostaglandin J$_2$ is a ligand for the adipocyte determination factor PPARg. *Cell*, **83**, 803–12.

Fukuoka, M., Ogino, Y., Sato, H., Ohta, T. and Komoriya, K. (1998). Regulation of RANTES and IL-8 production in normal human dermal fibroblasts by active vitamin D3 (tacalcitol). *Br. J. Pharmacol.*, **124**, 1433–8.

Gallay, P., Jongeneel, C. V., Barras, C., Burnier, M., Baumgartner, J.-D., Glauser, M. P. *et al.* (1993). Short time exposure to lipopolysaccharide is sufficient to activate human monocytes. *J. Immunol.*, **150**, 5086–93.

Galley, H. F., Davies, M. J. and Webster, N. R. (1996). Xanthine oxidase activity and free radical generation in patients with sepsis syndrome. *Critical Care Medicine*, **24**, 1649–53.

Geng, Y., Zhang, B. and Lotz, M. (1993). Protein tyrosine kinase activation is required for lipopolysaccharide induction of cytokines in human blood monocytes. *J. Immunol.*, **151**, 6692–700

Gessani, S., McCandless, S. and Baglioni, C. (1988). The glucocorticoid dexamethasone inhibits synthesis of interferon by decreasing level of its mRNA. *J. Biol. Chem.*, **263**, 7454–7.

Ghezzi, P. and Dinarello, C. A. (1988). Interleukin-1 induces interleukin-1. III. Specific inhibition of IL-1 production by IFN-γ. *J. Immunol.*, **140**, 4238–44.

Ghezzi, P., Bianchi, M., Mantovani, A., Spreafico, F. and Salmona, M. (1984). Enhanced xanthine oxidase activity in mice treated with interferon and interferon inducers. *Biochem. Biophys. Res. Commun.*, **119**, 144–9.

Ghezzi, P., Saccardo, B. and Bianchi, M. (1986a). Induction of xanthine oxidase and heme oxyge-nase and depression of liver drug metabolism by interferon: a study with different recombinant interferons. *J. Interferon Res.*, **6**, 251–6.

Ghezzi, P., Saccardo, B. and Bianchi, M. (1986b). Recombinant tumor necrosis factor depresses cytochrome P450-dependent microsomal drug metabolism in mice. *Biochem. Biophys. Res. Commun.*, **136**, 316–21.

Ghezzi, P., Saccardo, B., Villa, P., Rossi, V. and Bianchi, M. (1986c). Role of interleukin-1 in the depression of liver drug metabolism by endotoxin. *Infect. Immun.*, **54**, 837–40.

Gimble, J. M., Hudson, J., Henthorn, J., Hua, X. X. and Burstein, S. A. (1991). Regulation of inter-leukin 6 expression in murine bone marrow stromal cells. *Exp. Hematol.*, **19**, 1055–60.

Gnocchi, P., Losa, C., Trizio, D. and Isetta, A. M. (1992). Development and application of a radioimmunoassay (RIA) for the *in vitro* and *in vivo* quantification of murine IL-1β. *Lymphokine Cytokine Res.*, **11**, 257–63.

Goldbach, J.-M., Roth, J., Störr, B. and Zeisberger, E. (1997). Influence of pentoxifylline on fevers induced by bacterial lipopolysaccharide and tumor necrosis factor-α in guinea pigs. *Eur. J. Pharmacol.*, **319**, 273–8.

Grazioli, L., Alzani, R., Ciomei, M., Mariani, M., Restivo, A., Cozzi, E. *et al.* (1992). Inhibitory effect of suramin on receptor binding and cytotoxic activity of tumor necrosis factor alpha. *Int. J. Immunopharmacol.*, **14**, 637–42.

Greten, T. F., Sinha, B., Haslberger, C., Eigler, A. and Endres, S. (1996). Cicaprost and the type IV phosphodiesterase inhibitor, rolipram, synergize in suppression of tumor necrosis factor-α syn-thesis. *Eur. J. Pharmacol.*, **299**, 229–33.

Griffin, D. E. (1997). Cytokines in the brain during viral infection: clues to HIV-associated demen-tia. *J. Clin. Invest.*, **100**, 2948–51.

Gronert, K., Gewirtz, A., Madara, J. L. and Serhan, C. N. (1998). Identification of a human entero-cyte lipoxin A4 receptor that is regulated by interleukin (IL)-13 and interferon gamma and inhibits tumor necrosis factor alpha-induced IL-8 release. *J. Exp. Med.*, **187**, 1285–94.

Group, T. H. S. (1993). Multicenter, randomized, placebo-controlled study of ditiocarb (Imuthiol) in human immunodeficiency virus-infected asymptomatic and minimally symptomatic patients. The HIV87 Study Group. *AIDS Res. Hum. Retroviruses*, **9**, 83–9.

Grum, C. M., Ragsdale, R. A., Ketai, L. H. and Simon, R. H. (1987). Plasma xanthine oxidase in patients with adulte respiratory distress syndrome. *J. Critical Care*, **2**, 22–6.

Grundmann, H. J., Hahnle, U., Hegenscheid, B., Sahlmuller, G., Bienzle, G. and Blitstein, W. E. (1992). Inhibition of endotoxin-induced macrophage tumor necrosis factor expression by a prostacyclin analogueue and its beneficial effect in experimental lipopolysaccharide intoxica-tion. *J. Infect. Dis.*, **165**, 501–5.

Gulick, T., Chung, M. K., Pieper, S. J., Lange, L. G. and Schreiner, G. F. (1989). Interleukin 1 and tumor necrosis factor inhibit cardiac myocyte beta- adrenergic responsiveness. *Proc. Natl. Acad. Sci. USA*, **86**, 6753–7.

Hadjiminas, D. J., McMasters, K. M., Robertson, S. E. and Cheadle, W. G. (1994). Enhanced sur-vival from cecal ligation and puncture with pentoxifylline is associated with altered neutrophil trafficking and reduced interleukin-1 beta expression but not inhibition of tumor necrosis factor synthesis. *Surgery*, **116**, 348–55.

Hall, E. D., McCall, J. M. and Means, E. D. (1994). Therapeutic potential of the lazaroids (21-aminosteroids) in acute central nervous system trauma, ischemia and subarachnoid hemorrage. *Advances in Pharmacology*, **28**, 221–68.

Hamilton, J. A., Piccoli, D. S., Cebon, J., Layton, J. E., Rathanaswani, P., McColl, S. R. *et al.* (1992). Cytokine regulation of colony-stimulating factor CSF) production in cultured human synovial fibroblasts. II. Similarities and differences in the control of interleukin-1 induction of granulocyte-macrophage CSF and granulocyte-CSF production. *Blood*, **79**, 1413–9.

Han, J., Lee, J. D., Bibbs, S. L. and Ulevitch, R. J. (1994). A MAP kinase targeted by endotoxin in mammalian cells. *Science*, **265**, 808–11.

Haraguchi, S., Good, R. A., Cianciolo, G. J., Engelman, R. W. and Day, N. K. (1997). Immunosuppressive retroviral peptides: immunopathological implications for immunosuppressive influences of retroviral infections. *J. Leukoc. Biol.*, **61**, 654–66.

Harant, H., Andrew, P. J., Reddy, G. S., Foglar, E. and Lindley, I. J. (1997). 1alpha,25-dihydroxyvitamin D3 and a variety of its natural metabolites transcriptionally repress nuclear-factor-kappaB-mediated interleukin-8 gene expression. *Eur. J. Biochem.*, **250**, 63–71.

Hart, P. H., Whitty, G. A., Burgess, D. R., Croatto, M. and Hamilton, J. A. (1990). Augmentation of glucocorticoid action on human monocytes by interleukin-4. *Lymphokine Res.*, **9**, 147–53.

Hasko, G., Szabo, C., Nemeth, Z. H., Kvetan, V., Pastores, S. M. and Vizi, E. S. (1996). Adenosine receptor agonists differentially regulate IL-10, TNF-alpha, and nitric oxide production in RAW 264.7 macrophages and in endotoxemic mice. *J. Immunol.*, **157**, 4634–40.

Hayaishi, O., Ryotaro, Y., Takikawa, O. and Yasui, H., 1994, Indoleamine dioxygenase. A possible biological function. In *Progress in Tryptophan and Serotonin Research*, (ed. H. G. Schlossberger), pp. 33–37. Dde Gruyter, Berlin, Germany.

Hazechi, K., Mori, Y. and Ui, M. (1986). Induction of refractoriness of cyclic AMP responses to prostaglandin E_1 and epinephrine by prior exposure of guinea pig macrophages to lipopolysaccharide. *Archives of Biochemistry and Biophysics*, **246**, 772–82.

Haziot, A., Ferrero, E., Köntgen, F., Hijiya, N., Yamamoto, S., Silver, J. *et al.* (1996). Resistance to endotoxin shock and reduced dissemination of gram-negative bacteria in CD14-deficient mice. *Immunity*, **4**, 407–14.

Heber-Katz, E. and Click, R. E. (1972). Immune responses *in vitro*. V. Role of mercaptoethanol in the mixed- leukocyte reaction. *Cell Immunol.*, **5**, 410–8.

Herzenberg, L. A., De Rosa, S. C., Dubs, J. G., Roederer, M., Anderson, M. T., Ela, S. W. *et al.* (1997). Glutathione deficiency is associated with impaired survival in HIV disease. *Proc. Natl. Acad. Sci. USA*, **94**, 1967–72.

Hetier, E., Ayala, J., Bousseau, A. and Prochiantz, A. (1991). Modulation of interleukin-1 and tumor necrosis factor expression by beta-adrenergic agonists in mouse ameboid microglial cells. *Exp. Brain Res.*, **86**, 407–13.

Heyes, M. P., Brew, B. J., Martin, A., Price, R. W., Salazar, A. M., Sidtis, J. J. *et al.* (1991). Quinolinic acid in cerebrospinal fluid and serum in HIV-1 infection: relationship to clinical and neurological status. *Ann. Neurol.*, **29**, 202–9.

Hinson, R. M., Williams, J. A. and Shacter, E. (1996). Elevated interleukin 6 is induced by prostaglandin E2 in a murine model of inflammation: possible role of cyclo-oxygenase-2. *Proc. Natl. Acad. Sci.USA*, **93**, 4885–90.

Hiralta, F., Schiffman, D., Venkatasubramanian, K., Salomon, D. and Axelrod, J. (1980). A phospholipase A_2 inhibitory protein in rabbit neutrophils induced by glucocorticoids. *Proc. Natl. Acad. Sci.USA*, **77**, 2533–6.

Honda, A., Sugimoto, Y., Namba, T., Watabe, A., Irie, A., Negishi, M. *et al.* (1993). Cloning and expression of a cDNA for mouse prostaglandin E receptor EP2 subtype. *J. Biol. Chem.*, **268**, 7759–62.

Hooper, D. C., Bagasra, O., Marini, J. C., Zborek, A., Ohnishi, S. T., Kean, R. *et al.* (1997). Prevention of experimental allergic encephalomyelitis by targeting nitric oxide and peroxynitrite: implications for the treatment of multiple sclerosis. *Proc. Natl. Acad. Sci. USA*, **94**, 2528–33.

Hortelano, S., Diaz-Guerra, M. J. M., Gonzalez-Garcia, A., Leonardo, E., Gamallo, C., Bosca, L. *et al.* (1997). Linomide administration to mice attenuates the induction of nitric oxide synthase elicited by lipopolysaccharide-activated macrophages and prevents nephritis in MRL/Mp-*lpr/lpr* mice. *J. Immunol.*, **158**, 1402–8.

Housby, J. N., Cahill, C. M., Chu, B., Prevelige, R., Bickford, K., Stevenson, M. A. *et al.* (1999). Non-steroidal anti-inflammatory drugs inhibit the expression of cytokines and induce HSP70 in human monocytes. *Cytokine*, **11**, 347–58.

Huizinga, T. W., Dijkmans, B. A., van der Velde, E. A., van de Pouw Kraan, T. C., Verweij, C. L. and Breedveld, F. C. (1996). An open study of pentoxyfylline and thalidomide as adjuvant therapy in the treatment of rheumatoid arthritis. *Ann. Rheum. Dis.*, **55**, 833–6.

Hunt, A. E., Lali, F. V., Lord, J. D., Nelson, B. H., Miyazaki, T., Tracey, K. J. *et al.* (1999). Role of interleukin (IL)-2 receptor beta-chain subdomains and Shc in p38 mitogen-activated protein (MAP) kinase and p54 MAP kinase (stress- activated protein Kinase/c-Jun N-terminal kinase) activation. IL-2- driven proliferation is independent of p38 and p54 MAP kinase activation. *J. Biol. Chem.*, **274**, 7591–7.

Hurme, M. (1990). Modulation of interleukin-1 by cyclic AMP in human monocytes. *FEBS Lett.*, **263**, 35–7.

Hurme, M., Serkkola, E., Ronni, T. and Silvennoinen, O. (1990). Control of interleukin-1β expression by protein kinase C and cyclic adenosine monophosphate in myeloid leukemia cells. *Blood*, **76**, 2198–2203.

Hurme, M., Siljande, P. and Anttila, H. (1991). Regulation of interleukin-1β production by glucocorticoids in human monocytes: the mechanism of action depends on the activation signal. *Biochem. Biophys. Res. Commun.*, **180**, 1383–9.

Iino, Y., Toriyama, M., Kudo, K., Natori, Y. and Yuo, A. (1992). Erythromycin inhibition of lipopolysaccharide-stimulated tumor necrosis factor alpha production by human monocytes *in vitro*. *Ann. Otol. Rhinol. Laryngol. Suppl.*, **157**, 16–20.

Inglot, A. D., Zielinska-Jenczylik, J., Piasecki, E., Syper, L. and Mlochowski, J. (1990). Organoselenides as potential immunostimulants and inducers of interferon gamma and other cytokines in human peripheral blood leukocytes. *Experientia*, **46**, 308–11.

Jacobson, J. M., Greenspan, J. S., Spritzler, J., Ketter, N., Fahey, J. L., Jackson, J. B. *et al.* (1997). Thalidomide for the treatment of oral aphthous ulcers in patients with human immunodeficiency virus infection. National Institute of Allergy and Infectious Diseases AIDS Clinical Trials Group. *N. Engl. J. Med.*, **336**, 1487–93.

Jansen, P. M., de Jong, I. W., Hart, M., Kim, K. J., Aarden, L. A., Hinshaw, L. B. *et al.* (1996). Release of leukemia inhibitory factor in primate sepsis. Analysis of the role of TNF-α. *J. Immunol.*, **156**, 4401–7.

Jiang, C., Ting, A. T. and Seed, B. (1998). PPAR-g agonists inhibit production of monocyte inflammatory cytokines. *Nature*, **391**, 82–6.

Jin, H., Yang, R., Marsters, S., Ashkenazi, A., Bunting, S., Marra, M. N. *et al.* (1995). Protection against endotoxic shock by bactericidal/permeability-increasing protein in rats. *J. Clin. Invest.*, **95**, 1947–52.

Jordan, N. J., Watson, M. L., Yoshimura, T. and Westwick, J. (1996). Differential effects of protein kinase C inhibitors on chemokine production in human synovial fibroblasts. *Br. J. Pharmacol.*, **117**, 1245–53.

Jörres, A., Dinter, H., Topley, N., Gahl, G. M., Frei, U. and Scholz, P. (1997). Inhibition of tumour necrosis factor production in endotoxin-stimulated human mononuclear leukocytes by the prostacyclin analogueue iloprost: cellular mechanisms. *Cytokine*, **9**, 119–25.

Joyce, D. A., Steer, J. H. and Kloda, A. (1996). Dexamethasone antagonizes IL-4 and IL-10-induced release of IL-1RA by monocytes but augments IL-4-, IL-10-, and TGF-beta-induced suppression of TNF-alpha release. *J Interferon Cytokine Res*, **16**, 511–7.

Jun, C. D., Choi, B. M., Kim, H. M. and Chung, H. T. (1995). Involvement of protein kinase C during taxol-induced activation of murine peritoneal macrophages. *J. Immunol.*, **154**, 6541–7.

Kagechika, H., Kawachi, E., Fukasawa, H., Saito, G., Iwanami, N., Umemiya, H. *et al.* (1997). Inhibition of IL-1-induced IL-6 production by synthetic retinoids. *Biochem. Biophys. Res. Commun.*, **231**, 243–8.

Kaissis, S., Lee, J. C. and Hanna, N. (1989). Effects of prostaglandins and cAMP levels on monocyte IL-1 production. *Agents Action*, **27**, 274–6.

Kalebic, T., Kinter, A., Poli, G., Anderson, M. E., Meister, A. and Fauci, A. S. (1991). Suppression of human immunodeficiency virus expression in chronically infected monocytic cells by glutathione, glutathione ester, and N-acetylcysteine. *Proc. Natl. Acad. Sci.USA*, **88**, 986–90.

Kambayashi, T., Jacob, C. O., Zhou, D., Mazurek, N., Fong, M. and Strassmann, G. (1995). Cyclic nucleotide phosphodiesterase type IV participates in the regulation of IL-10 and in the subsequent inhibition of TNF-α and IL-6 release by endotoxin-stimulated macrophages. *J. Immunol.*, **155**, 4909–16.

Karussis, D. M., Meiner, Z., Lehmann, D., Gomori, J.-M., Schwarz, A., Linde, A. *et al.* (1996). Treatment of secondary progressive multiple sclerosis with the immunomodulator linomide: a double-blind, placebo-controlled pilot study with monthly magnetic resonance imaging evaluation. *Neurology*, **47**, 341–6.

Keller, E. T., Chang, C. and Ershler, W. B. (1996). Inhibition of NFkB activity through manteinance of the IkBα levels contributes to dihydrotestosterone-mediated repression of the interleukin-6 promoter. *J. Biol. Chem.*, **271**, 26267–75.

Kelly, S. A., Goldschmidt-Clermont, P. J., Milliken, E. E., Arai, T., Smith, E. H. and Bulkley, G. B. (1998). Protein tyrosine phosphorylation mediates TNF-induced endothelial- neutrophil adhesion *in vitro*. *Am. J. Physiol.*, **274**, H513–9.

Kerlund, K., Erlandsson Harris, H., Tracey, K. J., Wang, H., Fehniger, T., Klareskog, L. *et al.* (1999). Anti-inflammatory effects of a new tumour necrosis factor-alpha (TNF- alpha) inhibitor (CNI-1493) in collagen-induced arthritis (CIA) in rats. *Clin. Exp. Immunol.*, **115**, 32–41.

Kern, J. A., Lamb, R. J., Reed, J. C., Daniele, R. P. and Nowell, P. C. (1988). Dexamethasone inhibition of interleukin 1 beta production by human monocytes. Post-transcriptional mechanisms. *J. Clin. Invest.*, **81**, 237–44.

Kerner, B., Teichmann, B. and Welte, K. (1992). Dexamethasone inhibits tumor necrosis factor-induced granulocyte colony-stimulating factor production in human endothelial cells. *Exp. Hematol.*, **20**, 334–8.

Kerr, S. J., Armati, P. J., Pemberton, L. A., Smythe, G., Tattam, B. and Brew, B. J. (1997). Kynurenine pathway inhibition reduces neurotoxicity of HIV-1-infected macrophages. *Neurology*, **49**, 1671–81.

Kilbourn, R. G., Gross, S. S., Jubran, A., Adams, J., Griffith, O. W., Levi, R. *et al.* (1990). N^G-methyl-L-arginine inhibits tumor necrosis factor-induced hypothension: implications for the involvement of nitric oxide. *Proc. Natl. Acad. Sci.USA*, **87**, 3629–32.

Kirschning, C. J., Wesche, H., Merrill Ayres, T. and Rothe, M. (1998). Human toll-like receptor 2 confers responsiveness to bacterial lipopolysaccharide. *J. Exp. Med.*, **188**, 2091–7.

Klemm, P., Harris, H. J. and Perretti, M. (1996). Effect of rolipram in a murine model of acute inflammation: comparison with the corticoid dexamethasone. *Eur. J. Pharmacol.*, **281**, 69–74.

Kliewer, S. A., Sundseth, S. S., Jones, S. A., Brown, P. J., Wisely, G. B., Koble, C. S. *et al.* (1997). Fatty acids and eicosanoids regulate gene expression through direct interactions with peroxisome proliferator-activated receptors α and g. *Proc. Natl. Acad. Sci.USA*, **94**, 4318–23.

Knowles, R. G., Salter, M., Brooks, S. L. and Moncada, S. (1990). Anti-inflammatory glucocorticoids inhibit the induction by endotoxin on nitric oxide synthase in the lung, liver and aorta of the rat. *Biochem. Biophys. Res. Commun.*, **172**, 1042–8.

Knudsen, P. J., Dinarello, C. A. and Strom, T. B. (1986). Prostaglandins posttranscriptionally inhibit monocyte expression of interleukin 1 activity by increasing intracellular cyclic adenosine monophosphate. *J. Immunol.*, **137**, 3189–94.

Knudsen, P. J., Dinarello, C. A. and Strom, T. B. (1987). Glucocorticoids inhibit transcriptional and post-transcriptional expression of interleukin 1 in U937 cells. *J. Immunol.*, **139**, 4129–34.

Kopp, E. and Ghosh, S. (1994). Inhibition of NF-kB by sodium salicylate and aspirin. *Science*, **265**, 956–9.

Kovacs, E. J., Radzioch, D., Young, H. A. and Varesio, L. (1988). Differential inhibition of IL-1 and TNF-α mRNA expression by agents which block second messengers pathways in murine macrophages. *J. Immunol.*, **141**, 3101–5.

Kovalovsky, D., Paez Pereda, M., Sauer, J., Perez Castro, C., Nahmod, V. E., Stalla, G. K. *et al.* (1998). The Th1 and Th2 cytokines IFN-gamma and IL-4 antagonize the inhibition of monocyte IL-1 receptor antagonist by glucocorticoids: involvement of IL-1. *Eur. J. Immunol.*, **28**, 2075–85.

Kramer, R. M., Roberts, E. F., Um, S. L., Borsch-Haubold, A. G., Watson, S. P., Fisher, M. J. *et al.* (1996). p38 mitogen-activated kinase phosphorylates cytosolic phospholipase A2 (cPLA2) in thrombin-stimulated platelets. *J. Biol. Chem.*, **271**, 27723–9.

Ku, G., Doherty, N. S., Schmidt, L. F., Jackson, R. L. and Dinerstein, R. J. (1990). *Ex vivo* lipopolysaccharide-induced interleukin-1 secretion from murine peritoneal macrophages inhibited by probucol, a hypocholesterolemic agent with antioxidant properties. *FASEB J.*, **4**, 1645–53.

Kubin, M., Chow, J. M. and Trinchieri, G. (1994). Differential regulation of interleukin-12 (IL-12), tumor necrosis factor, and IL-1 beta production in human myeloid leukemia cell lines and peripheral blood mononuclear cells. *Blood*, **83**, 1847–55.

Kuhn, D. C., Stauffer, J. L., Gaydos, L. J., Lacey, S. L. and Demers, L. M. (1993). An inhibitor of thromboxane production attenuates tumor necrosis factor release by activated human alveolar macrophages. *Prostaglandins.*, **46**, 195–205.

Kunicka, J. E., Talle, M. A., Denhardt, G. H., Brown, M., Prince, L. A. and Goldstein, G. (1993). Immunosuppression by glucocorticoids: inhibition of production of multiple lymphokines by *in vivo* administration of dexamethasone. *Cell. Immunol.*, **149**, 39–49.

Kunkel, S. L., Chensue, S. W. and Phan, S. H. (1986). Prostaglandins as endogenous mediators of interleukin 1 production. *J. Immunol.*, **136**, 186–92.

Kunkel, S. L., Spengler, M., May, M. A., Spengler, R., Larrick, J. and Remick, D. (1988). Prostaglandin E2 regulates macrophage-derived tumor necrosis factor gene expression. *J. Biol. Chem.*, **263**, 5380–4.

Kuppen, P. J., Eggermont, A. M., Marinelli, A., de Heer, E., van de Velde, C. J. and Fleuren, G. J. (1991). Induction of lymphokine-activated killer activity in rat splenocyte cultures: the importance of 2-mercaptoethanol and indomethacin. *Cancer Immunol. Immunother.*, **33**, 28–32.

Laliberte, R. D., Perragaux, D., Svensson, L., Pazoles, C. J. and Gabel, C. A. (1994). Tenidap modulates cytoplasmic pH and inhibits anion transport *in vitro*. II. Inhibition of IL-1β production from ATP-treated monocytes and macrophages. *J. Immunol.*, **153**, 2168–79.

Lander, H. M., Sehajpal, P., Levine, D. M. and Novogrodsky, A. (1993). Activation of human peripheral blood mononuclear cells by nitric oxide-generating compounds. *J. Immunol.*, **150**, 1509–16.

Lang, F., Robert, J.-M., Boucrot, P., Welin, L. and Petit, J.-V. (1995). New antiinflammatory compounds that inhibit tumor necrosis factor production: probable interaction with protein kinase C activation. *J. Pharmacol. Exp. Ther.*, **275**, 171–6.

Lang, J. M., Touraine, J. L., Trepo, C., Choutet, P., Kirstetter, M., Falkenrodt, A. *et al.* (1988). Randomised, double-blind, placebo-controlled trial of ditiocarb sodium ('Imuthiol') in human immunodeficiency virus infection. *Lancet*, **2**, 702–6.

Langemann, H., Kabiersch, A. and Newcombe, J. (1992). Measurement of low-molecular-weight antioxidants, uric acid, tyrosine and tryptophan in plaques and white matter from patients with multiple sclerosis. *European Neurology*, **32**, 248–52.

Larrik, J. W., Morgan, J. C., Palings, I., Hirata, M. and Yen, M. H. (1991). Complementary DNA sequence of rabbit CAP-18, a unique lipopolysaccharide-binding protein. *Biochem. Biophys. Res. Commun.*, **179**, 170–5.

Laubach, V. E., Sheseley, E. G., Smithies, O. and Sherman, P. A. (1995). Mice lacking inducible nitric oxide synthase are not resistant to lipopolysaccharide-induced death. *Proc. Natl. Acad. Sci.USA*, **92**, 10688–92.

Le Moine, O., Stordeur, P., Schandené, L., Marchant, A., de Groote, D., Goldman, M. *et al.* (1996). Adenosine enhances IL-10 secretion by human monocytes. *J. Immunol.*, **156**, 4408–14.

Leal-Berumen, I., O'Byrne, P., Gupta, A., Richards, C. D. and Marshall, J. S. (1995). Prostanoid enhancement of interleukin-6 production by rat peritoneal mast cells. *J. Immunol.*, **154**, 4759–67.

Lee, J. C., Griswold, D. E., Votta, B. and Hanna, N. (1988). Inhibition of monocyte IL-1 production by the anti-inflammatory compound, SK&F 86002. *Int. J. Immunopharmacol.*, **10**, 835–43.

Lee, J. C., Badger, A. M., Griswold, D. E., Dunnington, D., Truneh, A., Votta, B. *et al.* (1993). Bicyclic imidazoles as a novel class of cytokine biosynthesis inhibitors. *Ann. NY Acad. Sci.*, **696**, 149–70.

Lee, J. C., Laydon, J. T., McDonnell, P. C., Gallagher, T. F., Kumar, S., Green, D. *et al.* (1994). A protein kinase involved in the regulation of inflammatory cytokine biosynthesis. *Nature*, **372**, 739–46.

Lee, S. W., Tsou, A.-P., Chan, H., Thomas, J., Petrie, K., Eugui, E. M. *et al.* (1988). Glucocorticoids selectively inhibit the transcription of the interleukin 1β gene and decrease the stability of interleukin 1 β mRNA. *Proc. Natl. Acad. Sci.USA*, **85**, 1204–8.

Lemire, J. M. and Archer, D. C. (1991). 1,25-dihydroxyvitamin D3 prevents the *in vivo* induction of murine experimental autoimmune encephalomyelitis. *J. Clin. Invest.*, **87**, 1103–7.

Lepper-Wooford, S. K., Carey, P. D., Byrne, K., Fisher, B. J., Blocher, C., Sugerman, H. J. *et al.* (1991). Ibuprofen attenuates plasma tumor necrosis factor activity during sepsis-induced acute lung injury. *J. Appl. Physiol.*, **71**, 915–23.

Leudke, C. J. and Cerami, A. (1990). Interferon-g overcomes glucocorticoid suppression of cachectin/tumor necrosis factor biosynthesis by murine macrophages. *J. Clin. Invest.*, **86**, 1234–40.

Levi, G., Patrizio, M., Bernardo, A., Petrucci, T. C. and Agresti, C. (1993). Human immunodeficiency virus coat protein gp120 inhibits the beta- adrenergic regulation of astroglial and microglial functions. *Proc. Natl. Acad. Sci. USA*, **90**, 1541–5.

Levin, J., Poore, T. E. and Zauber, N. P. (1970). Detection of endotoxin in the blood of patients with sepsis due to the gram-negative bacteria. *New Engl. J. Med.*, **283**, 1313–6.

Levine, S. J., Benfield, T. and Shelhamer, J. H. (1996). Corticosteroids induce intracellular interleukin-1 receptor antagonist type I expression by a human airway epithelial cell line. *Am. J. Respir. Cell Mol. Biol.*, **15**, 245–51.

Lew, W., Oppenheim, J. J. and Matsushima, K. (1988). Analysis of the suppression of IL-1 alpha and IL-1 beta production in human peripheral blood mononuclear adherent cells by a glucocorticoid hormone. *J. Immunol.*, **140**, 1895–902.

Littman, B. H., Drury, C. E., Zimmerer, R. O., Stack, C. B. and Law, C. G. (1995). Rheumatoid arthritis treated with tenidap and piroxicam. Clinical associations with cytokine modulation by tenidap. *Arthritis Rheum*, **38**, 29–37.

Liu, M. K., Herrera-Velit, P., Brownsey, R. W. and Reiner, N. E. (1994). CD14-dependent activation of protein kinase C and mitogen-activated protein kinases (p42 and p44) in human monocytes treated with bacterial lipopolysaccharide. *J. Immunol.*, **153**, 2642–52.

Luedke, C. E. and Cerami, A. (1990). Interferon-gamma overcomes glucocorticoid suppression of cachectin/tumor necrosis factor biosynthesis by murine macrophages. *J. Clin. Invest.*, **86**, 1234–40.

Lyte, M. (1988). *In vitro* production of interleukin-2 by lymphocytes in whole blood and isolated culture. *J. Clin. Lab. Immunol.*, **26**, 189–93.

Maeda, H. (1997). [Deleterious pathogenic mechanism involving host response in influenza virus infection in mice]. *Nippon. Rinsho.*, **55**, 2676–81.

Marchant, A., Amraoui, Z., Gueydan, C., Bruyns, C., Le Moine, O., Vandenabeele, P. *et al.* (1996). Methylprednisolone differentially regulates interleukin-10 and tumor necrosis factor production during endotoxemia. *Clin. Exp. Immunol.*, **106**, 91–6.

Marra, M. N., Wilde, C. G., Collins, M. S., Snable, J. L., Thornton, M. B. and Scott, R. W. (1992). The role of bactericidal permeability-increasing protein as a natural inhibitor of bacterial endotoxin. *J. Immunol.*, **148**, 532–7.

Marriott, J. B., Westby, M., Cookson, S., Guckian, M., Goodbourn, S., Muller, G. *et al.* (1998). CC-3052: a water-soluble analogue of thalidomide and potent inhibitor of activation-induced TNF-alpha production. *J. Immunol.*, **161**, 4236–43.

Martich, G. D., Danner, R. L., Ceska, M. and Suffredini, A. F. (1991). Detection of interleukin 8 and tumor necrosis factor in normal humans after intavenous endotoxin: the effect of antiinflammatory agents. *Journal of Experimental Medicine*, **173**, 1021–4.

Martin, C. A. and Dorf, M. E. (1991). Differential regulation of interleukin-6, macrophage inflammatory protein-1, and JE/MCP-1 cytokine expression in macrophage cell lines. *Cell. Immunol.*, **135**, 245–58.

McCord, J. M. and Fridovich, I. (1968). The reduction of cytochrome c by milk xanthine oxidase. *J. Biol. Chem.*, **243**, 5753–60.

Meisel, C., Vogt, K., Platzer, C., Randow, F., Liebenthal, C. and Volk, H.-D. (1996). Differential regulation of monocytic tumor necrosis factor-α and interleukin-10 expression. *Eur. J. Immunol.*, **26**, 1580–6.

Meistrell III, M. E., Cockroft, K. M., Botchinka, G. I., Di Santo, E., Bloom, O., Murthy, J. *et al.* (1997). TNF is a brain damaging cytokine in stroke. *Shock*, **8**, 341–8.

Mengozzi, M., Sironi, M., Gadina, M. and Ghezzi, P. (1991). Reversal of defective IL-6 production in lipopolysaccharide-tolerant mice by phorbol myristate acetate. *J. Immunol.*, **147**, 899–902.

Mengozzi, M., Fantuzzi, G., Faggioni, R., Marchant, A., Goldman, M., Orencole, S. *et al.* (1994). Chlorpromazine specifically inhibits peripheral and brain TNF production, and up-regulates interleukin 10 production in mice. *Immunology*, **82**, 207–10.

Michie, H. R., Manogue, K. R., Spriggs, D. R., Revhaug, A., O'Dwyer, S., Dinarello, C. A. *et al.* (1988). Detection of circulating tumor necrosis factor after endotoxin administration. *New Engl. J. Med.*, **318**, 1481–6.

Miesel, R. and Zuber, M. (1993). Elevated levels of xanthine oxidase in serum of patients with inflammatory and autoimmune rheumatic diseases. *Inflammation*, **17**, 551–61.

Miesel, R., Zuber, M., Sanocka, D., Graetz, R. and Kroeger, H. (1994). Effects of allopurinol on *in vivo* suppression of arthritis in mice and ex vivo modulation of phagocytic production of oxygen radicals in whole human blood. *Inflammation*, **18**, 597–612.

Miyachi, H., Azuma, A., Hioki, E., Iwasaki, S., Kobayashi, Y. and Hashimoto, Y. (1996a). Inducer-specific bidirectional regulation by thalidomide and phenylphthalimides of tumor necrosis factor-alpha production. *Biochem. Biophys. Res. Commun.*, **224**, 426–30.

Miyachi, H., Azuma, A., Hioki, E., Iwasaki, S., Kobayashi, Y. and Hashimoto, Y. (1996b). Cell type-/inducer-specific bidirectional regulation by thalidomide and phenylphthalimides of tumor necrosis factor-alpha production and its enantio-dependence. *Biochem. Biophys. Res. Commun.*, **226**, 439–44.

Mohri, M., Spriggs, D. R. and Kufe, D. (1990). Effects of lipopolysaccharide on phospholipase A2 activity and tumor necrosis factor expression in HL-60 cells. *J. Immunol.*, **144**, 2678–82.

Molnar-Kimber, K. L., Yonno, L., Heaslip, R. J. and Weichman, B. M. (1992). Differential regulation of TNF-α and IL-1β production from endotoxin stimulated human monocytes by phosphodieaterase inhibitors. *Mediators of Inflammation*, **1**, 411–17.

Moncada, S. and Higgs, E. A. (1995). Molecular mechanisms and therapeutic strategies related to nitric oxide. *FASEB J.*, **9**, 1319–30.

Moreira, A. L., Sampaio, E. P., Zmuidzinas, A., Frindt, P., Smith, K. A. and Kaplan, G. (1993). Thalidomide exerts its inhibitory action on tumor necrosis factor alpha by enhancing mRNA degradation. *J. Exp. Med.*, **177**, 1675–80.

Morrison, D. C. and Jacobs, D. M. (1976). Binding of polymyxin B to the lipd A portion of bacterial lipopolysaccharide. *Immunochemistry*, **13**, 813–8.

Morrison, D. C. and Ryan, J. L. (1987). Endotoxins and disease mechanisms. *Annual Review of Medicine*, **38**, 417–32.

Muller, K., Gram, J., Bollerslev, J., Diamant, M., Barington, T., Hansen, M. B. *et al.* (1991). Down-regulation of monocyte functions by treatment of healthy adults with 1 alpha,25 dihydroxyvitamin D3. *Int J Immunopharmacol*, **13**, 525–30.

Muller, K., Haahr, P. M., Diamant, M., Rieneck, K., Kharazmi, A. and Bendtzen, K. (1992). 1,25-Dihydroxyvitamin D3 inhibits cytokine production by human blood monocytes at the post-transcriptional level. *Cytokine*, **4**, 506–12.

Munn, D. H., Zhou, M., Attwood, J. T., Bondarev, I., Conway, S. J., Marshall, B. *et al.* (1998). Prevention of allogeneic fetal rejection by tryptophan catabolism. *Science*, **281**, 1191–3.

Munoz, C., Pascual-Salcedo, D., Castellanos, M., Alfranca, A., Aragonés, J., Vara, A. *et al.* (1996). Pyrrolidine dithiocarbamate inhibits the production of interleukin-6, interleukin-8, and granulocyte-macrophage colony-stimulating factor by human endothelial cells in response to inflammatory mediators: modulation of NFkB and AP-1 transcription factors activity. *Blood,* **88**, 3482–90.

Muñoz, E., Zubiaga, A., Huang, C. and Huber, B. (1992). Interleukin-1 induces protein tyrosine phosphorylation in T cells. *Eur. J. Immunol.,* **22**, 1391–6.

Muranjan, M., Wang, Q., Li, Y. L., Hamilton, E., Otieno-Omondi, F. P., Wang, J. *et al.* (1997). The trypanocidal Cape buffalo serum protein is xanthine oxidase. *Infect. Immun.,* **65**, 3806–14.

Muzio, M., Natoli, G., Saccani, S., Levrero, M. and Mantovani, A. (1998). The human toll signaling pathway: divergence of nuclear factor kappaB and JNK/SAPK activation upstream of tumor necrosis factor receptor- associated factor 6 (TRAF6). *J. Exp. Med.,* **187**, 2097–101.

Nassar, G. M., Morrow, J. D., Roberts, L. J. d., Lakkis, F. G. and Badr, K. F. (1994). Induction of 15-lipoxygenase by interleukin-13 in human blood monocytes. *J. Biol. Chem.,* **269**, 27631–4.

Nataf, S., Louboutin, J. P., Chabannes, D., Feve, J. R. and Muller, J. Y. (1993). Pentoxifylline inhibits experimental allergic encephalomyelitis. *Acta Neurol. Scand.,* **88**, 97–9.

Nathan, C. and Xie, Q.-W. (1994). Nitric oxide synthases: role, tolls, and controls. *Cell,* **78**, 915–8.

Neihörster, M., Inoue, M. and Wendel, A. (1992). A link between extracellular reactive oxygen and endotoxin-induced release of tumour necrosis factor *in vivo. Biochem. Pharmacol.,* **43**, 1151–4.

Neurath, M. F., Pettersson, S., Meyer zum Büschenfelde, K.-H. and Strober, W. (1996). Local administration of the antisense phosphorothioate oligonucleotides to the p65 subunit of NF-kB abrogates established experimental colitis in mice. *Nature Medicine,* **2**, 998–1004.

Newton, R. C. and Decicco, C. P. (1999). Therapeutic potential and strategies for inhibiting tumor necrosis factor-alpha. *J. Med. Chem.,* **42**, 2295–314.

Nightingale, S. L. (1998). From the Food and Drug Administration. *Jama,* **280**, 872.

Nishida, T., Takano, M., Kawakami, T., Nishino, N., Nakai, S. and Hirai, Y. (1988). The transcription of the interleukin beta gene is induced with PMA and inhibited with dexamethasone in U937 cells. *Biochem. Biophys. Res. Commun.,* **156**, 269–74.

Nishida, T., Nakai, S., Kawakami, T., Aihara, K., Nishino, N. and Hirai, Y. (1989). Dexamethasone regulation of the expression of cytokine mRNAs induced by interleukin-1 in the astrocytoma cell line U937MG. *FEBS Lett.,* **243**, 25–9.

Nishimura, K., Hashimoto, Y. and Iwasaki, S. (1994). Enhancement of phorbol ester-induced production of tumor necrosis factor alpha by thalidomide. *Biochem. Biophys. Res. Commun.,* **199**, 455–60.

Noel, P., Nelson, S., Bokulic, R., Bagby, G., Lippton, H., Lipscomb, G. *et al.* (1990). Pentoxifylline inhibits lipopolysaccharide-induced serum tumor necrosis factor and mortality. *Life Sci.,* **47**, 1023–9.

Novogrodsky, A., Vanichkin, A., Patya, M., Gazit, A., Osherov, N. and Levitzki, A. (1994). Prevention of lipopolysaccharide-induced lethal toxicity by tyrosine kinase inhibitors. *Science,* **264**, 1319–22.

Ohmori, Y., Strassman, G. and Hamilton, G. A. (1990). cAMP differentially regulates expression of mRNA encoding IL-1 α and IL-1 β in murine peritoneal macrophages. *J. Immunol.,* **145**, 3333–9.

Oishi, K., Sonoda, F., Kobayashi, S., Iwagaki, A., Nagatake, T., Matsushima, K. *et al.* (1994). Role of interleukin-8 (IL-8) and an inhibitory effect of erythromycin on IL-8 release in the airways of patients with chronic airway diseases. *Infect. Immun.,* **62**, 4145–52.

Okamoto, H., Oh, C. and Nakano, K. (1990). Possible involvement of adenosine 3′:5′-cyclic monophosphate and extracellular calcium in histamine stimulation of interleukin-1 release from macrophage-like P388D1 cells. *Immunology*, **70**, 186–90.

Okamoto, M., Sasano, M., Goto, M., Nishioka, K., Aotsuka, S., Nakamura, K. *et al.* (1991). Suppressive effect of anti-rheumatic drugs on interleukin-1β release from human peripheral blood monocytes. *Int. J. Immunopharmacol.*, **13**, 39–43.

Okonogi, K., Gettys, T. W., Uhing, R. J., Tarry, W. C., Adams, D. O. and Prpic, V. (1991). Inhibition of prostaglandin E_2-stimulated cAMP accumulation by lipopolysaccharide in murine peritoneal macrophages. *J. Biol. Chem.*, **266**, 10305–12.

Olah, T., Regely, K. and Mandi, Y. (1994). The inhibitory effects of allopurinol on the production and cytotoxicity of tumor necrosis factor. *Naunyn-Schmiedebergs Arch. Pharmacol.*, **350**, 96–9.

Ollivier, V., Parry, G. C. N., Cobb, R. R., de Prost, D. and Mackman, N. (1996). Elevated cyclic AMP inhibits NF-kappaB-mediated transcription in human monocytic cells and endothelial cells. *J. Biol. Chem.*, **271**, 20828–35.

Oppenheim, J. J., Koopman, W. J., Wahl, L. M. and Dougherty, S. F. (1980). Prostaglandin E2 rather than lymphocyte activating factor produced by activated human mononuclear cells stimulates increases in murine thymocyte cAMP. *Cell. Immunol.*, **49**, 64–73.

Osnes, L. T. N., Foss, K. B., Jo, G. B., Okkenhaug, C., Westwik, Ovstebo, R., and Kierulf, P. (1996). Acetylsalicylic acid and sodium salicylate inhibit LPS-induced NF-kB/c-Rel nuclear translocation, and synthesis of tissue factor (TF) and tumor necrosis factor alfa (TNF-α) in human monocytes. *Thromb. Haemost.*, **76**, 970–6.

Panina-Bordignon, P., Mazzeo, D., Lucia, P. D., D'Ambrosio, D., Lang, R., Fabbri, L. *et al.* (1997). Beta2-agonists prevent Th1 development by selective inhibition of interleukin 12. *J. Clin. Invest.*, **100**, 1513–9.

Penton-Rol, G., Cota, M., Polentarutti, N., Luini, W., Bernasconi, S., Borsatti, A. *et al.* (1999). Up-regulation of CCR2 chemokine receptor expression and increased susceptibility to the multitropic HIV strain 89.6 in monocytes exposed to glucocorticoid hormones [In Process Citation]. *J. Immunol.*, **163**, 3524–9.

Peristeris, P., Clark, B. D., Gatti, S., Faggioni, R., Mantovani, A., Mengozzi, M. *et al.* (1992). N-acetylcysteine and glutathione as inhibitors of tumor necrosis factor production. *Cell. Immunol.*, **140**, 390–9.

Perretti, M., Solito, E. and Parente, L. (1992). Evidence that endogenous intereukin-1 is involved in leukocyte migration in acute experimental inflammation in rats and mice. *Agents Actions*, **35**, 71–8.

Petros, A., Bennett, D. and Vallance, P. (1991). Effect of nitric oxide synthase inhibitors on hypotension in patients with septic shock. *Lancet*, **338**, 1557–8.

Pettipher, E. R. and Wimberly, D. J. (1994). Cyclo-oxygenase inhibitors enhance tumour necrosis factor production and mortality in murine endotoxic shock. *Cytokine*, **6**, 500–3.

Platzer, C., Meisel, C., Vogt, K., Platzer, M. and Volk, H. D. (1995). Up-regulation of monocytic IL-10 by tumor necrosis factor-alpha and cAMP elevating drugs. *Int. Immunol.*, **7**, 517–23.

Poli, V., Balena, R., Fattori, E., Markatos, A., Yamamoto, M., Tanaka, H. *et al.* (1994). Interleukin-6 deficient mice are protected from bone loss caused by estrogen depletion. *EMBO J.*, **13**, 1189–0.

Poltorak, A., He, X., Smirnova, I., Liu, M. Y., Huffel, C. V., Du, X. *et al.* (1998). Defective LPS signaling in C3H/HeJ and C57BL/10ScCr mice: mutations in Tlr4 gene. *Science*, **282**, 2085–8.

Porro, M. (1994). Structural basis of endotoxin recognition by natural polypeptides. *Trends Microbiol.*, **2**, 65–6.

Porro, M., Rustici, A., Velucchi, M., Agnello, D., Villa, P. and Ghezzi, P. (1998). Natural and synthetic polypeptides that recognize the conserved lipid a binding site of lipopolysaccharides. *Prog. Clin. Biol. Res.*, **397**, 315–25.

Portanova, J. P., Zhang, Y., Anderson, G. D., Hauser, S. D., Masferrer, J. L., Seibert, K. *et al.* (1996). Selective neutralization of prostaglandin E2 blocks inflammation, hyperalgesia, and interleukin 6 production *in vivo. J Exp. Med.*, **184**, 883–91.

Pottratz, S. T., Bellido, T., Mocharla, H., Crabb, D. and Manolagas, S. C. (1994). 17β etradiol inhibits expression of human IL-6 promoter-reporter construct by a receptor-dependent mechanism. *J. Clin. Invest.*, **93**, 944–50.

Pouliot, M., Baillargeon, J., Lee, J. C., Cleland, L. G. and Jaes, M. J. (1997). Inhibition of prostaglandin endoperoxide synthase-2 expression in stimulated human monocytes by inhibitors of p38 mitogen-activated protein kinase. *J. Immunol.*, **158**, 4930–7.

Poynter, M. E. and Daynes, R. A. (1998). Peroxisome proliferator-activated receptor alpha activation modulates cellular redox status, represses nuclear factor-kappaB signaling, and reduces inflammatory cytokine production in aging. *J. Biol. Chem.*, **273**, 32833–41.

Prabhakar, U., Brooks, D. P., Lipshlitz, D. and Esser, K. M. (1995). Inhibition of LPS-induced TNF alpha production in human monocytes by adenosine (A2) receptor selective agonists. *Int. J. Immunopharmacol.*, **17**, 221–4.

Radomski, M. W., Palmer, R. M. and Moncada, S. (1990). Glucocorticoids inhibit the expression of an inducible, but not the constitutive, nitric oxide synthase in vascular endothelial cells. *Proc. Natl. Acad. Sci.USA*, **87**, 10043–7.

Raetz, C. R. H., Ulevitch, R. J., Wright, S. D., Sibley, C. H., Ding, A. and Nathan, C. F. (1991). Gram-negative endotoxin: an extraordinary lipid with profound effects on eukaryotic signal transduction. *FASEB J.*, **5**, 2652–60.

Ramirez, F., Fowell, D. J., Puklavec, M., Simmonds, S. and Mason, D. (1996). Glucocorticoids promote a Th2 cytokine response by CD4+ T cells *in vitro. J. Immunol.*, **156**, 2406–12.

Ray, A. and Prefontaine, K. E. (1994). Physical association and functional antagonism between the p65 subunit of transcription factor NF-kB and the glucocorticoid receptor. *Proc. Natl. Acad. Sci.USA*, **91**, 752–6.

Re, F., Muzio, M., De Rossi, M., Polentarutti, N., Giri, J. G., Mantovani, A. *et al.* (1994). The type II 'receptor' as a decoy target for interleukin 1 in polymorphonuclear leukocytes: characterization of induction by dexamethasone and ligand binding properties of the released decoy receptor. *J. Exp. Med.*, **179**, 739–43.

Read, M. A., Whitley, M. Z., Gupta, S., Pierce, J. W., Best, J., Davis, R. J. *et al.* (1997). Tumor necrosis factor α-induced E-selectin expression is activated by the nuclear factor-kB and c-JUN N-terminal kinase/p38 mitogen-activated protein kinase pathways. *J. Biol. Chem.*, **272**, 2753–61.

Rees, D. D., Cellek, S., Pamer, R. M. and Moncada, S. (1990). Dexamethasone prevents the induction by endotoxin of a nitric oxide synthase and the associated effects on vascular tone: an insight into endotoxin shock. *Biochem. Biophys. Res. Commun.*, **173**, 541–7.

Remick, D. G. and Villarete, L. (1996). Regulation of cytokine gene expression by reactive oxygen and reactive nitrogen intermediates. *J. Leukoc. Biol.*, **59**, 471–5.

Renz, H., Gong, J.-H., Schmidt, A., Nain, M. and Gemsa, D. (1988). Release of tumor necrosis factor-α from macrophages. Enhancement and suppression are dose-dependently regulated by prostaglandin E$_2$ and cyclic nucleotides. *J. Immunol.*, **141**, 2388–93.

Ridley, S. H., Sarsfield, S. J., Lee, J. C., Bigg, H. F., Cawston, T. E., Taylor, D. J. *et al.* (1997). Actions of IL-1 are selectively controlled by p38 mitogen-activated protein kinase. Reguylation of prostaglandin H synthase-2, metalloproteinases, and IL-6 at different levels. *J. Immunol.*, **158**, 3165–73.

Rifkind, D. (1967). Prevention by polymyxin B of endotoxin lethality in mice. *J. Bacteriol.*, **93**, 1463–4.

Ritchie, P. K., Spangelo, B. L., Krzymowski, D. K., Rossiter, T. B., Kurth, E. and Judd, A. M. (1997). Adenosine increases interleukin 6 release and decreases tumour necrosis factor release from rat adrenal zona glomerulosa cells, ovarian cells, anterior pituitary cells, and peritoneal macrophages. *Cytokine*, **9**, 187–98.

Rock, C. S., Coyle, S. M., Keogh, C. V., Lazarus, D. D., Hawes, A. S., Leskiw, M. *et al.* (1992). Influence of hypercortisolemia on the acute-phase protein response to endotoxin in humans. *Surgery*, **112**, 467–74.

Roederer, M., Staal, F. J. T., Raju, P. A., Ela, S. W. and Herzenberg, L. A. (1990). Cytokine-stimulated human immunodeficiency virus replication is inhibited by N-acetylcysteine. *Proc. Natl. Acad. Sci.USA*, **87**, 4884–8.

Rojas, A., Padròn, J., Caveda, L., Palacios, M. and Moncada, S. (1993). Role of nitric oxide pathway in the protection against lethal endotoxemia afforded by low doses of lipopolysaccharide. *Biochem. Biophys. Res. Commun.*, **191**, 441–6.

Rola-Pleszczynski, M. and Lemaire, I. (1985). Leukotrienes augment interleukin-1 production by human monocytes. *J. Immunol.*, **135**, 3958–91.

Rola-Pleszczynski, M., Gagnon, L. and Chavaillaz, P. A. (1988). Immune regulation by leukotriene B4. *Ann. NY Acad. Sci.*, **524**, 218–26.

Romano, M., Faggioni, R., Sironi, M., Sacco, S., Echtenacher, B., Di Santo, E. *et al.* (1997a). Carrageenan-induced acute inflammation in the mouse air pouch synovial model. Role of tumor necrosis factor. *Mediators of Inflammation*, **6**, 1–7.

Romano, M., Sironi, M., Toniatti, C., Polentarutti, N., Fruscella, P., Ghezzi, P. *et al.* (1997b). Role of IL-6 and its soluble receptor in induction of chemokines and leukocyte recruitment. *Immunity (Cell press)*, **6**, 315–325.

Rook, G. A. W., Hernandez-Pando, R. and Lightman, S. L. (1994). Hormones, peripherally activated prohormones and regulation of the Th1/Th2 balance. *Immunol. Today*, **15**, 301–3.

Rossi, A., Elia, G. and Santoro, M. G. (1997). Inhibition of nuclear factor kB by prostaglandin A1: an effect associated with heat shock transcription factor activation. *Proc. Natl. Acad. Sci.USA*, **94**, 746–50.

Rouse, J., Cohen, P., Trigon, S., Morange, M., Alonso-Llamazares, A., Zamanillo, D. *et al.* (1994). Identification of a novel protein kinase cascade stimulated by chemical stress and heat-shock which activates MAP kinase-activated MAPKAP kinase-2 and induces phosphorylation of the small heat shock proteins. *Cell*, **78**, 1027–37.

Rustici, A., Velucchi, M., Faggioni, R., Sironi, M., Ghezzi, P., Quataert, S. *et al.* (1993). Molecular mapping and detoxification of the lipid A binding site by synthetic peptides. *Science*, **259**, 361–5.

Sacco, S., Agnello, D., Sottocorno, M., Lozza, G., Monopoli, A., Villa, P. *et al.* (1998a). Non-steroidal antiinflammatory drugs (NSAID) increase TNF production in the periphery but not in the central nervous system. *J. Neurochem.*, **71**, 2063–70.

Sacco, S., Aquilini, L., Ghezzi, P., Pinza, M. and Guglielmotti, A. (1998b). Mechanism of the inhibitory effect of melatonin on TNF production *in vivo* and *in vitro*: independence on adrenal steroids and possible role of antioxidant action. *Eur. J. Pharmacol.*, **343**, 249–55.

Saez-Llorens, X., Ramilo, O., Mustafa, M. M., Mertsola, J., de Alba, C., Hansen, E. *et al.* (1990). Pentoxifylline modulates meningeal inflammation in experimental bacterial meningitis. *Animicrob. Agents Chemother.*, **34**, 837–43.

Saito, K., Chen, C. Y., Masana, M., Crowley, J. S., Markey, S. P. and Heyes, M. P. (1993). 4-Chloro-3-hydroxyanthranilate, 6-chlorotryptophan and norharmane attenuate quinolinic acid formation by interferon-gamma-stimulated monocytes (THP-1 cells). *Biochem. J.*, **291**, 11–4.

Sakai, S., Ochiai, H., Nakajima, K. and Terasawa, K. (1997). Inhibitory effect of ferulic acid on macrophage inflammatory protein-2 production in a murine macrophage cell line, RAW264.7. *Cytokine*, **9**, 242–8.

Sakurai, H., Hisada, Y., Ueno, M., Sugiura, M., Kawashima, K. and Sugita, T. (1996). Activation of transcription factor NF-kB in experimental glomerulonephritis in rats. *Biochim. Biophys. Acta*, **1316**, 132–8.

Salari, H. P., Braquet, P. and Borgeat, P. (1985). Stimulation of lipoxygenase product synthesis in human leukocytes and platelets by melittin. *Mol. Pharmacol.*, **28**, 546–8.

Sampaio, E. P., Kaplan, G., Miranda, A., Nery, J. A., Miguel, C. P., Viana, S. M. *et al.* (1993). The influence of thalidomide on the clinical and immunologic manifestation of erythema nodosum leprosum. *J. Infect. Dis.*, **168**, 408–14.

Santos, A. A., Scheltinga, M. R., Lynch, E., Brown, E. F., Lawton, P., Chambers, E. *et al.* (1993). Elaboration of interleukin 1-receptor antagonist is not attenuated by glucocorticoids after endotoxemia. *Arch Surg*, **128**, 138–43; discussion 143–4.

Santos, L. and Tipping, P. G. (1994). Attenuation of adjuvant arthritis in rats by treatment with oxygen radical scavengers. *Immunol. Cell. Biol.*, **72**, 406–14.

Sathe, S. S., Tsigler, D., Sarai, A. and Kumar, P. (1995). Pentoxifylline impairs macrophage defense against Mycobacterium avium complex. *J. Infect. Dis.*, **172**, 863–6.

Satoh, M., Adachi, K., Suda, T., Yamazaki, M. and Mizuno, D. (1991). TNF-driven inflammation during mouse liver regeneration after partial hepatectomy and its role in growth regulation of liver. *Mol. Biother.*, **3**, 136–47.

Sauer, J., Castren, M., Hopfner, U., Holsboer, F., Stalla, G. K. and Arzt, E. (1996). Inhibition of lipopolysaccharide-induced monocyte interleukin-1 receptor antagonist synthesis by cortisol: involvement of the mineralocorticoid receptor. *J. Clin. Endocrinol. Metab.*, **81**, 73–9.

Schaad, N. C., Magistretti, P. J. and Schorderet, M. (1991). Prostanoids and their role in cell-cell interactions in the central nervous system. *Neurochem. Int.*, **18**, 303–22.

Schade, U. F., Ernst, M., Reinke, M. and Wolter, D. T. (1989). Lipoxygenase inhibitors suppress formation of tumor necrosis factor *in vitro* and *in vivo*. *Biochem. Biophys. Res. Commun.*, **159**, 748–54.

Schade, U. F., Engel, R. and Jakobs, D. (1991). Differential protective activities of site specific lipoxygenase inhibitors in endotoxic shock and production of tumor necrosis factor. *Int. J. Immunopharmacol.*, **13**, 565–71.

Scheinman, R. I., Cogswell, P. C., Lofquist, A. K. and Baldwin Jr., A. S. (1995). Role of transcriptional activation of IkBα in mediation of immunosuppression by glucocorticoids. *Science*, **270**, 283–6.

Schmidt, H., Rush, B., Simonian, G., Murphy, T., Hsieh, J. and Condon, M. (1996). Thalidomide inhibits TNF response and increases survival following endotoxin injection in rats. *J. Surg. Res.*, **63**, 143–6.

Schreck, R., Rieber, P. and Baeuerle, P. A. (1991). Reactive oxygen intermediates as apparently widely used messengers in the activation of the NF-kappa B transcription factor and HIV-1. *EMBO J.*, **10**, 2247–58.

Schreck, R., Meier, B., Mannel, D., Dröge, W. and Baeuerle, P. A. (1992). Dithiocarbamates as potent inhibitors of nuclear factor kB activation in intact cells. *J. Exp. Med.*, **175**, 1181–94.

Schulze-Osthoff, K., Bakker, A. C., Vanhaesenbroeck, B., Beyaert, R., Jacob, W. A. and Fiers, W. (1992). Cytotoxic activity of tumor necrosis factor is mediated by early damage of mitochondrial function. Evidence for the involvement of mitochondrial radical generation. *J. Biol. Chem.*, **267**, 5317–23.

Schwartz, M. D., Repine, J. E. and Abraham, E. (1995). Xanthine oxidase-derived oxygen radicals increase lung cytokine expression in mice subjected to hemorrhagic shock. *Am. J. Respir. Cell. Mol. Biol.*, **12**, 434–40.

Seitz, M., Dewald, B., Gerber, N. and Baggiolini, M. (1991). Enhanced production of neutrophil-activating peptide-1/interleukin-8 in rheumatoid arthritis. *J. Clin. Invest.*, **87**, 463–9.

Serafin, W. E., 1996, Drugs used in the treatment of asthma. In *Goodman & Gilman's The Pharmacological Basis Of Therapeutic.* (9th edn), (ed. J. G. Hardman, L. E. Limbird, P. B. Molinoff, R. W., Ruddon, A. Goodman Gilman), pp. 659–81. McGraw–Hill, New York.

Serhan, C. N., Haeggström, J. Z. and Leslie, C. C. (1996). Lipid mediator networks in cell signaling: update and impact of cytokines. *FASEB J.*, **10**, 1147–58.

Serkkola, E., Hurme, M. and Palkama, T. (1992). Prolonged elevation of intracellular cyclic AMP activates interleukin-1 production in human peripheral blood monocytes. *Scand. J. Immunol.*, **35**, 203–8.

Severn, A., Rapson, N. T., Hunter, C. A. and Liew, F. Y. (1992). Regulation of tumor necrosis factor production by adrenaline and beta- adrenergic agonists. *J. Immunol.*, **148**, 3441–5.

Sevransky, J. E., Shaked, G., Novogrodsky, A., Levitzki, A., Gazit, A., Hoffman, A. *et al.* (1997). Tyrphostin AG556 improves survival and reduces multiorgan failure in canine *Escherichia coli* peritonitis. *J. Clin. Invest.*, **99**, 1966–73.

Shacter, E., Arzadon, G. K. and Williams, J. (1992). Elevation of interleukin-6 in response to a chronic inflammatory stimulus in mice: inhibition by indomethacin. *Blood*, **80**, 194–202.

Shannon, E. J. and Sandoval, F. (1996). Thalidomide can be either agonistic or antagonistic to LPS evoked synthesis of TNF-alpha by mononuclear cells. *Immunopharmacol. Immunotoxicol*, **18**, 59–72.

Shapira, L., Takashiba, T., Champagne, C., Amar, S. and Van Dyke, T. E. (1994). Involvement of protein kinase C and protein tyrosine kinase in lipopolysaccharide-induced TNF-α and IL-1β production by human monocytes. *J. Immunol.*, **153**, 1818–24.

Shenkar, R. and Abraham, E. (1995). Effects of treatment with the 21-aminosteroid, U7438F, on pulmonary cytokine expression following hemorrhage and resuscitation. *Critical Care Medicine*, **23**, 132–9.

Shimizu, T., Nomiyama, S., Hirata, F. and Hayaishi, O. (1978). Indoleamine 2,3-dioxygenase. Purification and some properties. *J. Biol. Chem.*, **253**, 4700–6.

Shimozato, T., Iwata, M., Kawada, H. and Tamura, N. (1991). Human immunoglobulin preparation for intravenous use induces elevation of cellular cyclic adenosine 3':5'-monophosphate levels, resulting in suppression of tumour necrosis factor alpha and interleukin-1 production. *Immunology*, **72**, 497–501.

Sinha, B., Semmler, J., Eisenhut, T., Eigler, A. and Endres, S. (1995). Enhanced tumor necrosis factor suppression and cyclic adenosine monophosphate accumulation by combination of phosphodiesterase inhibitors and prostanoids. *Eur. J. Immunol.*, **25**, 147–53.

Sipe, J. D., Bartle, L. M. and Loose, L. D. (1992). Modification of proinflammatory cytokine production by the antirheumatic agents tenidap and naproxen: a possible correlate with clinical acute phase response. *J. Immunol.*, **148**, 480–4.

Sirko, S. P., Shindler, R., Doyle, M. J., Weisman, S. M. and Dinarello, C. A. (1991). Transcription, translation and secretion of interleukin 1 and tumor necrosis factor: effects of tebufelone, a dual cyclo-oxygenase/5-lipooxygenase inhibitor. *Eur. J. Immunol.*, **21**, 243–50.

Sironi, M., Breviario, F., Proserpio, P., Biondi, A., Vecchi, A., Van Damme, J. *et al.* (1989). IL-1 stimulates IL-6 production in endothelial cells. *J. Immunol.*, **142**, 549–53.

Sironi, M., Gadina, M., Kankova, M., Riganti, F., Mantovani, A., Zandalasini, M. *et al.* (1992). Differential sensitivity of *in vivo* TNF and IL-6 production to modulation by antiinflammatory drugs in mice. *Int. J. Immunopharmacol.*, **14**, 1045–50.

Sironi, M., Bianchi, M., Riganti, F. and Ghezzi, P. (1993). Suppression of interleukin 6 production in endotoxin tolerance in a mouse glioma cell line: reversal by phorbol ester. *Lymphokine Cytokine Res.*, **12**, 39–43.

Sironi, M., Pozzi, P., Polentarutti, N., Benigni, F., Coletta, I., Guglielmotti, A. *et al.* (1996). Inhibition of inflammatory cytokine production and protection against endotoxin toxicity by benzidamine. *Cytokine*, **8**, 910–6.

Snyder, D. S. and Unanue, E. R. (1982). Corticosteroids inhibit murine macrophage Ia expression and interleukin 1 production. *J. Immunol.*, **129**, 1803–5.

Sommer, N., Löschmann, P.-A., Northoff, G. H., Weller, M., Steinbrecher, A., Steinbach, J. P. *et al.* (1995). The antidepressant rolipram suppresses cytokine production and prevents autoimmune encephalomyelitis. *Nature Medicine*, **1**, 244–8.

Sousa, A. R., Trigg, C. J., Lane, S. J., Hawksworth, R., Nakhosteen, J. A., Poston, R. N. *et al.* (1997). Effect of inhaled glucocorticoids on IL-1 beta and IL-1 receptor antagonist (IL-1 ra) expression in asthmatic bronchial epithelium. *Thorax*, **52**, 407–10.

Spangelo, B. L., Isakson, P. C. and MacLeod, R. M. (1990). Production of interleukin-6 by anterior pituitary cells is stimulated by increased intracellular adenosine 3,5′-monophosphate and vasoactive intestinal peptide. *Endocrinology*, **127**, 403–9.

Spengler, R. N., Spengler, M. L., Lincol, P., Remick, D. G., Strieter, R. M. and Kunkel, S. L. (1989). Dynamics of dibutyryl cyclic AMP- and prostaglandin E_2-mediated suppression of lipopolysaccharide-induced tumor necrosis factor alpha gene expression. *Infect. Immun.*, **57**, 2837–41.

Spinas, G. A., Bloeash, D., Keller, U., Zimmerli, W. and Cammisuli, S. (1991). Pretreatment with ibuprofen augments circulating tumor necrosis factor-α, interleukin-6, and elastase during acute endotoxemia. *J. Infect. Dis.*, **163**, 89–95.

Sprenger, H., Beck, J., Nain, M., Wesemann, W. and Gemsa, D. (1991). The lack of receptors for atrial natriuetic peptides on human monocytes prevents a rise of cGMP and induction of tumor necrosis factor-α synthesis. *Immunobiol.*, **183**, 94–101.

Spriggs, E. J., Sherman, M. L., Imamura, K., Mohri, M., Rodriguez, C., Robbins, G. *et al.* (1990). Phospholipase A_2 activation and autoinduction of tumor necrosis factor gene expression by tumor necrosis factor. *Cancer Res.*, **50**, 7101–7.

Staal, F. J. T., Roederer, M. and Herzenberg, L. A. (1990). Intracellular thiols regulate activation of nuclear factor kB and transcription of human immunodeficiency virus. *Proc. Natl. Acad. Sci.USA*, **87**, 9943–7.

Staal, F. J., Anderson, M. T., Staal, G. E., Herzenberg, L. A. and Gitler, C. (1994). Redox regulation of signal transduction: tyrosine phosphorylation and calcium influx. *Proc. Natl. Acad. Sci. USA*, **91**, 3619–22.

Staruch, M. J. and Wood, D. D. (1985). Reduction of serum interleukin-1-like activity after treatment with dexamethasone. *J. Leuk. Biol.*, **37**, 193–207.

Stefanova, I., Corcoran, M. L., Horak, E. M., Wahl, L. M., Bolen, J. B. and Horak, I. D. (1993). Lipopolysaccharide induces activation of CD14-associated protein tyrosine kinase p53/56^{lyn}. *J. Biol. Chem.*, **268**, 20725–8.

Steube, K. G. and Drexler, H. G. (1995). The protein kinase C activator Bryostatin-1 induces the rapid release of TNF alpha from MONO-MAC-6 cells. *Biochem. Biophys. Res. Commun.*, **214**, 1197–203.

Stirling, D., Sherman, M. and Strauss, S. (1997). Thalidomide. A surprising recovery. *J. Am. Pharm. Assoc. (Wash.)*, **NS37**, 306–13.

Strassmann, G., Patil-Koota, V., Finkelman, F., Fong, M. and Kambayashi, T. (1994). Evidence for the involvement of interleukin 10 in the differential deactivation of murine peritoneal macrophages by prostaglandin E2. *J Exp. Med.*, **180**, 2365–70.

Strieter, R. M., Remick, D. G., Ward, P. A., Spengler, R. M., Lynch, J. P., Larrick, J. *et al.* (1988). Cellular and molecular regulation of tumor necrsis factor-alpha production by pentoxifylline. *Biochem. Biophys. Res. Commun.*, **155**, 1230–6.

Stuehr, D. J. and Marletta, M. A. (1985). Mammalian nitrate biosynthesis: mouse macrophages produce nitrite and nitrate in response to *Escherichia coli* lipopolysaccharide. *Proc. Natl. Acad. Sci.USA*, **82**, 7738–42.

Stuhlmeier, K. M., Tarn, C., Csizmadia, V. and Bach, F. H. (1996). Selective suppression of endothelial cell activation by arachidonic acid. *Eur. J. Immunol.*, **26**, 1417–23.

Sudlow, A. W., Carey, F., Forder, R. and Rothwell, N. J. (1996). The role of lipocortin-1 in dexamethasone-induced suppression of PGE2 and TNF alpha release from human peripheral blood mononuclear cells. *Br. J. Pharmacol.*, **117**, 1449–56.

Sugama, K., Namba, Y., Hatanaka, M. and Hanaoka, M. (1987). 2-Mercaptoethanol acts as a potentiating factor of interleukin-2- dependent lymphocyte proliferation. *Microbiol. Immunol.*, **31**, 691–700.

Sugimoto, Y., Namba, T., Honda, A., Hayashi, Y., Negishi, M., Ichikawa, A. *et al.* (1992). Cloning and expression of a cDNA for mouse prostaglandin E receptor EP3 subtype. *J. Biol. Chem.*, **267**, 6463–6.

Sugimoto, Y., Shigemoto, R., Namba, T., Negishi, M., Mizuno, N., Narumiya, S. *et al.* (1994). Distribution of the mRNA for the PGE receptor subtype EP3 in the mouse nervous system. *Neuroscienc*, **62**, 919–28.

Sullivan, G. W., Carper, H. T., Novick, W. J., Jr. and Mandell, G. L. (1988). Inhibition of the inflammatory action of interleukin-1 and tumor necrosis factor (alpha) on neutrophil function by pentoxifylline. *Infect. Immun.*, **56**, 1722–9.

Sung, S. J. and Walters, J. A. (1991). Increased cyclic AMP levels enhance IL-1 α and IL-1 β mRNA expression and protein production in human myelomonocytic cell lines and monocytes. *J. Clin. Invest.*, **88**, 1915–23.

Sunyer, T., Lewis, J., Collin-Osdoby, P. and Osdoby, P. (1999). Estrogen's bone-protective effects may involve differential IL-1 receptor regulation in human osteoclast-like cells. *J. Clin. Invest.*, **103**, 1409–18.

Taffet, S. M., Singhel, K. J., Overholtzer, J. F. and Shurtleff, S. A. (1989). Regulation of tumor necrosis factor expression in a macrophage-like cell line by lipopolysaccharide and cyclic AMP. *Cell. Immunol.*, **120**, 291–300.

Takano, T., Fiore, S., Maddox, J. F., Brady, H. R., Petasis, N. A. and Serhan, C. N. (1997). Aspirin-triggered 15-epi-lipoxin A4 (LXA4) and LXA4 stable analogues are potent inhibitors of acute inflammation: evidence for anti-inflammatory receptor. *J. Exp. Med.*, **185**, 1693–704.

Tannenbaum, C. S. and Hamilton, T. A. (1989). Lipopolysaccharide-induced gene expression in murine peritoneal macrophages is selectively suppressed by agents that elevate intracellular cAMP. *J. Immunol.*, **142**, 1274–80.

Tavares, J. L., Wangoo, A., Dilworth, P., Marshall, B., Kotecha, S. and Shaw, R. J. (1997). Thalidomide reduces tumour necrosis factor-alpha production by human alveolar macrophages. *Respir. Med.*, **91**, 31–9.

Theisen-Popp, P., Pape, H. and Muller-Peddinghaus, R. (1992). Interleukin-6 (IL-6) in adjuvant arthritis of rat and its pharmacological modulation. *Int. J. Immunopharmacol.*, **14**, 565–71.

Tobler, A., Meier, R., Seitz, M., Dewald, B., Baggiolini, M. and Fey, M. F. (1992). Glucocorticoids downregulate gene expression of GM-CSF, NAP-1/IL-8 and IL-6 but not of M-CSF in human fibroblast. *Blood*, **79**, 45–51.

Tracey, D. E., Hardee, M. M., Richard, K. A. and Paslay, J. W. (1988). Pharmacological inhibition of interleukin-1 activity on T cells by hydrocortisone, cyclosporine, prostaglandins and cyclic nucleotides. *Immunopharmacology*, **15**, 47–62.

Tramontana, J. M., Utaipat, U., Molloy, A., Akarasewi, P., Burroughs, M., Makonkawkeyoon, S. *et al.* (1995). Thalidomide treatment reduces tumor necrosis factor alpha production and enhances weight gain in patients with pulmonary tuberculosis. *Mol. Med.*, **1**, 384–97.

Tsuboi, I., Tanaka, H., Nakao, M., Shichijo, S. and Itoh, K. (1995). Nonsteroidal antiinflammatory drugs differentially regulate cytokine production in human lymphocytes: up-regulation of TNF, IFN-g and IL-2, in contrast to down-regulation of IL-6 production. *Cytokine*, **7**, 372–9.

Ulich, T. R., Guo, K. Z., Irwin, B., Remick, D. G. and Davantelis, G. N. (1990). Endotoxin-induced cytokine gene expression *in vivo*. II. Regulation of tumor necrosis factor and interleukin-1 α/β expression and suppression. *Am. J. Pathol.*, **137**, 1173–85.

van Deventer, S. J., Buller, H. L., ten Cate, J. W., Sturk, A. and Pauw, W. (1988). Endotoxaemia: an early predictor of septicaemia in febrile patients. *Lancet*, **1**, 605–609.

Vane, J. R. (1971). Inhibition of prostaglandin synthesis as a mechanism of action for aspirin-like drugs. *Nature*, **231**, 232–5.

Vanichkin, A., Patya, M., Gazit, A., Levitzki, A. and Novogrodsky, A. (1996). Late administration of a lipophilic tyrosine kinase inhibitor prevents lipopolysaccharide and Escherichia coli-induced lethal toxicity. *J. Infect. Dis.*, **173**, 927–33.

van Leenen, D., van der Poll, T., Levi, M., ten Cate, H., van Deventer, S. J. H., Hack, C. E. *et al.* (1993). Pentoxifylline attenuates neutrophil activation in experimental endotoxemia in chimpanzees. *J. Immunol.*, **151**, 2318–25.

Velucchi, M., Rustici, A. and Porro, M., 1994, Molecular requirements of peptide structures binding to the lipid A region of bacterial endotoxin. In *Vaccines '94*, (ed. E. Norrby, F. Brown, R. M. Chanock and A. Ginsderg), pp. 141–146. Cold Spring Harbor Laboratory, Cold Sprin Harbor, NY.

Veterans Administration Systemic Sepsis Cooperative Study Group (1987). Effects of high-dose glucocorticoid therapy on mortality in patients with clinical signs of systemic sepsis. *New Engl. J. Med.*, **317**, 659–65.

Villa, P., Sartor, G., Angelini, M., Sironi, M., Conni, M., Gnocchi, P. *et al.* (1995). Pattern of cytokines and pharmacomodulation in sepsis induced by cecal ligation and puncture and endotoxin. *Clin. Diagn. Lab. Immunol.*, **2**, 549–53.

Villiger, P. M., Terkeltaub, R. and Lotz, M. (1992). Monocyte chemoattractant protein-1 (MCP-1) expression in human articular cartilage. Induction by peptide regulatory factors and differential effects of dexamethasone anf retinoic acid. *J. Clin. Invest.*, **90**, 489–96.

Volterra, A., Trotti, D., Cassutti, P., Tromba, C., Selvaggo, A., Melcangi, R. C. *et al.* (1992). High sensitivity of glutamate uptake to extracellular free arachidonic acid levels in rat cortical synaptosomes and astrocytes. *J. Neurochem.*, **59**, 600–6.

von der Möhlen, M. A. M., Kimmings, N. A., Wedel, N. I., Mevissen, M. L. C. M., Jansen, J., Friedmann, N. *et al.* (1995). Inhibition of endotoxin-induced cytokine release and neutrophil activation in humans by use of recombinant bactericidal/permeability-increasing protein. *J. Infect. Dis.*, **172**, 144–51.

Waage, A. (1987). Production and clearance of tumor necrosis factor in rats exposed to endotoxin and dexamethasone. *Clin. Immunol. Immunopathol.*, **45**, 348–55.

Waage, A., Slupphaug, G. and Shalaby, R. (1990). Glucocorticoids inhibit the production of IL6 from monocytes, endothelial cells and fibroblasts. *Eur. J. Immunol.*, **20**, 2439–43.

Wagner, D. R., McTiernan, C., Sanders, V. J. and Feldman, A. M. (1998). Adenosine inhibits lipopolysaccharide-induced secretion of tumor necrosis factor-alpha in the failing human heart. *Circulation*, **97**, 521–4.

Wang, H., Zhang, M., Bianchi, M., Sherry, B., Sama, A. and Tracey, K. J. (1998). Fetuin (alpha2-HS-glycoprotein) opsonizes cationic macrophage deactivating molecules. *Proc. Natl. Acad. Sci. USA*, **95**, 14429–34.

Wang, J., Harada, A., Matsushita, S., Matsumi, S., Zhang, Y., Shioda, T. *et al.* (1998). IL-4 and a glucocorticoid up-regulate CXCR4 expression on human CD4+ T lymphocytes and enhance HIV-1 replication. *J. Leukoc. Biol.*, **64**, 642–9.

Wang, S., Yan, L., Wesley, R. A. and Danner, R. L. (1997). Nitric oxide increases tumor necrosis factor production in differentiated U937 cells by decreasing cyclic AMP. *J. Biol. Chem.*, **272**, 5959–65.

Warren, H. S., Daner, R. L. and Munford, R. S. (1991). Anti-endotoxin monoclonal antibodies (sounding board). *New Engl. J. Med.*, **326**, 1153–6.

Watabe, A., Sugimoto, Y., Honda, A., Irie, A., Namba, T., Negishi, M. *et al.* (1993). Cloning and expression of cDNA for a mouse EP1 subtype of prostaglandin E receptor. *J. Biol. Chem.*, **268**, 20175–8.

Watson, W. C., Pucevich, C. L., Cremer, M. A., Pinals, R. S. and Townes, A. S. (1985). Analysis of dimethyl sulfoxide immunosuppression in the rat model of collagen II autoimmune arthritis: an effect dependent upon intraperitoneal administration and associated with toxicity. *Agents Actions*, **17**, 84–8.

Weinstein, S. L., June, C. H. and DeFRanco, A. L. (1993). Lipopolysaccharide-induced protein tyrosine phosphorylation in human macrophages is mediated by CD14. *J. Immunol.*, **151**, 3829–38.

Weiss, J. P., Elsbach, P., Olsson, I. and Odeberg, H. (1978). Purification and characterization of a potent bactericidal and membrane active protein from the granules of human polymorphonuclear leukocytes. *J. Biol. Chem.*, **253**, 2664–72.

Wiegers, G. J. and Reul, J. M. (1998). Induction of cytokine receptors by glucocorticoids: functional and pathological significance. *Trends Pharmacol. Sci.*, **19**, 317–21.

Winter, B. K., Fiskum, G. and Gallo, L. L. (1995). Effects of L-carnitine on serum triglyceride and cytokine levels in rat models of cachexia and septic shock. *Br. J. Cancer*, **72**, 1173–9.

Wnendt, S., Finkam, M., Winter, W., Ossig, J., Raabe, G. and Zwingenberger, K. (1996). Enantioselective inhibition of TNF-alpha release by thalidomide and thalidomide-analogues. *Chirality.*, **8**, 390–96.

Wright, S. D., Ramos, R. A., Tobias, P. S., Ulevitch, R. J. and Mathison, J. C. (1990). CD14, a receptor for complexes of lipopolysaccharide (LPS) and LPS binding protein. *Science*, **249**, 1431–3.

Wurfel, M. M., Monks, B. G., Ingalls, R. R., Dedrick, R. L., Delude, R., Zhou, D. *et al.* (1997). Targeted disruption of the lipopolysaccharide (LPS)-binding protein gene leads to profound suppression of LPS responses ex vivo, whereas *in vivo* responses remain intact. *J. Exp. Med.*, **186**, 2051–6.

Wylie, G., Appelboom, T., Bolten, W., Breedveld, F. C., Feely, J., Leeming, M. R. *et al.* (1995). A comparative study of tenidap, a cytokine-modulating anti-rheumatic drug, and diclofenac in rheumatoid arthritis: a 24-week analysis of a 1-year clinical trial. *Br. J. Rheumatol.*, **34**, 554–63.

Yamauchi, A. and Bloom, E. T. (1993). Requirement of thiol compounds as reducing agents for IL-2-mediated induction of LAK activity and proliferation of human NK cells. *J. Immunol.*, **151**, 5535–44.

Yan, L., Wang, S., Rafferty, S. P., Wesley, R. A. and Danner, R. L. (1997). Endogenously produced nitric oxide increases tumor necrosis factor-α production in transfected human U937 cells. *Blood*, **90**, 1160–7.

Yang, R. B., Mark, M. R., Gray, A., Huang, A., Xie, M. H., Zhang, M. *et al.* (1998). Toll-like receptor-2 mediates lipopolysaccharide-induced cellular signalling. *Nature*, **395**, 284–8.

Yoshida, R., Urade, Y., Tokuda, M. and Hayaishi, O. (1979). Induction of indoleamine 2,3-dioxygenase in mouse lung diring virus infection. *Proc. Natl. Acad. Sci.USA*, **76**, 4084–6.

Yoshimura, T., Kurita, C., Yamazaki, F., Shindo, J., Morishima, I., Machida, K. *et al.* (1995). Effects of roxithromycin on proliferation of peripheral blood mononuclear cells and production of lipopolysaccharide-induced cytokines. *Biol. Pharm. Bull.*, **18**, 876–81.

Zabel, P., Schonharting, M. M., Wolter, D. T., and Shade, U. F. (1989). Oxpentifylline in endotoxemia. *Lancet*, **316**, 379–85.

Zabel, P., Horst, H. J., Kreiler, C. and Schlaak, M. (1990). Circadian rhythm of interleukin-1 production of monocytes and the influence of endogenous and exogenous glucocorticoids in man. *Klin. Wochenschr.*, **68**, 1217–21.

Zeni, F., Pain, P., Vindimian, M., Gay, J.-P., Gery, P., Bertrand, M. *et al.* (1996). Effects of pentoxifylline on circulating cytokine concentrations and hemodynamics in patients with septic shock: results from a double-blind, randomized, placebo-controlled study. *Critical Care Medicine*, **24**, 207–14.

Zhang, F. X., Kirschning, C. J., Mancinelli, R., Xu, X. P., Jin, Y., Faure, E. *et al.* (1999). Bacterial lipopolysaccharide activates nuclear factor-kappaB through interleukin-1 signaling mediators in cultured human dermal endothelial cells and mononuclear phagocytes. *J. Biol. Chem.*, **274**, 7611–4.

Zhang, Y., Lin, J.-X. and Vilcek, J. (1988). Synthesis of interleukin 6 (interferon-beta2/B cell stimulatory factor 2) in human fibroblasts is triggered by an increase in intracellular cyclic AMP. *J. Biol. Chem.*, **263**, 6177–82.

Zheng, H., Crowley, J. J., Chan, J. C., Hoffmann, H., Hatherill, J. R., Ishizaka, A. *et al.* (1990). Attenuation of tumor necrosis factor-induced endothelial cell cytotoxicity and neutrophil chemiluminescence. *Am. Rev. Respir. Dis.*, **142**, 1073–8.

Zimmerman, R. J., Marafino, B. J., Jr., Chan, A., Landre, P. and Winkelhake, J. L. (1989). The role of oxidant injury in tumor cell sensitivity to recombinant human tumor necrosis factor *in vivo*. Implications for mechanisms of action. *J. Immunol.*, **142**, 1405–9.

Zinetti, M., Fantuzzi, G., Delgado, R., Di Santo, E., Ghezzi, P. and Fratelli, M. (1995). Endogenous nitric oxide production by human monocytic cells regulates LPS-induced TNF production. *Eur. Cytokine Netw.*, **6**, 45–8.

Zitnik, R. J., Kotloff, R. M., Latifpour, J., Zheng, T., Whiting, N. L., Schwalb, J. *et al.* (1994). Retinoic acid inhibition of IL-1-induced IL-6 production by human lung fibroblasts. *J. Immunol.*, **152**, 1419–27.

Zuckerman, S. H., Shellhaas, J. and Butler, L. D. (1989). Differential regulation of lipopolysaccharide-induced interleukin 1 and tumor necrosis factor synthesis: effects of endogenous and exogenous glucocorticoids and the role of the pituitary-adrenal axis. *Eur. J. Immunol.*, **19**, 301–5.

Zuckerman, S. H., Evans, G. F. and Butler, L. D. (1991). Endotoxin tolerance: independent regulation of interleukin 1 and tumor necrosis factor expression. *Infect. Immun.*, **59**, 2774–80.

Zurier, R. B. and Quagliata, F. (1971). Effect of prostaglandin E1 on adjuvant arthritis. *Nature*, **234**, 304–6.

Zurier, R. B., Damjanov, I., Sayadoff, D. M. and Rothfield, N. F. (1977). Prostaglandin E1 treatment of NZB/NZW F1 hybrid mice. *Arthritis Rheum.*, **20**, 1449–56.

3 *Inhibitors of cytokine processing*

A classical approach in pharmacology has always been to identify and develop inhibitors of enzymes. Enzyme inhibitors are powerful therapeutic tools for diseases ranging from cancer to infection and inflammation. In the field of inflammation, suffice it to mention acetylsalicylic acid and cyclo-oxygenase inhibitors, which have been revisited in the light of the recognition of cyclo-oxygenase-2 as the main prostaglandin-producing enzyme induced in inflammation. Proteolytic enzymes are involved in processing TNFα and IL-1β to the mature soluble protein. Therefore, considerable effort has focused on inhibiting TNF processing and IL-1 converting enzyme. As discussed in the chapter on chemokines (Chapter 7), these molecules may be processed extracellularly by dipeptidyl peptidase IV/CD26 and by other undefined proteases.

3.1 Cysteine protease inhibitors

IL-1β converting enzyme (ICE) is the obligate enzyme for processing the inactive pro-IL-1β (31 kD) to the biologically active secreted cytokine IL-1β (17 kD). ICE (now called caspase-1) is the first member of the caspase family, molecules involved in inflammation and in the regulation of mammalian programmed cell death (apoptosis) (Kumar, 1995; Alnemri *et al.*, 1996). The term caspase (Fig. 3.1) comes from the catalytic properties of these enzymes. The 'c' shows that they are cysteine proteases, and 'aspase' refers to their ability to cleave after aspartic acid, this being the most distinctive catalytic property of this protease family.

Caspases are synthesized as pro-enzymes, which are proteolytically activated to form a heterodymeric catalytic domain. Caspase-1/ICE cleaves pro-IL-1β at Asp116–Ala117. The mature active form of human caspase-1 derives from a 404 amino acid precursor (p45) by proteolytic cleavage at Asp103, Asp119, Asp297, and Asp316. Caspase-1 itself is involved in the cleavage of p45. The active enzyme is made of two subunits: p20 (amino acid 120–297) and p10 (317–404). Cysteine 285 serves as the catalytic residue and mutation of this amino acid results in complete loss of enzyme activity. Crystallization of caspase-1 shows that the catalytically active form is a tetramer consisting of a (p20–p10)$_2$ homodimer. The p20 and p10 subunits are both involved in generating the active site of caspase-1, and are required for catalysis.

The minimum peptide substrate for caspase-1 contains four amino acids before the cleavage site, the optimal peptide sequence being Ac–YVAD (amino acids are identified by the single letter code: Tyr Val Ala Asp). A classical caspase-1 inhibitor is

THE HUMAN CASPASE FAMILY

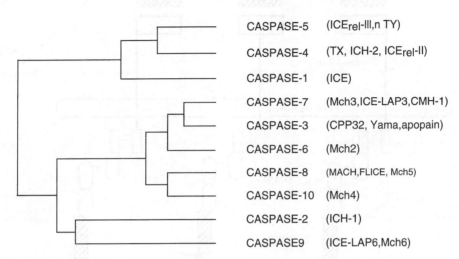

CASPASE-5	(ICE$_{rel}$-III,n TY)
CASPASE-4	(TX, ICH-2, ICE$_{rel}$-II)
CASPASE-1	(ICE)
CASPASE-7	(Mch3,ICE-LAP3,CMH-1)
CASPASE-3	(CPP32, Yama,apopain)
CASPASE-6	(Mch2)
CASPASE-8	(MACH,FLICE, Mch5)
CASPASE-10	(Mch4)
CASPASE-2	(ICH-1)
CASPASE9	(ICE-LAP6,Mch6)

Fig. 3.1 The caspase family. Phylogenetic relationships among caspases with, in parentheses, alternative designations. (Reproduced with kind permission from Alnemri *et al.*, 1996.)

Ac–YVAD–chloromethylketone. Caspases show no sequence similarity with granzymes, serine proteases that induce apoptosis. However, both caspase-1 and granzyme-B require Asp in p1 position for biological activity.

Monocytes express caspase-1 but most of it is in the inactive 45 kDa precursor form. Monocyte activation results in increased ICE activity, and activity is also increased under conditions that promote apoptosis. Although to date the only known substrates of caspase-1 are pro-IL-1β and IL-18, this enzyme has been detected in various cell types that do not seem to produce substantial amounts of IL-1β and IL-18. There may, therefore, be other substrates too, possibly important in certain pathways of apoptosis. IL-1β does not have a leader peptide and caspase-1 associated with the internal surface of the plasma membrane serves as a transport mechanism for the export of IL-1β.

A discussion of the role of caspases in programmed cell death is beyond the scope of this chapter (Thornberry and Lazebnik, 1998). ICE/caspase-related protease cascades are involved in apoptotic cell death and one of the best studied pathways *in vitro* is that triggered by the fas receptor (APO-1, CD95) (Chinnaiyan and Dixit, 1996). Proteases of the caspase/ICE family, specifically CPP32 (caspase-3), are activated after engagement of fas by the fas ligand or by appropriate antibodies. Schematically, the intracellular domain of the fas receptor, through an adaptor protein known as FADD or MORT, engages a cysteine protease (caspase-8) known as FLICE-MACH. Caspase 3-like proteases are subsequently activated in this proteolytic cascade (Fig. 3.2).

A substantial proportion of current understanding of the genetic regulation of apoptosis has come from studies with a nematode, *Caenorhabditis elegans*, as a model system. Studies with this worm have shown that three genes, known as ced-3, ced-4 and ced-9, play a crucial role in regulating cell death. Ced-4 is similar to the mammalian bcl2 protein, but the ced-4 gene encodes a protein whose function in apoptosis is not clear.

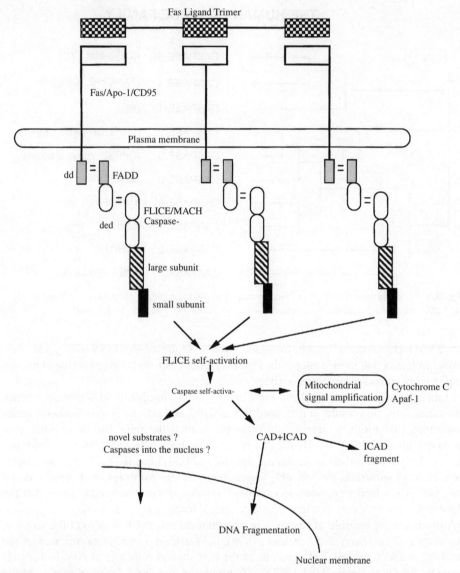

Fig. 3.2 Caspases involved in signaling cell death. The death receptor fas/Apo1/CD95 is taken as an example. Through the FADD adapter, caspase-8 (FLICE/MACH) is recruited; this enzyme activates a caspase cascade, leading to cell death: dd, death domain; ded, death effector domain.

Ced-3 is similar to the mammalian cysteine protease ICE/caspase-1, a strong indication of the evolutionary conservation of the apoptotic pathways.

Based on the recognition of the caspases sequence-specificity, it has been, and presumably will be, relatively straightforward to generate specific inhibitors (Miller *et al.,* 1995; Nicholson *et al.,* 1995; Dolle *et al.,* 1997). A widely used inhibitor is the three-peptide benzyloxycarbonyl–Val–Ala–Asp fluoromethylketone (z-VAD.fmk). An inhibitor more specific for caspase-1/ICE-like proteases is acetyl–Tyr–Val–Ala–Asp chloromethylketone (ac-YVAD.cmk).

IL-1β is not the only substrate of caspase-1. IL-18 was originally described as an IFNγ inducing factor (IGIF), a co-stimulus for IFNγ production (Okamura *et al.*, 1998). IL-18 is produced by mononuclear phagocytes and is structurally reminiscent of IL-1β, having a unique all-β-plated structure. Similarly to IL-1β, it is synthesized as pro-IL-18, without a signal peptide and has no biological activity. Caspase-1 processes pro-IL-18 at the p1 position, producing a mature, active peptide, which is released from cells (Ghayur *et al.*, 1997; Gu *et al.*, 1997). Therefore, the *in vivo* activity of caspase-1 inhibitors needs to be considered in the perspective of two molecular targets: IL-1β and IL-18. Also, caspase-3 has been shown to process IL-16.

An obvious general issue in the design of caspase inhibitors is combining activity on the enzyme with cell permeability. These agents inhibit the production of IL-1β and IL-18 and inhibit inflammatory responses *in vivo*. Apoptosis is involved in a variety of pathophysiological processes and caspase inhibitors may, therefore, be useful in various pathologies (Miller *et al.*, 1995). For instance, fulminating hepatitis is believed to be mediated by the cytotoxic action of T cells against liver cells. Cytotoxic T cells kill through the perforine/granzyme pathway, as well as the fas ligand pathway. Caspase inhibitors have shown protective activity against fas-mediated fulminating liver distruction and death in a mouse model (Miller *et al.*, 1995).

Analysis of the crystal structure showed that the ac-YVAD-cmk inhibitor binds covalently at Cys285, consistently with the notion that caspase-1 is a cysteine protease. A search is now in progress for potent, selective, irreversible inhibitors of ICE, which would mimic peptides' structure. For instance, piridazino-diazepines have been reported as a high-affinity peptidomimetic class of caspase-1 inhibitors (Dolle *et al.*, 1997). These incorporate an aspartic acid-derived α-substituted metylketone as the essential recognition element.

3.2 Inhibitors of TNFα converting enzyme (TACE)

TNFα is synthesized as a 26 kD precursor protein, which is processed to a secreted 17 kD mature form by cleavage of an Ala–Val bond between residues 76 and 77. The enzyme involved is a metalloprotease, an endopeptidase requiring Zn for its activity (Gearing *et al.*, 1995). TACE has recently been cloned molecularly (Moss *et al.*, 1997; Black *et al.*, 1997; Maskos *et al.*, 1998). Matrix metalloproteases are proteolytic enzymes vital for tissue remodeling, and are important in the pathogenesis of inflammatory diseases such as rheumatoid arthritis. The search for matrix metalloprotease inhibitors has, therefore, been vigorous. Several inhibitors that block the processing of pro-TNFα to mature soluble TNFα have been identified (McGeehan *et al.*, 1994; Mohler *et al.*, 1994; Gearing *et al.*, 1997; Hattori *et al.*, 1997). These inhibitors are generally hydroxammic acid-based. They specifically interfere with the release of TNFα and have no effect on the production of other pro-inflammatory cytokines such as IL-1, IL-6 and chemokines. Peptide-hydroxammate broad-spectrum metalloprotease inhibitors were shown to protect mice against lethal shock caused by bacterial endotoxin and acute graft versus host disease (McGeehan *et al.*, 1994; Mohler *et al.*, 1994; Gearing *et al.*, 1997; Hattori *et al.*, 1997).

Table 3.1   Inhibition of cytokine and cytokine receptor release by metalloprotease inhibitors

Cytokines	TNFα, TGFα, SCF, M-CSF
Cytokine receptors	IL-1 (type II, decoy), TNF (type I and II), IL-6
Adhesion molecules	L-selectin
Other	Fas ligand

Data compiled from (Crowe *et al.*, 1995; Kayagaki *et al.*, 1995; Mullberg *et al.*, 1995; Williams *et al.*, 1996; Gallea-Robache *et al.*, 1997; Solorzano *et al.*, 1997; Orlando, *et al.*, 1997).

However, the action of these inhibitors is not restricted to the processing of TNFα (Table 3.1). Other soluble cytokines are produced from a transmembrane domain membrane-anchored precursor. Metalloprotease inhibitors inhibited the release of membrane-anchored precursor cytokines, such as transforming growth factor α (TGFα), stem cell factor (STC), and macrophage colony stimulating factor (M-CSF). Release of the fas ligand is also mediated by a matrix metalloprotease. As discussed in detail in Chapter 5, cytokine receptors are also released by proteolytic processing mediated by a matrix metalloprotease. Matrix metalloprotease inhibitors block the release of various cytokine receptors, including the TNF p55 type I receptor, the TNF p75 type II receptor, the IL-1 type II receptor, and the IL-6 receptor, as well as shedding of surface adhesion molecules, such as L-selectin (Crowe *et al.*, 1995; Kayagaki *et al.*, 1995; Mullberg *et al.*, 1995; Williams *et al.*, 1996; Gallea-Robache *et al.*, 1997; Orlando *et al.*, 1997; Solorzano *et al.*, 1997). Since at least some of these receptors block cytokine action, including that of TNF (see Chapter 4), these broad-spectrum matrix metalloprotease inhibitors are in a way self-defeating.

TACE was found to be resistant to natural endogenous polypeptides, which inhibit the action of classical matrix metalloproteases, known as tissue inhibitors of matrix metalloprotease-1 (TIMP) and 2. Finally, the 26-kD cell-associated TNFα precursor is biologically active and serves as the specific ligand for the p75 type II receptor. As a consequence of the precursor's biological activity and the high levels associated with blockade by matrix metalloprotease inhibitors, exacerbation of liver injury was observed in an experimental model of hepatitis after treatment with these agents (Solorzano *et al.*, 1997).

Metalloproteases appear to be important regulators of membrane expression and secretion of cytokines and cytokine receptors. Possibly a family of enzymes is involved in processing. It is, therefore, important to identify enzymes and design specific inhibitors that only affect the release of those molecules, which offer a target for pharmacological intervention, such as TNFα.

References

Alnemri, E. S., Livingston, D. J., Nicholson, D. W., Salvesen, G., Thornberry, N. A., Wong, W. W. *et al.* (1996). Human ICE/CED-3 protease nomenclature. *Cell*, **87**, 171.

Black, R. A., Rauch, C. T., Kozlosky, C. J., Peschon, J. J., Slack, J. L., Castner, B. J. *et al.* (1997). A metalloproteinase disintegrin that releases tumour-necrosis factor-alpha from cells. *Nature*, **385**, 729–33.

Chinnaiyan, A. M. and Dixit, V. M. (1996). The cell-death machine. *Curr. Biol.*, **6**, 555–62.

Crowe, P. D., Walter, B. N., Mohler, K. M., Otten-Evans, C., Black, R. A., and Ware, C. F. (1995). A metalloprotease inhibitor blocks shedding of the 80-kD TNF receptor and TNF processing in T lymphocytes. *J. Exp. Med.*, **181**, 1205–10.

Dolle, R. E., Prasad, C. V. C., Prouty, C. P., Salvino, J. M., Awad, M. M. A., Schmidt, S. J. *et al.* (1997). Pyridazinodiazepines as a high-affinity, P2-P3 peptidomimetic class of interleukin-1beta-converting enzyme inhibitor. *J. Med. Chem.*, **40**, 1941–6.

Gallea-Robache, S., Morand, V., Millet, S., Bruneau, J-M., Bhatnagar, N., Chouaib, S. *et al.* (1997). A metalloproteinase inhibitor blocks the shedding of soluble cytokine receptors and processing of transmembrane cytokine precursors in human monocytic cells. *Cytokine*, **9**, 340–346.

Gearing, A. J. H., Beckett, P., Christodoulou, M., Churchill, M., Clements, J. M., Crimmin, M. *et al.* (1995). Matrix metalloproteinases and processing of pro-TNF-α. *J. Leukoc. Biol.*, **57**, 774–7.

Gearing, A. J. H., Beckett, P., Christodoulou, M., Churchill, M., Clement, J., Davidson, A. H. *et al.* (1997). Processing of tumour necrosis factor-alfa precursor by metalloproteinases. *Nature*, **370**, 555–7.

Ghayur, T., Banerjee, S., Hugunin, M., Butler, D., Herzog, L., Quintal, L. *et al.* (1997). Caspase-1 processes IFN-gamma-inducing factor and regulates LPS-induced IFN-gamma production. *Nature*, **386**, 619–23.

Gu, Y., Kuida, K., Tsutsui, H., Ku, G., Hsiao, K., Fleming, M. A. *et al.* (1997). Activation of interferon-gamma inducing factor mediated by interleukin-1beta converting enzyme. *Science*, **275**, 206–9.

Hattori, K., Hirano, T., Ushiyama, C., Miyajima, H., Yamakawa, N., Ebata, T. *et al.* (1997). A metalloproteinase inhibitor prevents lethal acute graft-versus-host disease in mice. *Blood*, **90**, 542–8.

Kayagaki, N., Kawasaki, A., Ebata, T., Ohmoto, H., Ikeda, S., Inoue, S. *et al.* (1995). Metalloproteinase-mediated release of human fas ligand. *J. Exp. Med.*, **182**, 1777–83.

Kumar, S. (1995). ICE-like proteases in apoptosis. *Trends. Biochem. Sci.*, **20**, 198–202.

Maskos, K., Fernandez-Catalan, C., Huber, R., Bourenkov, G. P., Bartunik, H., Reddy, P. *et al.* (1998). Crystal structure of the catalytic domain of human tumor necrosis factor-alpha-converting enzyme. *Proc. Natl. Acad. Sci. USA.*, **95**, 3408–12.

McGeehan, G. M., Becherer, J. D., Bast Jr, R. C., Boyer, C. M., Champion, B., Conolli, K. M. *et al.* (1994). Regulation of tumour necrosis factor-alfa processing by a metalloproteinase inhibitor. *Nature*, **370**, 558–61.

Miller, B. E., Krasney, P. A., Gauvin, D. M., Holbrook, K. B., Koonz, D. J., Abruzzese, R. V. *et al.* (1995). Inhibition of mature IL-1beta production in murine macrophages and a murine model of inflammation by WIN 67694, an inhibitor of IL-1beta converting enzyme. *J. Immunol.*, **154**, 1331–8.

Mohler, K. M., Sleath, P. R., Fitzner, J. N., Cerretti, D. P., Alderson, M., Kerwar, S. S. *et al.* (1994). Protection against a lethal dose of endotoxin by an inhibitor of tumour necrosis factor processing. *Nature*, **370**, 218–20.

Moss, M. L., Jin, S. L., Milla, M. E., Bickett, D. M., Burkhart, W., Chen, W. J. *et al.* (1997). Cloning of a disintegrin metalloproteinase that processes precursor tumour-necrosis factor-α. *Nature*, **385**, 733–6.

Mullberg, J., Durie, F. H., Otten-Evans, C., Alderson, M. R., Rose-John, S., Cosman, D. *et al.* (1995). A metalloprotease inhibitor blocks shedding of the IL-6 receptor and the p60 TNF receptor. *J. Immunol.*, **155**, 5198–205.

Nicholson, D. W., Ali, A., Thornberry, N. A., Vaillancourt, J. P., Gallant, M., Gareau, Y. *et al.* (1995). Identification and inhibition of the ICE/CED-3 protease necessary for mammalian apoptosis. *Nature*, **376**, 37–43.

Okamura, H., Kashiwamura, S., Tsutsui, H., and Yoshimoto, T. (1998). Regulation of interferon-gamma production by IL-12 and IL-18. *Curr. Opin. Immunol.*, **10**, 259–64.

Orlando, S., Sironi, M., Bianchi, G., Drummond, A. H., Boraschi, D., Yabes, D. *et al.* (1997). Role of the metalloproteases in the release of the IL-1 type II decoy receptor. *J. Biol. Chem.*, **272**, 31764–9.

Solorzano, C. C., Ksontini, R., Pruitt, J. H., Hess, P. J., Edwards, P. D., Kaibara, A. *et al.* (1997). Involvement of 26-kDa cell-associated TNF-alfa in experimental hepatitis and exacerbation of liver injury with a matrix metalloproteinase inhibitor. *J. Immunol.*, **158**, 414–9.

Thornberry, N. A., and Lazebnik, Y. (1998). Caspases: enemies within. *Science*, **281**, 1312–6.

Williams, L. M., Gibbons, D. L., Gearing, A., Maini, R. N., Feldmann, M., and Brennan, F. M. (1996). Paradoxical effects of a synthetic metalloproteinase inhibitor that blocks both P55 and P75 TNF receptor shedding and TNFalfa processing in RA synovial membrane cell cultures. *J. Clin. Invest.*, **12**, 2833–41.

4 *Interleukin-1 receptor antagonist*

4.1 Introduction

Interleukin-1 receptor antagonist (IL-1ra) has been administered to healthy human volunteers, patients with septic shock, rheumatoid arthritis, graft versus host disease and multiple sclerosis. IL-1ra is clearly safe and is without significant impairment of natural host defenses. Although there is only a modest benefit in patients with septic shock, IL-1ra reduces disease activity and progression of joint destruction in patients with rheumatoid arthritis. This chapter updates the current knowledge on IL-1ra, with particular emphasis on human disease and the effect of IL-1ra in clinical trials.

IL-1ra appears to be a unique situation in cytokine biology (see Chapter 1). If one considers the number of cytokines that have been described, most appear to be unique gene products with unique structural and biological characteristics. However, there is also increasing evidence that some cytokines can be 'grouped' into mini-families in which both ligands and their receptors are structurally related. For example, the 'TNF family' has several related ligands and receptors, and share some of the biological properties. In the case of IL-1, there are three structurally related gene products: IL-1α, IL-1β, and IL-1ra. Each of these unique gene products bind the same receptors, albeit with different affinities. However, the binding of IL-1ra to the IL-1R type I has a rather slow off-rate and prevents the formation of the heterodimer with the IL-1R-AcP (Greenfeder *et al.*, 1995). As such, IL-1ra functions as a receptor antagonist but unlike the general category of receptor-antagonists in pharmacology, there is no agonist activity across a rather large range of concentrations. Healthy humans, who are exquisitely sensitive to the systemic effect of IL-1 (see below), have no biochemical, hematological or physiological responses to intravenous administration of 100–1000 mg doses IL-1ra that are 10 000–100 000 greater than the amount of IL-1α or IL-1β. For example, volunteers and patients receiving intravenous IL-1ra, do not experience clinical symptoms at these doses (Granowitz *et al.*, 1992; Antin *et al.*, 1994) whereas headache, chills, and fever occur following 10 ng/kg of IL-1. Thus, one can conclude that the mechanism for binding to the IL-1R type I, without detectable signal transduction, is a highly effective and unique situation in pharmacology.

Given the structural requirements for ligand-receptor specificity, the nature of IL-1ra is also unique because no other cytokine 'family' contains such a member, despite a growing number of family members. In the case of the 'IL-1 mini-family', the cytokine IL-18 is closely related to IL-1β but is an agonist (Dinarello, 1999). Rat IL-18 does have a deletion mutant, which may serve as a receptor antagonist (Conti *et al.*, 1997). However, this deletion mutant has not been tested for receptor binding or antagonism. Interestingly, splice variants encoding intracellular isoforms of IL-1ra have been described and may act as a reservoir of anti-IL-1 molecules (Arend *et al.*, 1998; Muzio *et al.*, 1995; 1999). Recent descriptions of four new members of the IL-1 family suggest that these may also function as IL-1 receptor antagonists (Kumar *et al.*, 2000; Smith D. E. *et al.*, 2000).

4.2 Systemic effects of IL-1

In order to understand the clinical utility of IL-1ra in disease, a summary of the systemic effects of IL-1 injected into humans is helpful. Although the systemic effects of IL-1 are studied in animals, IL-1α or IL-1β has been injected in patients with various solid tumors or as part of a reconstitution strategy in bone marrow transplantation. Acute toxicities of either IL-1α or IL-1β were greater following intravenous, compared to subcutaneous, injection; subcutaneous injection was associated with significant local pain, erythema, and swelling (Kitamura and Takaku, 1989; Laughlin *et al.*, 1993). Chills and fever are observed in nearly all patients, even in the 1 ng/kg dose group (Tewari *et al.*, 1990). The febrile response increases in magnitude with increasing doses (Crown *et al.*, 1991, 1993; Smith *et al.*, 1992, 1993; Nemunaitis *et al.*, 1994) and chills and fever were abated with indomethacin treatment (Iizumi *et al.*, 1991). In patients receiving IL-1α, (Smith *et al.*, 1992, 1993) or IL-1β (Crown *et al.*, 1991; Nemunaitis *et al.*, 1994), nearly all subjects experienced significant hypotension at doses of 100 ng/kg or greater. Systolic blood pressure fell steadily and reached a nadir of 90 mmHg or less 3–5 h after the infusion of IL-1. At doses of 300 ng/kg, most patients required intravenous pressors. By comparison, in a trial of 16 patients given from 4 to 32 ng/kg IL-1β subcutaneously, there was only one episode of hypotension at the highest dose level (Laughlin *et al.*, 1993). These results suggest that the hypotension is probably due to induction of NO, and elevated levels of serum nitrate have been measured in patients with IL-1-induced hypotension (Smith *et al.*, 1992).

At 30–100 ng/kg of IL-1β, patients exhibited a sharp increase in cortisol levels 2–3 h after the injection. Similar increases were noted in patients given IL-1α. In 13 of 17 patients given IL-1β, there was a fall in serum glucose within the first hour of administration, and in 11 patients, glucose fell to 70 mg/100 ml or lower (Crown *et al.*, 1991). In addition, there were increases in ACTH and thyroid stimulating hormone but a decrease in testosterone (Smith *et al.*, 1992). No changes were observed in coagulation parameters such as prothrombin time, partial thromboplastin, or fibrinogen degradation products. This latter finding is to be contrasted to TNFα infusion into healthy humans, which results in a distinct coagulopathy syndrome (van der Poll *et al.*, 1990).

Not unexpectedly, IL-1 infusion into humans significantly increased circulating IL-6 levels in a dose-dependent fashion (Smith *et al.*, 1992). At a dose of 30 ng/kg, mean IL-6 levels were 500 pg/ml 4 h after IL-1 (baseline <50 pg/ml) and 8000 pg/ml after a dose of 300 ng/kg. In another study, infusion of 30 ng/kg of IL-1α induced elevated IL-6 levels within 2 h (Tilg *et al.*, 1994). These elevations in IL-6 are associated with a rise in C-reactive protein and a decrease in albumin. In two studies, one with IL-1α (Tilg *et al.*, 1994) and one with IL-1β (Bargetzi *et al.*, 1993), a rapid increase in circulating IL-1ra and TNF soluble receptors (p55 and p75) were observed following a 30-min intravenous infusion.

4.3 How does IL-1ra bind to the type I IL-1R but not trigger a biological response?

The primary amino acid homology of mature human IL-1β, compared to IL-1ra, is 26%, which is greater than that between IL-1α and IL-1β. Each member of the human IL-1 family is comprised of an all-β strand molecule, which forms an open barrel-like structure closely related to structure of FGF (Murzin *et al.*, 1992). Since each member of the IL-1 family binds to the IL-1RI, it is not surprising that IL-1α, IL-1β, and IL-1ra share structural similarities. How does IL-1ra bind to IL-1RI with a high affinity yet not trigger a response? Crystal structural analysis of the IL-1R/IL-1ra complex reveals that IL-1ra contacts all three domains of the IL-1RI (Schreuder *et al.*, 1997).

IL-1β has two sites of binding to IL-1RI. There is a primary binding site located at the open top of its barrel shape (Gruetter *et al.*, 1994), which is similar but not identical to that of IL-1α (Lambriola-Tomkins *et al.*, 1993); and a second site on the back side of the IL-1β molecule (Gruetter *et al.*, 1994). IL-1ra also has two binding sites similar to those of IL-1β (Evans *et al.*, 1994; Vigers *et al.*, 1994). However, the back side site in IL-1ra is more homologous to that of IL-1β than the primary binding site (Evans *et al.*, 1994). Thus, the present interpretation is that the back side site of IL-1ra binds to IL-1RI and occupies the receptor. Lacking the second binding site, IL-1ra does not trigger a signal. The crystal structure of complexes of IL-1ra with soluble IL-1RI reveals that the second binding site is the 'trigger' site for IL-1 signaling and is not in contact with the IL-1RI (Schreuder *et al.*, 1997) (see below for discussion of IL-1 receptor dimerization). After IL-1ra binds to IL-1RI-bearing cells, there is no phosphorylation of the epidermal growth factor receptor (Dripps *et al.*, 1991), a well-established and sensitive assessment of IL-1 signal transduction (Bird and Saklatvala, 1989).

The formation of the heterodimer consisting of the IL-1RI and IL-1R accessory protein (IL-1R-AcP) (Greenfeder *et al.*, 1995), probably explains the failure of IL-1ra to trigger a signal (see Chapter 1). From the structural differences, described above, between IL-1β and IL-1ra, one can propose that the second binding site missing from the IL-1ra is, in fact, the site that binds the accessory protein. The cross-linked complex of radiolabeled IL-1ra to the type I receptor was not precipitated by a specific antibody to the accessory protein (Greenfeder *et al.*, 1995). As discussed in Chapter 1, IL-1ra binds to the type I receptor with the same affinity as that of IL-1 but, lacking the second binding site, the IL-1R-AcP does not dock to the IL-1ra and the heterodimer is not formed. The binding of IL-1ra to the type I receptor probably prevents or disrupts the complex between IL-1 and the type I receptor. This model implies that signal transduction takes place only when the heterodimer is formed. A triple mutation in IL-1ra (Greenfeder *et al.*, 1995) may have partially reconstituted the second binding domain, so that a degree of dimerization takes place between the cytosolic domains of IL-1RI and IL-1R-AcP, resulting in increased agonist activity of the mutated IL-1ra (Greenfeder *et al.*, 1995).

Like other models of two chain receptors, IL-1 binds first to the IL-1RI with a low affinity. The crystal structure of the IL-1RI complexed with IL-1β has been reported and sheds light on the changes that take place after the low affinity binding (Vigers *et al.*, 1997). The two receptor binding sites of IL-1β have been reported using specific mutations. The crystal structure reveals that both receptor binding sites contact the IL-1RI at the first and third domains (Vigers *et al.*, 1997). Upon contact with the first domain, there appears to be a change in the rigidity of the third domain to encounter contact with the second binding site of IL-1β. IL-1β itself does not undergo a structural change. Since IL-1ra has only one binding site (Evans *et al.*, 1994), the absence of the second binding site prevents contact with the third domain. Hence the critical contact point appears to be at the third domain. Since this contact is likely to be absent in complexes with the IL-1ra (Schreuder *et al.*, 1997), the structural change in the IL-1RI third domain may allow docking of the IL-1R-AcP with the IL-1RI/IL-1β complex. Without the complex of IL-1R-AcP/IL-1RI/IL-1β, there is no signal transduction (Greenfeder *et al.*, 1995).

Several investigations have focused on finding a low-molecular-weight compound that would act as an IL-1 receptor antagonist. In fact, it is estimated that several hundred thousand compounds in various chemical libraries have been screened using cell binding assays, in which the cell expressed IL-1RI and the ligand was radiolabeled IL-1α. To date, none have been reported. Others have used the amino acid sequence of IL-1ra itself to synthesize small peptides that could act as IL-1 receptor antagonists. A series of peptides, derived from three regions of IL-1ra, were synthesized (N-terminal residues 5–9, central 90–98 and C-terminal 143–148). The ability of these peptides to inhibit IL-1-induced IL-2 production was evaluated, each peptide possessed some inhibitory activity, particularly the peptide VTKFYF from the C-terminal part of IL-1ra. (Wieczorek *et al.*, 1996). Other studies screened large numbers of small peptides, generated from recombinatorial peptide display libraries, for their ability to bind to IL-1RI immobilized on a chip, and screened with a laser beam for displacement or change in the refraction of the laser light. In doing so, over 10 million small peptides were screened and one was discovered that blocked the binding of IL-1α to human IL-1R type I with an inhibitory concentration of 45–150 μM (Yanofsky *et al.*, 1996). Variants of this peptide were synthesized and effectively blocked IL-1 responses in human and monkey cells at 2 nM but did not affect IL-1 responses on mouse cells. Thus, small peptides can effectively block IL-1, as well as the bona fide IL-1ra.

4.4 IL-1 receptor antagonist in preclinical studies

4.4.1 Overall concepts

Blocking IL-1 receptors with IL-1ra has increased our understanding of IL-1 as a mediator of disease. Numerous animal studies have employed IL-1ra to demonstrate a role for IL-1 in disease processes. These animal studies are listed in Table 4.1. In addition to administration of IL-1ra, synoviocytes have been transfected with IL-1ra and when expressed in the joint, a decrease in arthritis has been observed (Makarov *et al.*, 1995). Hence, these studies form the basis for gene therapy with IL-1ra. In mice with a null mutation for the IL-1ra gene, there is increased death to lethal endotoxemia (Hirsch *et al.*, 1996). In transgenic mice overproducing IL-1ra, increased protection against lethal endotoxemia has been reported (Hirsch *et al.*, 1996). Other methods, such as neutralizing anti-IL-1 antibodies, antibodies to IL-1RI, and soluble IL-1 receptors, are equally effective, although limited by their animal specificity. In contrast, IL-1ra exhibits little species specificity and the human recombinant molecule is often used in animal studies. In most disease models, other cytokines are produced in addition to IL-1. Therefore, the data depicted in Table 4.1 reveal that IL-1 plays an important role in the pathogenesis of inflammatory and immunologically mediated-disease.

Table 4.1   Effects of IL-1ra *in vivo*

Models of infection
Improved survival in LPS-induced shock in primates, mice, rats and rabbits
Improved survival in *Klebsiella pneumoniae* infection in newborn rats
Reduction in shock and mortality in rabbits and baboons from *E. coli* or *Staphylococcus epidermidis* bacteremia
Amelioration of shock and reduction in death after cecal ligation and puncture
Attenuation of LPS-induced lung nitric oxide activity
Decreased hypoglycemia, production of CSF and early tolerance in mice after administration of endotoxin
Reduction in LPS-induced hyperalgesia
Protection against TNF-induced lethality in D-galactosamine treated mice
Reduction in nematode-induced intestinal nerve dysfunction
Decreased circulating or cellular TNF production in models of sepsis
Decreased IL-6 production after LPS or enteric LPS administration
Protection from *Bacillus anthracis* toxin-induced lethality in mice
Decreased intestinal inflammation and bacterial invasion in shigellosis
Reversal of decreased survival by insulin-like growth factor-1 in sepsis
Decreased in live *E.coli*-induced thrombin, tissue plasminogen activator, plasminogen activator inhibitor and elastase elevations

Models of local inflammation
Decreased neutrophil accumulation in inflammatory peritonitis in mice
Reduction in immune complex-induced neutrophil infiltration, eicosanoid production and tissue necrosis in rabbit colitis
Reduction in acid-induced neutrophil infiltration and enterocolitis in rats
Decreased endotoxin-induced intestinal secretory diarrhea in mice
Inhibition of permanganate-induced granulomas in rats
Inhibition of LPS-induced intra-articular neutrophil infiltration
Decreased IL-1-induced synovitis and loss of cartilage proteoglycan
Reduced myocardial neutrophil accumulation after coronary occlusions in dogs
Reduced inflammation and mortality in acute pancreatitis
Decreased hepatic inflammation following hemorrhagic shock
Modest reduction in acetomenophen-induced liver damage
Decreased IL-8 and MCP-1 levels induced by intravitreal LPS
Reduction in hapten-induced intestestinal motor dysfunction and intestinal myeloperoxidase levels
Decreased cerulean-induced pancreatic inflammation
95% reduction in expression of macrophage chemokine osteopontin and renal injury

Models of acute or chronic lung injury
Decreased local LPS-induced neutrophil infiltration in rats
Inhibition of antigen-induced pulmonary eosinophil accumulation and airway hyperactivity in guinea pigs
Prevention of bleomycin or silica-induced pulmonary fibrosis
Reduction in hypoxia-induced pulmonary hypertension
Reduction in carrageenan-induced pleurisy in rats
Decreased intratracheal IL-1-induced fluid leak (systemic administration)
Decreased albumin leak after systemic LPS
Inhibition of antigen-induced eosinophil accumulation in guinea pigs

Models of central nervous system functions
Decreased stress-induced hypothalamic-pituitary axis
Decreased immobilization-induced stress on hypothalamic-pituitary axis
Decreased LiCl-induced hyperalgesia in rats
Decreased LPS-induced fever
Reduced astrocytosis after spinal cord transection
Increased survival after heat stroke in rats
Protection against NMDA-mediated neurotoxicity
Decreased cerebral ischemia-induced edema and inforact size
Reduced astrocytosis-mediated wound closure after brain damage
Decreased LPS-induced brain monoamine levels
Reduction in ischemia and excitotoxic-induced brain damage in rats
Decreased in number of necrotic neurons in cerebral artery occlusion

Table 4.1   *continued*

Models of metabolic dysfunction
Reduction in fatty streak formation in apolipoprotein E-deficient mice
Reduction in hepatocellular damage following ischemia-reperfusion
Improved survival after hemorrhagic shock in mice
Inhibition of SAA gene expression and synthesis in high dose IL-2 toxicity
Decreased muscle protein breakdown in rats with peritonitis due to cecal ligation
Reduced muscle protein breakdown in rats with chronic septic peritonitis
Inhibition of weight loss following muscle tissue injury
Decrease in bone loss in ovariectomized rats
Decreased multinucleated osteoclasts in ovariectomized rats
Reversal of LPS-induced CRF gene expression in the hypothalamus
Prevention of LPS-induced ACTH release

Models of autoimmune disease
Diminution of *Streptococcus* wall-induced arthritis in rats
Reduction in collagen-induced arthritis in mice
Suppression of anti-basement membrane glomerulonephritis
Delayed hyperglycemia in the diabetic BB rat
Decreased hyperglycemia in non-obese diabetic mice
Reduction in autoimmune myelin basic protein-induced encephalomyelitis
Reduction in elevated cortisone levels in allergic encephalomyelitis
Enhanced suppression of cyclosporin A on IgG synthesis induced by complete Freund's adjuvant

Models of immune-mediated disease
Prevention of graft versus host disease in mice
Prolongation of islet allograft survival
Reduction in skin contact hypersensitivity to haptens
Decrease in coronary artery fibronectin deposition in heterotopic cardiac transplant
Decreased adjuvant arthritis in rats
Reduction in streptozotocin-induced diabetes
Increased survival of corneal transplants

Models of malignant disease
Reduction in the number and size of metastatic melanoma
Reduction in growth of subcutaneous melanoma tumors
Reduced LPS-induced augmentation of metastatic melanoma
Reduction in tumor-mediated cachexia (intratumoral injection)

Effect of models of angiogenesis
Decreased new blood vessel growth following sciatic nerve injury in mice
Decreased vascularization of inflammatory polymers implanted subcutaneously in mice

Impairment of host responses
Increased mortality to *Klebsiella pneumoniae* in newborn rats (high dose)
Increased mortality to *Listeria* infection
Enhanced growth of *Mycobacterium avium* in organs
Worsening of infectious arthritis (late administration)
Increased vascular leak in mice given high dose IL-2

Reports without an effect of IL-1ra
Antigen-induced arthritis in rabbits
LPS-and *Staphylococcus epidermidis* bacteremia-induced fever in rabbits
Fever after LPS injection into the brain
Leukopenia in rats after LPS
Hypertriglyceridemia after LPS in mice
LPS-induced increase in skin blood flow

Leukemic cells
Reduced spontaneous proliferation, colony formation and cytokine production of human AML, CML
  (adult and juvenile) leukemia cells
Reduced spontaneous IL-6 and PGE_2 production in multiple myeloma cells
Decreased spontaneous release of serotonin and histamine in rat basophilic leukemia cells
Decreased spontaneous blast proliferation and cytokine production

Table 4.2   Effect of IL-1ra *in vitro*

Immune-mediated responses
No effect on mitogen- or antigen-induced T-cell proliferation
Decreased IL-2-induced LAK cell generation
Decreased in IL-2-induced LAK cell TNF production
Decreased phorbol ester-induced B-cell proliferation and IgG synthesis

Effects on bone cells
Decreased *E. coli*-induced chaperone proetin-induced osteolytic activity in rat calvarium
Decreased LPS-induced bone resorption in mouse calvarium

Production of cytokines and other molecules
Reduced LPS-induced monocyte production of IL-1β, IL-1α, IL-6, IL-6
Decreased LPS-induced fibroblast production of IL-6
Decreased asbestos-stimulated IL-8 from mesothelial cells
Reduced spontaneous production of substance P by cultured neurons
Enhanced natural killer cell activity[a]
Increased spontaneous PGE$_2$ production by cutured decidual cells
Increased smooth muscle cell proliferation*

Other effects *in vitro*
Reduction in *Actinobacillus* LPS -induced bone resorption
Reduction in spleen cell colony forming units after radiation
Decreased LPS-induced nitric oxide synthase in glial cells
Decreased *Clostridia dificile*-toxin activity on hepatocytes
Reduced VCAM-1 and ICAM expresson induced by Rickettsia LPS on HUVEC
Decreased TSH-stimulated cAMP release in thyroid cells
Decreased *Clostridia dificile*-toxin A-induced intestinal secretory factor release
Decreased NO release and insulin production in rat islets following TNF
Decreased PDGF receptor expression in rat lung myofibroblasts following exposure to particulates

---

[a] This effect may be due to a reduction in the suppressive effects of PGE2 which is induced by IL-1 in these cells.

In these studies, a reduction of at least 50% is observed, but in many, the amelioration of pathological changes can be complete. One consistent observation is the reduction in the number of infiltrating neutrophils associated with local inflammation, and this effect of IL-1ra may be due to preventing IL-1-induced synthesis of IL-8 and related chemokines (Porat *et al.*, 1992). For example, intravitreal injection of LPS into rabbits induces IL-8 and macrophage chemotactic protein-1 in the aqueous humor. The concentrations of the two chemokines at 24 h were inhibited by both anti-TNFα and IL-1ra. A combination of anti-TNFα and IL-1ra had an additive effect and inhibited up to 90% chemokine production (Mo *et al.*, 1999).

There is, however, one important caveat: in the majority of these studies: IL-1ra has been administered just prior to the challenging event. This is particularly the case in models of infection where injecting IL-1ra before a lethal challenge has significantly reduced mortality but when injected shortly after the challenge, IL-1ra had little or no effect on reducing death. On the other hand, in acute pancreatitis, a dose-dependent administration of IL-1ra later in the disease reduced the severity of tissue damage (Norman *et al.*, 1995a, 1995b). In some models of chronic disease, administration of IL-1ra after the onset of disease can still dramatically reduce severity (Vidal-Vanaclocha *et al.*, 1994).

Since triggering so few IL-1 receptors results in a biological response, it is necessary to sustain a high level of IL-1ra to block unoccupied receptors. When exogenous IL-1 is injected intravenously into animals, pretreatment with a 100-fold molar excess of IL-1ra is necessary to prevent the response to IL-1. For example, injecting rabbits with 100 ng/kg of IL-1β produces fever; while a pre-injection of 10 μg/kg of IL-1ra prevents the fever (Dinarello *et al.*, 1992). However, under natural conditions, where endogenous IL-1 and other cytokines are released, an IL-1ra plasma level of 10–20 μg/ml is needed before one observes a reduction in disease. In humans, similar levels of IL-1ra are needed to block the hematological response to LPS. *In vitro*, considerably lower concentrations of IL-1ra are needed (Arend *et al.*, 1990). For example, a one-to-one molar ratio of IL-1ra to IL-1 blocks 50% of the IL-1-induced response in blood monocytes (Granowitz *et al.*, 1992) and a concentration of 100 ng/ml of IL-1ra reduces the spontaneous proliferation, colony formation, and cytokine production of AML or CML cells (Estrov *et al.*, 1991; Rambaldi *et al.*, 1991; Schirò *et al.*, 1993).

IL-1ra is rapidly excreted into the urine and its plasma levels rise and fall dramatically after an intravenous injection. In humans, the plasma half-life is approximately 6 min. Although the binding of IL-1ra to the type 1 IL-1R is considered irreversible, continued expression of unoccupied surface IL-1 receptors probably continues during disease and, therefore, continued high levels of IL-1ra are required to suppress IL-1 activity. Some models have used continuous infusion of IL-1ra. For example, osteopontin is a macrophage chemotactic and adhesion molecule that facilitates macrophage infiltration in rat anti-glomerular basement membrane glomerulonephritis. A constant infusion of IL-1ra over 14 days (induction phase), or days 7 to 21 (established disease), significantly reduced expression of this chemokine in either the induction phase of disease or established disease ($P< 0.001$) with significant inhibition of macrophage accumulation and progressive renal injury (Yu *et al.*, 1999).

4.4.2 Effect of IL-1ra in models of rheumatoid arthritis

The best model for human rheumatoid arthritis appears to be collagen-induced arthritis in the mouse, whereas rat adjuvant arthritis is considered a better model for non-steroidal anti-inflammatory drugs (NSAID). Nevertheless, administration of IL-1ra to rats with adjuvant arthritis has reduced bone erosions and joint destruction. Rats with developing adjuvant arthritis were treated with IL-1ra by continuous infusion. The results were a modest but significant reduction in swelling of the ankle joints, paw weights, and histologic evaluation of bone and cartilage lesions. However, marked inhibition of bone resorption was observed, even at doses with which anti-inflammatory activity was not seen. In contrast, IL-1ra treatment of rats with established collagen-induced arthritis resulted in a near complete suppression of all parameters of the disease (Bendele *et al.*, 1999).

Using transplantation of 3T3 fibroblasts transfected with human IL-1ra, paws and knee joints were inspected to evaluate inflammation and cartilage destruction in a model of murine collagen type II arthritis. The onset of the collagen arthritis was almost nearly prevented in joints with the transfected IL-1ra expressing cells, whereas joints containing cells transfected with the empty vector showed severe inflammation and destruction of cartilage. In the ipsilateral paws of the IL-1ra gene-expressing knees, reduced inflammation and joint destruction was observed (Bakker *et al.*, 1997). There are several studies on the ability of IL-1ra to reduce the severity of rheumatoid arthritis-like disease in animals, which have been reviewed by Arend (Arend *et al.*, 1998).

4.4.3 Effect of IL-1ra on intestinal inflammation

Ulcerative colitis and Crohn's disease are chronic, relapsing inflammatory processes in the gastro-intestinal tract that account for a large number of patients with autoimmune disease, often termed inflammatory bowel disease (IBD). Elevation of IL-1, IL-6, IL-8, IL-12, and IFN and GM-CSF have been implicated. IL-1 has been implicated as a target for therapeutic intervention. Animal studies support a role for IL-1, since IL-1ra reduces intestinal inflammation in various models. In the rabbit, administration of IL-1ra reduces PGE_2, necrosis and infiltration of inflammatory cells (Cominelli *et al.*, 1990, 1992). A subserosal injection of streptococcal peptidoglycan induces granulomatous enterocolitis and systemic inflammation in rats. IL-1ra reduced acute and chronic enterocolitis, adhesions, and arthritis (McCall *et al.*, 1994). Production of toxin A from *Clostridium difficile* causes enterocolitis in animals and humans. Using a model of isolated rabbit ileal mucosa, supernatants from macrophages stimulated with toxin A induced intestinal secretion, which was inhibited (72%) by a monoclonal anti-IL-1β interleukin but not anti-IL-1α. IL-1ra treatment inhibited 80%; $P < 0.01$) of the secretory activated induced by the toxin-A stimulated macrophages (Rocha *et al.*, 1998).

4.4.4 Effect of IL-1ra on brain function

In rats, the intraperitoneal injection of LPS increases brain concentrations of norepinephrine, dopamine, and serotonin. Preteatment with IL-1ra completely blocked the LPS-induced changes in brain monoamines (Mohankumar *et al.*, 1999). Since IL-1β has been found in human brain (Breder *et al.*, 1988), its role in ischemic and infectious brain damage has been the focus of investigation. Using a model of ischemic brain damage in rats, pretreatment with IL-1ra reduces the area of necrosis (Loddick and Rothwell, 1996). Intrastriatal infusion of IL-1ra markedly inhibited striatal neuronal damage caused by N-methyl-D-aspartate or alpha-amino-3-hydroxy-5-methyl-4-isoxazolepropionate (AMPA) receptor activation in the rat (Lawrence *et al.*, 1998). These data reveal selective actions of IL-1 and IL-1ra in the striatum, which influence cortical neuronal loss and suggest that IL-1 selectively enhances damage caused by AMPA receptor activation.

4.4.5 Role of IL-1 and IL-1ra in neovascularization

IL-1β has angiogenic properties, in part by inducing angiogenic factors such as IL-8 and vascular endothelial growth factor (VEGF). In a model of sciatic nerve injury, local application of IL-1ra reduced new blood vessel growth (Guénard *et al.*, 1991). The role of IL-1 and TNF in the pathogenesis of atherosclerosis has been considered in the context of inducing a local inflammatory reaction within the vessel. The stimulant for the response may be, in part, due to the ability of oxidized low-density lipoproteins to induce these cytokines in human blood monocytes (Ku *et al.*, 1992; Thomas *et al.*, 1994). Mice deficient in apolipoprotein E develop pathologic fatty acid streaks in blood vessels when fed a high lipid diet. In these mice, treatment with a constant infusion of IL-1ra administered by minipump, reduced the incidence of the fatty acid streak formation to the same degree as did estradiol implants.

4.4.6 Topical IL-1ra

Topical IL-1ra has been used to increase the survival of orthotopic corneal allografts. Using topical application of IL-1ra three times per day, there was neither donor-specific delayed-type hypersensitivity ($P<.001$) nor the capacity to reject orthotopic donor-type skin allografts, suggesting that IL-1 plays a key role in promoting allosensitization when corneal allografts are placed orthotopically (Yamada *et al.*, 1998).

4.5 Transgenic mice overexpressing IL-1ra

Mice overexpressing IL-1ra have been generated and examined for phenotypic changes. The first studies focused on challenge to LPS, which resulted in greater survival rates compared to wild-type controls (Hirsch *et al.*, 1996). These results are similar to those reported for the survival benefit of exogenous IL-1ra administered to mice (Alexander *et al.*, 1991) or rats (Alexander *et al.*, 1992) given a lethal dose of LPS. In transgenic mice overexpressing IL-1ra under the control of the murine glial fibrillary acidic protein promoter, the febrile response to intracerebroventricular IL-1β was absent, suggesting that receptors in the CNS were blocked by IL-1ra (Lundkvist *et al.*, 1999). However, following intraperitoneal LPS, a febrile response and elevations in circulating IL-6 were observed, consistent with studies on LPS responses in IL-1β-deficient mice (Alheim *et al.*, 1997; Fantuzzi *et al.*, 1997).

4.6 Studies in IL-1ra-deficient mice

Three groups have reported that mice deficient in IL-1ra exhibit spontaneous phenotypes. These mice have been initially bred from C57Bl6 genetic backgrounds, which affects their phenotype. The manifestations of disease, however, are dependent on the genetic background of the mice. Mice deficient in IL-1ra have low litter numbers and exhibit growth retardation in adult life (Hirsch *et al.*, 1996). Injection of LPS into IL-1ra-deficient mice results in increased lethality (Hirsch *et al.*, 1996). This is consistent with the protective effect of IL-1ra on endotoxin lethality in mice (Alexander *et al.*, 1991). It is also consistent with the observation that mice overexpressing IL-1ra are protected against the lethal effects of endotoxin (Hirsch *et al.*, 1996).

Higher antibody levels spontaneously develop in IL-1ra-deficient mice (Horai *et al.*, 1998). In addition, Duff has observed that mice deficient in IL-1ra develop spontaneous arteritis characterized by infiltrating macrophages and neutrophils (Nicklin *et al.*, 2000).

The most dramatic phenotype has been observed in IL-1ra-deficient mice crossed from a C57Bl6 to a BALB C genetic background (Horai *et al.*, 2000). In these mice, spontaneous arthritis developed in both males and females starting at 5 weeks of age. By 13 weeks of age, all mice were affected. The disease was characterized by multiple joint involvement showing bone erosions, osteoclast activation, and infiltration of neutrophils. In addition, enlarged spleens and lymph nodes were noted. Compared to the wild-type, there was marked increased gene expression of IL-1β, IL-6, TNFα, Cox-2, and type I receptor. In addition, circulating levels of IgG, G1, but not IgM, were observed. Rheumatoid factor and anti-double stranded DNA antibodies were elevated. One can conclude from these studies that endogenous IL-1ra plays a role in the development of this generalized spontaneous inflammatory arthritis, since the wild-type controls living in the same environment do not develop this disease. The genetic background is important in that spontaneous disease does not occur in IL-1ra deficient mice with a C57BL6 genetic background.

Consistent with the observation of joint bone erosions in IL-1ra-deficient mice, mice deficient in the type I IL-1R exhibit no significant trabecular bone loss following ovariectomy compared to wild-type controls (Lorenzo *et al.*, 1998). As discussed below, patients with rheumatoid arthritis treated for 24 weeks with daily injections of IL-1ra, exhibit reduced bone erosions compared to patients injected with placebo (Bresnihan *et al.*, 1998).

4.7 Effects of IL-1ra in healthy humans

As stated above, healthy humans are highly sensitive to IL-1 agonist activities; for example, 1 ng/kg of intravenous IL-1β produces symptoms (Tewari *et al.*, 1990). In contrast, the intravenous infusion of 10 mg/kg of IL-1ra, a 10 million-fold molar excess, is without effects (Granowitz *et al.*, 1992). IL-1ra given intravenously to healthy volunteers is without side-effects or changes in biochemical, hematologic, or endocrinologic parameters, even when peak blood levels reach 30 μg/ml and are sustained above 10 μg/ml for several hours (Granowitz *et al.*, 1992). These studies support the concept that there is no role for IL-1 in the regulation of body temperature, blood pressure, or hematopoiesis in health. It is also consistent with the failure to observe spontaneous expression of the IL-1β gene in circulating blood cells from healthy persons using sensitive PCR methods (Mileno *et al.*, 1995). Interestingly, PBMC taken from these volunteers after receiving IL-1ra failed to produce IL-6 when stimulated ex vivo with LPS (Granowitz *et al.*, 1992).

In order to evaluate the effect of IL-1 receptor blockade in clinical disease under controlled experimental conditions, healthy volunteers were challenged with intravenous endotoxin and administered an infusion of IL-1ra at the same time. Even at 10 mg/kg IL-1ra, there was no effect on endotoxin-induced fever, although blood levels of IL-1ra were not significantly elevated until one hour after the bolus injection of endotoxin. Since IL-1ra does not cross the blood–brain barrier, this may account for the inability of IL-1ra to diminish endotoxin fever (Dinarello *et al.*, 1992). However, IL-1R blockade was accomplished, since there was a 50% reduction in the endotoxin-induced neutrophilia and a reduction in the circulating levels of G-CSF compared to subjects injected with endotoxin plus saline (Granowitz *et al.*, 1993).

Endotoxin injection suppresses the mitogen-induced proliferative response of peripheral blood mononuclear cells *in vitro*. However, in volunteers injected with endotoxin plus IL-1ra, there was no suppression of the response (Granowitz *et al.*, 1993). Mitogen- and antigen- induced proliferation is a well-established parameter of immunocompetence and is associated with decreased production of IL-2. Similar to experimental endotoxin injection, this suppression is observed in patients with multiple trauma, sepsis, and cardiopulmonary bypass. In experimental endotoxemia, and the above clinical conditions, treatment with cyclo-oxygenase inhibitors restores these cell-mediated immune responses (Markewitz *et al.*, 1993). This effect of cyclo-oxygenase inhibitors is consistent with the well-known suppressive effects of PGE$_2$ on IL-2 production and T-cell proliferation.

Since IL-1 is a potent inducer of COX-2, it is not surprising that blocking IL-1 receptors during endotoxemia would reduce IL-1-induced PGE_2 production during endotoxemia. Thus, these studies establish that under conditions of low-dose endotoxemia, it is possible to block IL-1-mediated responses with IL-1ra. Those host–response parameters that were unaffected by IL-1ra are likely due to other cytokines such as TNF or IL-6 or the combination of these cytokines with IL-1.

What are the structural requirements of the respective molecules that account for this dramatic difference? The ability of IL-1β to optimally trigger cell signaling requires stability of the overall tertiary structure of the cytokine, so that mutations in one amino acid may unfold the molecule resulting in a several hundred-fold loss in activity but without a loss in receptor binding. This suggests that biological activity requires binding of IL-1β to a relatively broad area on the receptor. The tertiary structure of IL-1ra, which is closely related to that of IL-1β, allows for tight binding to the IL-1RI but IL-1ra clearly lacks the second binding site that allows docking of the IL-1R-AcP to form the heterodimer. Without dimerization, no signal is transduced but occupancy of the IL-1RI by IL-1ra results in a very effective prevention of IL-1 signal transduction. Small molecules may mimic the near perfect receptor antagonism of IL-1ra but to date, none have been reported.

4.8 Therapeutic effects of IL-1ra in humans

4.8.1 Treating septic shock

IL-1ra has been in given to patients with septic shock, rheumatoid arthritis, and steroid-resistant graft versus host disease. A phase II, randomized, placebo-controlled, open-label trial of 99 patients with septic shock was carried-out. Patients received either placebo or a loading bolus of 100 mg followed by a 3-day infusion of 17, 67, or 133 mg/h IL-1ra (Fisher *et al.*, 1993). A dose-dependent improvement in 28-day mortality was observed; mortality was reduced from 44% in the placebo group to 16% in the group receiving the highest dose of IL-1ra ($P = 0.015$). In that study, there was a dose-related fall in the circulating levels of IL-6 24 h after the initiation of IL-1ra infusion. This fall in IL-6 levels is consistent with the well-established control of circulating IL-6 levels by IL-1, and the correlation of disease severity and outcome with IL-6 levels.

This phase II trial was followed by a large placebo-controlled, double blind study. In this phase III trial, 893 patients were randomized to receive placebo or a loading bolus of 100 mg followed by a 3-day infusion of 1 or 2 mg/kg/h IL-1ra or placebo. There was no statistically significant reduction in all-cause mortality in the entire group (Fisher *et al.*, 1994). However, a retrospective analysis of patients with a predicted risk of mortality of 24% or greater, revealed a significant reduction in 28-day mortality (45% in the placebo group and 35% in patients receiving 2 mg/kg/h for 72 h, $P = 0.005$) (Fisher *et al.*, 1994). In addition, the post-study analysis of data revealed an increase in survival time with IL-1ra in patients with one or more organ failures ($n = 563$, $P = 0.009$). Although there was no overall statistically significant benefit in 28-day all-cause mortality, the results revealed a trend in the group receiving IL-1ra and warranted another trial with the primary endpoint targeted to patients with a high risk of mortality (Fisher *et al.*, 1994).

This first phase III study was analyzed by Knaus (Knaus *et al.*, 1993). Although the mortality rate in the placebo group was 41.8%, and 41.5% in the IL-1ra group, in patients who were bacteremic at study entry, the mortality was 37% in the placebo group and 28% in the IL-1ra group ($P = 0.071$). In patients without bacteremia, a 36% mortality rate was observed in both groups. Also, patients who had a documented pathogen identified at study entry, had a lower mortality rate if they had received IL-1ra (31.5%) compared to placebo (37.5%) ($P = 0.12$). Patients without a documented infection had a slightly higher mortality rate than the placebo group but this difference did not reach statistically significant levels ($P = 0.21$).

A second phase III trial in 91 academic centers in the North America and in Europe was initiated, with the intention of randomizing 1300 patients to either placebo or IL-1ra. The IL-1ra was administered as an intravenous bolus injection of 100 mg followed by 3 days of constant infusion of 2.0 mg/kg/h. The primary end-point was survival time in patients with end-organ dysfunction and/or shock at the time of entry. There were 512 patients who met these entry criteria. However, there were 184 patients who had been enrolled and randomized but who did not meet the primary end-points. The mortality was 24.2% in the placebo group and 18.3% in the IL-1ra group ($P = 0.33$). A mid-trial analysis was undertaken after 696 patients had been enrolled. The study was terminated during an interim analysis because a reduction in overall 28-day mortality was unlikely to reach statistical significance. The patient groups were well matched in that 52.9% of the placebo patients were in shock at the time of study entry and 50.9% of the IL-1ra group. There was no excess mortality in patients receiving IL-1ra. The 28-day all-cause mortality was 33.1% in the IL-1ra group (116/350) compared to 36.4% (126/346) in the placebo group ($P = 0.36$), a 9% reduction in mortality ($P = 0.36$). However, as in each of the IL-1ra trials in patients with septic shock, subgroups appeared to have benefited. For example, patients with gram-positive infection had a mortality rate of 35.4% compared to 28.9% in the IL-1ra treated group ($P = 0.40$). This was off-set by increased mortality in the group receiving IL-1ra for unknown organism(s) (41.8% versus 28.6%, $P = 0.21$). Nevertheless, unless such a hypothesis is retested in another prospective trial, the subgroup analysis remains unproven.

A survival analysis was made in those patients who had major organ dysfunction (target population) and, like the overall group, there was no difference in probability of survival. These analyses support the view that:

(1) IL-1ra administration in patients with life-threatening sepsis is safe;

(2) there is a consistent but small improvement in survival with IL-1ra;

(3) there are patients with particular presentations at trial entry that clearly benefit from IL-1ra treatment; and

(3) the overall patient group, although with improved survival, is too heterogeneous to show statistically significant differences.

Are we asking too much from monotherapy in sepsis? Similar results have been reported for antiTNF based therapy in these patients (Abraham *et al.*, 1995, 1996, 1998; Fisher *et al.*, 1996). One concept is to combine IL-1ra with anti-TNF strategies for treating septic shock.

4.8.2 IL-1ra in patients with rheumatoid arthritis

IL-1ra was initially tested in a trial in 25 patients with rheumatoid arthritis. In the group receiving a single subcutaneous dose of 6 mg/kg, there was a fall in the mean number of tender joints ($P<0.05$) (Lebsack *et al.*, 1991). In patients receiving 4 mg/kg per day for 7 days, there was a reduction in the number of tender joints from 24 to 10, the erythrocyte sedimentation rate fell from 48 to 31, and C-reactive protein decreased from 2.9 to 1.9 μg/ml. In this group, the mean plasma concentration of IL-1ra was 660 ±240 ng/ml.

In an expanded double-blind trial, IL-1ra was given to 175 patients (Campion *et al.*, 1996). The patients enrolled into the study had active disease and were taking non-steroidal anti-inflammatory drugs and/or up to 10 mg/day of prednisone. There was an initial phase of 3 weeks of either 20, 70, or 200 mg, one, three, or seven times per week. Thereafter, patients received the same dose once a week for 4 weeks. Placebo was given to patients once a week for the entire 7-week study period. To maintain the blindness of the study, patients received daily injections of either IL-1ra or placebo on the days IL-1ra was not administered.

Four measurements of efficacy were used: number of swollen joints, number of painful joints, patient and physician assessment of disease severity. A reduction of 50% or greater in these scores from baseline was considered significant in the analysis. After 3 weeks, a statistically significant reduction in the total number of parameters was observed with the optimal improvement in patients receiving 70 mg per day. Daily dosing appeared more effective than weekly dosing when assessed by the number of swollen joints, the investigator and patient assessments of disease activity, pain score, and C-reactive protein levels.

A large double-blind, placebo-controlled multicenter trial of IL-1ra in 472 patients with rheumatoid arthritis has been reported (Bresnihan *et al.*, 1998). The study was comprised of patients who had discontinued use of disease-modifying agents, such as gold and methotrexate, 6 weeks prior to entry. Patients had active and severe RA (disease duration 8 years) and were recruited into a 24-week course of therapy into placebo or one of 3 IL-1ra groups. Patients had stable disease of two or more years duration, which was controlled by non-steroidal anti-inflammatory agents. Some were taking less than 10 mg of prednisone daily. There were three doses of IL-1ra administered subcutaneously: 30, 75, and 150 mg/day for 24 weeks. At entry, age, sex, disease duration, and percentage of patients with rheumatoid factor and joint bone erosions were similar in each of the groups. After 24 weeks, 43% of the patients receiving 150 mg/day of IL-1ra met the American College of Rheumatology criteria for response (the primary efficacy measure), 44% met the Paulus criteria, and statistically significant ($P = 0.048$) improvements were seen in the number of swollen joints, number of tender joints, investigator's assessment of disease activity, patient's assessment of disease activity, pain score on a visual analogue scale, duration of morning stiffness and Health Assessment score. In addition, there was a dose-dependent reduction in C-reactive protein level, and erythrocyte sedimentation rate.

Importantly, the rate of radiologic progression in the patients receiving IL-1ra was significantly less than in the placebo group at 24 weeks, as evidenced by the Larsen score and the erosive joint count. The reduction in new bone erosions was assessed by two radiologists who were blinded to the patient treatment, as well as blinded to the chronology of the X-ray films. This finding suggests that IL-1ra is blocking the osteoclast-activating factor property of IL-1, as has been reported in myeloma cell cultures (Torcia *et al.*, 1996). This study confirmed both the efficacy and the safety of IL-1ra in a large cohort of patients with active and severe rheumatoid arthritis.

The only side-effect was local skin rash, which was observed primarily during the first 2 weeks of therapy. After 24 weeks, there were no statistically significant increases in infection in the IL-1ra arm compared to placebo. When the trial was extended another 24 weeks, there was also no statistically significant increases in infection. Some patients have now been treated with IL-1ra for over 3 years and there are no reports of increased infection or cancer. Another trial of IL-1ra in patients with rheumatoid arthritis has been carried out in patients randomized to receive treatment with methotrexate or different doses of IL-1ra plus methotrexate treatment. 419 patients were randomized to receive either placebo or increasing doses of IL-1Ra. Patients were also being treated with methotrexate (mean 17 mg/week). After 24 weeks, patients taking IL-1Ra (1.0 mg/kg) had significantly decreased parameters of disease compared to the placebo (Cohen *et al.*, 1999). For example, the percent of patients with a reduction of 50% in disease activity was 24% with IL-1Ra compared to 4% for placebo (P<0.003). These studies suggest that the addition of IL-1Ra to optimal methotrexate results in a further decrease in disease (Cohen *et al.*, 1999).

4.8.3 Graft versus host disease

A phase I/II trial of escalating doses of IL-1ra in 17 patients with steroid-resistant graft versus host disease has been completed (Antin *et al.*, 1994). IL-1ra (400–3400 mg/day) was given as a continuous intravenous infusion every 24 h for 7 days. Using an organ-specific, acute-disease scale, there was improvement in 16 of the 17 patients. Moreover, a decrease in the steady state mRNA for TNFα in peripheral blood mononuclear cells correlated with improvement ($P = 0.001$) (Antin *et al.*, 1994). These studies in humans are similar to the use of IL-1ra in animal models of graft versus host disease.

For clinical efficacy, IL-1ra in patients with rheumatoid arthritis exhibits a dose-dependent response. Even the reduction of endotoxin-induced neutrophilia in healthy subjects is dose-dependent. Animal studies support these clinical observations. The requirement for such high plasma levels of IL-1ra is not completely understood because IL-1ra levels are already several logs higher than measurable IL-1 levels in the most severe cases of septic shock. Rapid renal clearance, binding to the soluble form of the type I receptor and the effect of acidosis in the local or systemic situation may explain a need for these high levels.

4.9 Do endogenous levels of IL-1ra reflect or affect the severity of human disease?

4.9.1 Overall concepts

Does endogenous production of IL-1ra affect disease outcome? There is little question that elevated production of IL-1ra is an excellent marker of disease, and certainly a better indicator than levels of IL-1 itself. In some clinical conditions, the elevation in IL-1ra, rather than IL-1 itself, may indicate the presence of a pathological condition. Detecting elevated IL-1ra production could indicate a natural compensatory mechanism to counter the activity of IL-1. For example, in rheumatoid arthritis (Chomarat *et al.*, 1995) or HIV-

1-infected persons (Thea *et al.*, 1996) IL-1ra levels are elevated. Is the amount of IL-1ra produced in disease sufficient to dampen the response to IL-1? Although the answer to this question remains unclear in humans, using specific, neutralizing antibodies to mouse IL-1ra, an increase in the formation of Schistosome egg granulomata was observed when endogenous IL-1ra was neutralized (Chensue *et al.*, 1993). In rabbits with immune complex colitis, infusion of a neutralizing antibody to rabbit IL-1ra resulted in exacerbation and prolongation of the colitis (Ferretti *et al.*, 1994). At the time of writing, the phenotype of the IL-1ra deficient mouse supports the concept that endogenous IL-1ra affords protection in some disease-prone animals. However, in other genetic backgrounds, IL-1ra deficient mice are nearly normal.

The molar 'ratio' of endogenous IL-1ra to IL-1β levels in body fluids from patients with infectious, inflammatory, or autoimmune disease is often 10–100-fold more IL-1ra than IL-1β. In some selected clinical conditions, that ratio is far less. If the molar ratio of endogenous IL-1ra to IL-1 falls, does this affect disease outcome? Some data provide important findings regarding this question. In AML cells, where IL-1β is spontaneously expressed, IL-1ra gene expression is suppressed even when stimulated with GM-CSF (Rambaldi *et al.*, 1991). In 81 patients with CML, cell lysates contained more IL-1β than cells from healthy subjects, whereas the levels of IL-1ra were the same for both groups (Wetzler *et al.*, 1991). In addition, the survival of 44 patients with elevated IL-1β was lower compared to patients with low IL-1β levels. During accelerated blast crisis, IL-1ra levels were lower compared to patients in a chronic-phase (Wetzler *et al.*, 1991). Stromal cultures established from bone marrow of patients with aplastic anemia produced less spontaneous, as well as induced, IL-1ra compared to stromal cells established from normal bone marrow (Holmberg *et al.*, 1994). Recently we have measured high levels of soluble IL-1R type II in the circulation of 25 patients with hairy cell leukemia, which correlate with high levels of IL-1β (Barak *et al.*, 1994, 1996); however, an increase in IL-1ra levels in these patients was associated with a response to treatment.

4.9.2 Measuring IL-1ra in disease states

Measurement of IL-1β in the circulation is not an easy task, even in clinical situations of overwhelming systemic inflammation (Cannon *et al.*, 1993; Casey *et al.*, 1993). This may be due to binding of IL-1β to soluble IL-1R type II, α-2 macroglobulin, or to other proteins. In addition, concentrations of IL-1β are in the low pg/ml range. In fact, various collection and extraction methods have been employed (Cannon *et al.*, 1988). When extracted, there have been positive correlations of circulating IL-1β with disease activity (Eastgate *et al.*, 1988; Casey *et al.*, 1993). On the other hand, measuring IL-1ra levels in the circulation is not associated with technical difficulties and the concentrations are in the nanogram per milliliter range. The relatively high levels of IL-1ra in the circulation, compared to IL-1β, is probably due to the signal peptide on the secreted isoform of IL-1ra (Arend *et al.*, 1998), its passage through the Golgi (Andersson *et al.*, 1992) and its efficient translation from polyadenylated RNA compared to that of IL-1β (Schindler *et al.*, 1990).

In healthy humans, IL-1β levels are undetectable or low. On the other hand, IL-1ra levels are 200–400 pg/ml. In human subjects injected with endotoxin, circulating IL-1β levels reach a peak level of 50–100 pg/ml, whereas IL-1ra rises to 6–10 ng/ml (Granowitz *et al.*, 1991; Fischer *et al.*, 1992). In patients and volunteers receiving IFNα treatment, IL-1ra levels are also elevated into the nanogram range (Tilg *et al.*, 1993), whereas saline-injected subjects have circulating 200–400 pg/ml of IL-1ra. IL-1ra can also be measured as spontaneous production from cultured human PBMC or in whole blood cultures (Nerad *et al.*, 1992). IL-1ra is present in brocho-alveolar lavage (BAL) fluid, peritoneal fluid, and cerebrospinal fluid.

4.9.3 Induction of circulating IL-1ra following IL-1α, IL-1β, IFNα, IFNγ, IL-6, IL-10, G-CSF and intravenous IgG infusion in humans

The therapeutic use of cytokines in disease is often associated with an increase in circulating IL-1ra, usually without a concomitant rise in circulating IL-1β. The role for increased IL-1ra in the therapeutic actions of these cytokines remains unclear, although it is possible that the increase in IL-1ra level is sufficient to reduce IL-1-mediated inflammation. IL-1α induces circulating IL-1ra levels in humans (Tilg *et al.*, 1994). Circulating levels of IL-1ra increased in patients infused with either IL-1α or IL-1β (Kopp *et al.*, 1996). Before the IL-1 infusion, mean circulating IL-1ra levels were 453 pg/ml, which increased dose-dependently with the dose of IL-1 and exceeded 1 µg/ml.

In one study, the administration of G-CSF to humans induced IL-1ra, and the increase of circulating IL-1ra was associated with decreased slow-wave sleep. It was proposed that IL-1ra had reduced the sleep-inducing property of endogenous IL-1 (Schuld *et al.*, 1999). Interferon therapy induces a rather rapid increase in circulating IL-1ra (Tilg *et al.*, 1993, 1994), as well as *in vitro* spontaneous production in whole blood cultures (Huang *et al.*, 1995; Reznikov *et al.*, 1998). In a study of 14 patients with chronic hepatitis type C, injection of IFNβ did not affect circulating TNF or IL-1β levels, but significant increases in circulating levels of IL-6 and IL-1ra were observed 180 min after IFNβ injection (Ohno *et al.*, 1998).

Intravenous IgG infusion in humans is associated with increases in circulating IL-1ra (Dinarello, 1994), although it remains unclear whether any of the therapeutic benefits of IgG therapy are due to IL-1ra increases. In patients with severe forms of IgA nephropathy, serum IL-1ra was low but increased to levels observed in healthy subjects following IgG therapy (Rostoker *et al.*, 1998).

4.9.4 IL-1ra reflects disease activity: IL-1ra as an acute phase protein

Several studies measuring IL-1ra in the circulation report a positive correlation with disease severity. In fact, when comparing disease severity to circulating factors, acute-phase proteins like C-reactive protein (CRP) and IL-1ra have nearly the same correlation coefficient. In patients with rheumatoid arthritis, the correlation of disease-severity scores, such as the Larsen score, with IL-1ra has an *r* value of 0.32 (*P*<0.0001) (Jouvenne *et al.*, 1998). Levels of IL-1ra are higher in patients with destructive joint disease than non-destructive disease (Jouvenne *et al.*, 1998). Circulating IL-1ra levels also correlate with CRP, erythrocyte sedimentation rate, and the Ritchie severity score (all *P*<0.0001). In a study of patients admitted to the hospital with symptoms of unstable angina, elevated IL-1ra and IL-6 correlated (Biasucci *et al.*, 1999). Although all patients were treated similarly, with low molecular weight heparin, aspirin, and intravenous nitrates, after 48 h approximately 50% of the patients progressed to require an intervention (graft by-pass surgery or angioplasty). The other 50% improved and were discharged home. At 48 h, the IL-1ra levels had all fallen in the discharged group, whereas the group requiring intervention exhibited rising levels of IL-1ra.

The severity of necrotizing enterocolitis and circulating concentrations of IL-1β and IL-1ra have been examined (Edelson *et al.*, 1999). Serial blood samples at onset, 8, 24, 48, and 72 h were obtained from newborn infants with predefined signs and symptoms of necrotizing enterocolitis. IL-1ra at a concentration of >130 000 pg/ml had a sensitivity of 100% and a specificity of 92%. The authors concluded that the severity of necrotizing enterocolitis are not due to a lack of IL-1ra.

Levels of IL-1ra appear to reflect levels of IL-1β and, indeed, IL-1 stimulates the production of IL-1ra in monocytes. Most importantly, IL-1 stimulates IL-1ra gene expression and synthesis in hepatocytes and hence can be considered to be an acute-phase protein (Gabay *et al.*, 1997). However, IL-1ra is devoid of direct biological activity and, therefore, is not similar to IL-6, which stimulates hepatocytes to produce CRP and other true acute-phase proteins. In general, IL-6 levels also correlate with disease severity and also with CRP levels in a variety of diseases. For example, in patients with burns, IL-1ra and IL-6 levels each reflect the severity and extent of the burn injury (Mandrup-Poulsen *et al.*, 1995).

4.9.5 Production of IL-1ra by PBMC in disease states

In a study of spontaneous production of IL-1ra from PBMC in over 450 elderly persons, elevated production of IL-1ra and IL-6 correlate with decreased albumin (Roubenoff *et al.*, 1998). This suggests that increased inflammation associated with some aging persons can be reflected in the levels of IL-1ra, as it does with IL-6. In patients with renal failure being treated with hemodialysis, elevated spontaneous IL-1ra production from PBMC was observed, compared to patients with renal failure without dialysis treatment (Pereira *et al.*, 1992). Again, this may reflect an ongoing inflammatory process associated with hemodialysis.

4.9.6 Endogenous IL-1ra production may affect disease activity

In patients with acute Lyme arthritis, the duration of joint inflammation is shortest in those patients with the highest joint fluid levels of IL-1ra, whereas it is prolonged in those patients with low levels of IL-1ra (Miller *et al.*, 1993). The reciprocal relationship was found for synovial fluid levels of IL-1β in the same patients. Similar findings were found in the relative production of IL-1ra and IL-1β in synovial tissue explants of patients with rheumatoid or osteoarthritis (Firestein *et al.*, 1992, 1994; Roux-Lombard *et al.*, 1992). In normal skin, an intracellular form of IL-1ra is present in higher concentrations compared to IL-1α (Hammerberg *et al.*, 1992) but in psoriatic lesions, the balance is in favor of IL-1α (Hammerberg *et al.*, 1992; Kristensen *et al.*, 1992). In the case of the soluble IL-1R type II, the higher the level of the soluble receptor in the circulation of patients with rheumatoid arthritis, the lower the disease activity (Jouvenne *et al.*, 1998). In the case of patients with hairy cell leukemia, circulating levels of IL-1ra are elevated during remission from the disease (Barak *et al.*, 1998). In the study cited above, in which spontaneous production of IL-1ra correlated with IL-6 and decreased albumin levels in elderly persons (Roubenoff *et al.*, 1998), wrist radiographs revealed that there was a negative correlation between production of IL-1ra and degree of osteoporosis (Fraenkel *et al.*, 1998). A similar negative correlation was made in patients with type I diabetes mellitus (Mandrup-Poulsen *et al.*, 1994).

The ratio of urinary excretion of IL-1ra to that of IL-1β was measured in 23 patients with acute renal graft rejection and in 17 patients with stable graft function. Patients with rejection had higher urinary IL-1β/creatinine ratios, lower IL-1ra/creatinine ratios, and consequently lower IL-1ra/IL-1β ratios (P<0.005), compared with patients without rejection. In patients with acute rejection, IL-1β/creatinine ratios increased from 3.5 to 8.1 (P<0.0005). The authors concluded that patients who produce high amounts of IL-1ra compared to IL-1β, are less likely to experience acute allograft rejection than patients with low IL-1ra/IL-1β ratios (Teppo *et al.*, 1998).

4.10 Polymorphisms in the IL-1ra gene and associations with disease states

There is a well-described polymorphism in intron-2 of the promoter of the IL-1ra gene termed the A1–5 allele. This polymorphism is due to a variable 86 base pair tandem repeat (Tarlow *et al.*, 1993). IL-1ra polymorphisms have been associated with lichen sclerosis (Clay *et al.*, 1994) and alopecia areata (Tarlow *et al.*, 1994). Fang and co-workers (Fang *et al.*, 1998) examined the frequency of this allele in 93 consecutive patients admitted to the surgical intensive care unit and compared the frequency to that in a cohort of 261 local blood donors in apparent good health. The results were surprising in that there was a high frequency of the IL-1raA2 allele in the cohort with severe sepsis compared to the healthy cohort (P<0.01). Although there was no association with outcome (survival or organ failure), the study suggests that persons homozygous for this allele were more likely to find themselves in a surgical intensive care unit with severe sepsis that those without the allele. The internal control for this study was the lack of clinical outcome associated with the Taq1 allele (Pociot *et al.*, 1992) of the IL-1β gene in this cohort of 93 patients.

Can we believe that this IL-1ra allele makes one more likely to develop severe sepsis? What is known about this allele and IL-1ra production? In one study, the amount of IL-1ra produced from patients with insulin-dependent diabetes mellitus was reduced (Mandrup-Poulsen *et al.*, 1994). In another study, granulocyte-macrophage colony-stimulating factor was used to stimulate IL-1ra production and persons with the IL-1raA2 allele exhibited increased production compared to those without this allele (Danis *et al.*, 1995). In addition, in that study, there was reduced production of IL-1α in these subjects. Clearly, these results need to be confirmed prospectively but the concept that a gene polymorphism is associated with a measurable difference in the amount of the gene product and an outcome to disease may help resolve the problems encountered in new therapeutic clinical trials in septic shock patients. As it now stands, it seems that persons with the IL-1raA2 allele synthesize more IL-1ra, which is a risk factor for developing severe sepsis following a surgical procedure.

Linkage of a particular cytokine gene polymorphism to disease is not always found in each population studied. For example, a predisposition to develop severe systemic lupus erythematosus was linked to the IL-1raA2 allele in a cohort of persons in the United Kingdom (Blakemore *et al.*, 1994). In a cohort living in Australia, this association was not found (Danis *et al.*, 1995). Similarly, the association of the IL-1ra allele and ulcerative colitis in England (Mansfield *et al.*, 1994) was not observed in a cohort of patients living in Southern Germany (Hacker *et al.*, 1997). The Fang study was on German patients and hence the importance of their observation concerning susceptibility to severe sepsis needs to be studied in a different population. A positive association with the IL-1ra allele has been reported in schizophrenic patients (Katila *et al.*, 1999). In a Danish study using the method of transmission disequilibrium test, the IL-1raA2 allele was studied for linkage and intrafamilial association with insulin dependent diabetes mellitus in 245 Danish families. There was no evidence of linkage or intrafamilial with the IL-1ra polymorphism.

IL-1ra allele of intron-2 was studied in a cohort of 827 healthy human subjects, 130 patients with angiographically normal coronary arteries, 98 patients with single-vessel coronary artery disease, and 328 with multivessel coronary disease (Francis *et al.*, 1999). The patients were part of a cohort being treated for coronary artery disease in Sheffield, England. IL-1ra intron-2 allele frequency in patient without disease was the same as in 827 healthy control subjects. Allele 2 was significantly over-represented in patients with single-vessel disease (34% versus 23% in controls). Patients with single-vessel disease that were homozygotes for allele 2 were highly significant ($P = 0.0036$). Using an independent London population, this association with single-vessel disease was present but less sigtnificant ($P = 0.0603$). Combining the two cohorts, there was a highly significant association between single-vessel disease and homozygousity for allele 2 in IL-1ra ($P = 0.0024$).

Altogether, 270 healthy controls, 74 patients with ulcerative colitis, 72 with Crohn's disease, 40 with primary sclerosing cholangitis for the allelic frequencies, and 60 healthy individuals were examined for the *ex vivo* stimulated production of IL-1β and IL-1ra (Stokkers *et al.*, 1998). Genotyping for five novel restriction fragment length polymorphisms in the genes for IL-1β and IL-1ra were performed. There were no significant differences in the allelic frequencies or allele carriage rates in the IL-1β and IL-1ra in Crohn's disease, ulcerative colitis, and healthy controls (Stokkers *et al.*, 1998). Patients with ulcerative colitis carried the combination of both the infrequent allele of the Taq1 polymorphism in the proIL-1β sequence (Pociot *et al.*, 1992) and the Mwo endonuclease polymorphism compared to controls; however, it remain unclear whether this association is responsible in the pathogenesis of ulcerative colitis.

Several cytokine genotypes were examined in 148 patients of white Dutch ancestory with mutiple sclerosis and compared to 98 healthy subjects. All the patients were unrelated, Dutch, and white. Although no significant differences in genotypes, allele frequencies, or carrier frequencies were found between patients and healthy controls, a specific IL-1ra allele 2 and IL-1β allele 2 combination was associated with disease severity as measured on the 'Expanded Disability Status Scale' when compared with the other possible combinations ($P = 0.007$). It was proposed that IL-1ra and IL-1β are disease severity genes, rather than disease susceptibility genes (Schrijver *et al.*, 1999).

References

Abraham, E., Wunderink, R., Silverman, H., Perl, T. M., Nasraway, S. *et al.* (1995). Efficacy and safety of monoclonal antibody to human tumor necrosis factor-α in patients with sepsis syndrome. *JAMA*, **273**, 934–41.

Abraham, E., Glauser, M. P., Butler, T., Garbino, J., Gelmont, D., Laterre, P. F. *et al.* (1997). p55 Tumor necrosis factor receptor fusion protein in the treatment of patients with severe sepsis and septic shock. A randomized controlled multicenter trial. Ro 45–2081 Study Group. *JAMA*, **277**, 1531–8.

Abraham, E., Anzueto, A., Gutierrez, G., Tessler, S., San Pedro, G., Wunderink, R. *et al.* (1998). Double-blind randomised controlled trial of monoclonal antibody to human tumour necrosis factor in treatment of septic shock. NORASEPT II Study Group. *Lancet*, **351**, 929–33.

Alexander, H. R., Doherty, G. M., Buresh, C. M., Venzon, D. J. and Norton, J. A. (1991). A recombinant human receptor antagonist to interleukin-1 improves survival after lethal endotoxemia in mice. *J. Exp. Med.*, **173**, 1029–32.

Alexander, H. R., Doherty, G. M., Venzon, D. J., Merino, M. J., Fraker, D. L. and Norton, J. A. (1992). Recombinant interleukin-1 receptor antagonist (IL-1ra): effective therapy against gram-negative sepsis in rats. *Surgery*, **112**, 188–94.

Alheim, K., Chai, Z., Fantuzzi, G., Hasanvan, H., Malinowsky, D., Di Santo, E *et al.* (1997). Hyperresponsive febrile reactions to interleukin (IL) 1alpha and IL-1beta, and altered brain cytokine mRNA and serum cytokine levels, in IL-1beta-deficient mice. *Proc. Natl. Acad. Sci. USA*, **94**, 2681–6.

Andersson, J., Björk, L., Dinarello, C. A., Towbin, H. and Andersson, U. (1992). Lipopolysaccharide induces human interleukin-1 receptor antagonist and interleukin-1 production in the same cell. *Eur. J. Immunol.*, **22**, 2617–23.

Antin, J. H., Weinstein, H. J., Guinan, E. C., McCarthy, P., Bierer, B. E., Gilliland, D. G. *et al.* (1994). Recombinant human interleukin-1 receptor antagonist in the treatment of steroid-resistant graft-versus-host disease. *Blood*, **84**, 1342–8.

Arend, W. P., Malyak, M., Guthridge, C. J. and Gabay, C. (1998). Interleukin-1 receptor antagonist: role in biology. *Ann. Rev. Immunol.*, **16**, 27–55.

Arend, W. P., Welgus, H. G., Thompson, R. C. and Eisenberg, S. P. (1990). Biological properties of recombinant human monocyte-derived interleukin-1 receptor antagonist. *J. Clin. Invest.*, **85**, 1694–7.

Bakker, A. C., Joosten, L. A., Arntz, O. J., Helsen, M. M., Bendele, A. M., van de Loo, F. A. *et al.* (1997). Prevention of murine collagen-induced arthritis in the knee and ipsilateral paw by local expression of human interleukin-1 receptor antagonist protein in the knee. *Arthritis Rheum.*, **40**, 893–900.

Barak, V., Nisman, B., Dann, E. J., Kalickman, I., Ruchlemer, R., Bennett, M. A. *et al.* (1994). Serum interleukin-1β levels as a marker in hairy cell leukemia: correlation with disease status and sIL-2R levels. *Leuk. Lymphom.*, **14**, 33–9.

Barak, V., Vannier, E., Nisman, B., Pollack, A. and Dinarello, C. A. (1996). Cytokines and their soluble receptors as markers for hairy cell leukemia. *Eur. Cytokine Netw.*, **7**, 536(absract).

Barak, V., Nisman, B., Polliack, A., Vannier, E. and Dinarello, C. A. (1998). Correlation of serum levels of interleukin-1 family members with disease activity and response to treatment in hairy cell leukemia. *Eur. Cytokine Netw.*, **9**, 33–9.

Bargetzi, M. J., Lantz, M., Smith, C. G., Torti, F. M., Olsson, I., Eisenberg, S. P. *et al.* (1993). Interleukin-1 beta induces interleukin-1 receptor antagonist and tumor necrosis factor binding proteins. *Cancer Res.*, **53**, 4010–3.

Bendele, A., McAbee, T., Sennello, G., Frazier, J., Chlipala, E. and McCabe, D. (1999). Efficacy of sustained blood levels of interleukin-1 receptor antagonist in animal models of arthritis: comparison of efficacy in animal models with human clinical data. *Arthritis Rheum.*, **42**, 498–506.

Biasucci, L. M., Liuzzo, G., Fantuzzi, G., Caligiuri, G., Rebuzzi, A. G., Ginnetti, F. *et al.* (1999). Increasing levels of interleukin (IL)-1Ra and IL-6 during the first 2 days of hospitalization in unstable angina are associated with increased risk of in-hospital coronary events. *Circulation,* **99**, 2079–84.

Bird, T. A. and Saklatvala, J. (1989). IL-1 and TNF transmodulate epidermal growth factor receptors by a protein kinase C-independent mechanism. *J. Immunol.,* **142**, 126–33.

Blakemore, A. I., Tarlow, J. K., Cork, M. J., Gordon, C., Emery, P. and Duff, G. W. (1994). Interleukin-1 receptor antagonist gene polymorphism as a disease severity factor in systemic lupus erythematosus. *Arthritis Rheum.,* **37**, 1380–5.

Breder, C. D., Dinarello, C. A. and Saper, C. B. (1988). Interleukin-1 immunoreactive innervation of the human hypothalamus. *Science,* **240**, 321–4.

Bresnihan, B., Alvaro-Gracia, J. M., Cobby, M., Doherty, M., Domljan, Z., Emery, P. *et al.* (1998). Treatment of rheumatoid arthritis with recombinant human interleukin-1 receptor antagonist. *Arthritis Rheum.,* **41**, 2196–204.

Campion, G. V., Lebsack, M. E., Lookabaugh, J., Gordon, G. and Catalano, M. (1996). Dose-range and dose-frequency study of recombinant human interleukin-1 receptor antagonist in patients with rheumatoid arthritis. *Arthritis Rheum.,* **39**, 1092–101.

Cannon, J. G., van der Meer, J. W., Kwiatkowski, D., Endres, S., Lonnemann, G., Burke, J. F. *et al.* (1988). Interleukin-1 beta in human plasma: optimization of blood collection, plasma extraction, and radioimmunoassay methods. *Lymphokine Res.,* **7**, 457–67.

Cannon, J. G., Nerad, J. L., Poutsiaka, D. D. and Dinarello, C. A. (1993). Measuring circulating cytokines. *J. Appl. Physiol.,* **75**, 1897–902.

Casey, L. C., Balk, R. A. and Bone, R. C. (1993). Plasma cytokines and endotoxin levels correlate with survival in patients with the sepsis syndrome. *Ann. Intern. Med.,* **119**, 771–8.

Chensue, S. W., Bienkowski, M., Eessalu, T. E., Warmington, K. S., Hershey, S. D., Lukas, N. W. *et al.* (1993). Endogenous IL-1 receptor antagonist protein (IRAP) regulates schistosome egg granuloma formation and the regional lymphoid response. *J. Immunol.,* **151**, 3654–62.

Chomarat, P., Vannier, E., Dechanet, J., Rissoan, M. C., Banchereau, J., Dinarello, C. A. *et al.* (1995). The balance of IL-1 receptor antagonist/IL-1β in rheumatoid synovium and its regulation by IL-4 and IL-10. *J. Immunol.,* **154**, 1432–9.

Clay, F. E., Cork, M. J., Tarlow, J. K., Blakemore, A. I., Harrington, C. I., Lewis, F. *et al.* (1994). Interleukin 1 receptor antagonist gene polymorphism association with lichen sclerosus. *Hum. Gen.,* **94**, 407–10.

Cohen, S., Hurd, E., Cush, J. J., Schiff, M. H., Weinblatt, M. E., Moreland, L. W., Bear, M., Rich, W., and McCabe, D. P. (1999). Treatment of interleukin-1 receptor antagonist in combination with methotrexate in rheumatoid arthritis patients. *Arthr. Rheumatol.* **42, (suppl)**: S273 (abstract).

Cominelli, F., Nast, C. C., Clark, B. D., Schindler, R., Llerena, R., Eysselein, V. E. *et al.* (1990). Interleukin-1 gene expression, synthesis and effect of specific IL-1 receptor blockade in rabbit immune complex colitis. *J. Clin. Invest.,* **86**, 972–80.

Cominelli, F., Nast, C. C., Duchini, A. and Lee, M. (1992). Recombinant interleukin-1 receptor antagonist blocks the proinflammatory activity of endogenous interleukin-1 in rabbit immune colitis. *Gastroenterology,* **103**, 65–71.

Conti, B., Jeong, J. W., Tinti, C., Son, J. H. and Joh, T. H. (1997). Induction of IFN-γ-inducing factor in the adrenal cortex. *J. Biol. Chem.,* **272**, 2035–7.

Crown, J., Jakubowski, A., Kemeny, N., Gordon, M., Gasparetto, C., Wong, G *et al.* (1991). A phase I trial of recombinant human interleukin-1β alone and in combination with myelosuppressive doses of 5-fluoruracil in patients with gastrointestinal cancer. *Blood*, **78**, 1420–27.

Crown, J., Jakubowski, A. and Gabrilove, J. (1993). Interleukin-1: biological effects in human hematopoiesis. *Leuk. Lymphoma*, **9**, 433–40.

Danis, V. A., Millington, M., Huang, Q., Hyland, V. and Grennan, D. (1995a). Lack of association between an interleukin-1 receptor antagonist gene polymorphism and systemic lupus erythematosus. *Dis. Markers*, **12**, 135–9.

Danis, V. A., Millington, M., Hyland, V. and Grennan, D. (1995b). Cytokine production by normal human monocytes: inter-subject variation and relationship to an IL-1 receptor antagonist (IL-1ra) gene polymorphism. *Clin. Exp. Immunol.*, **99**, 303–10.

Dinarello, C. A. (1994). Is there a role for interleukin-1 blockade in intravenous immunoglobulin therapy? *Immunol. Rev.*, **139**, 173–88.

Dinarello, C. A. (1999). IL-18: A Th1-inducing, proinflammatory cytokine and new member of the IL-1 family. *J. Allergy Clin. Immunol.*, **103**, 11–24.

Dinarello, C. A., Zhang, X. X., Wen, H. D., Wolff, S. M. and Ikejima, T. (1992). The effect of interleukin-1 receptor antagonist on IL-1, LPS, *Staphylococcus epidermidis* and tumor necrosis factor fever. In *Neuro-immunology of fever*, (ed. T. Bartfai and D. Ottoson), pp. 11–18. Pergamon Press, Oxford.

Dripps, D. J., Brandhuber, B. J., Thompson, R. C. and Eisenberg, S. P. (1991). Effect of IL-1ra on IL-1 signal transduction. *J. Biol. Chem.*, **266**, 10331–6.

Eastgate, J. A., Symons, J. A., Wood, N. C., Grinlinton, F. M., di Giovine, F. S. and Duff, G. W. (1988). Correlation of plasma interleukin 1 levels with disease activity in rheumatoid arthritis. *Lancet*, **2**, 706–9.

Edelson, M. B., Bagwell, C. E. and Rozycki, H. J. (1999). Circulating pro- and counterinflammatory cytokine levels and severity in necrotizing enterocolitis. *Pediatrics*, **103**, 766–71.

Estrov, Z., Kurzrock, R., Wetzler, M., Kantarjian, H., Blake, M., Harris, D. *et al.* (1991). Suppression of chronic myelogenous leukemia colony growth by IL-1 receptor antagonist and soluble IL-1 receptors: a novel application for inhibitors of IL-1 activity. *Blood*, **78**, 1476–84.

Evans, R. J., Bray, J., Childs, J. D., Vigers, G. P. A., Brandhuber, B. J., Skalicky, J. J. *et al.* (1994). Mapping receptor binding sites in the IL-1 receptor antagonist and IL-1β by site-directed mutagenesis: identification of a single site in IL-1ra and two sites in IL-1β. *J. Biol. Chem.*, **270**, 11477–83.

Fang, X.-M., Schröder, S., Hoeft, A. and Stüber, F. (1999). Comparison of two polymorphisms of the interleukin-1 gene family: interleukin-1 receptor antagonist polymorphism contributyes to susceptibility to severe sepsis. *Crit. Care Med.*, **27**, 1330–4.

Fantuzzi, G., Ku, G., Harding, M. W., Livingston, D. L., Sipe, J. D., Kuida, K. *et al.* (1997). Response to local inflammation of IL-1β converting enzyme-deficient mice. *J. Immunol.*, **158**, 1818–24.

Ferretti, M., Casini-Raggi, V., Pizarro, T. T., Eisenberg, S. P., Nast, C. C. and Cominelli, F. (1994). Neutralization of endogenous IL-1 receptor antagonist exacerbates and prolongs inflammation in rabbit immune colitis. *J. Clin. Invest.*, **94**, 449–53.

Firestein, G. S., Berger, A. E., Tracey, D. E., Chosay, J. G., Chapman, D. L., Paine, M. M. *et al.* (1992). IL-1 receptor antagonist protein production and gene expression in rheumatoid arthritis and osteoarthritis synovium. *J. Immunol.*, **149**, 1054–62.

Firestein, G. S., Boyle, D. L., Yu, C., Paine, M. M., Whisenand, T. D., Zvaifler, N. J. *et al.* (1994). Synovial IL-1 receptor antagonist and interleukin-1 balance in rheumatoid arthritis. *Arthrit. Rheumat.*, **37**, 644–52.

Fischer, E., van Zee, K. J., Marano, M. A., Rock, C. S., Kenney, J. S., Poutsiaka, D. D. *et al.* (1992). Interleukin-1 receptor antagonist circulates in experimental inflammation and in human disease. *Blood*, **79**, 2196–200.

Fisher, C. J. J., Dhainaut, J. F., Pribble, J., Knaus, W. and Catalano, M. A. (1993). In *A study evaluating the efficacy of human recombinant interleukin-1 receptor antagonist in the treatment of patients with sepsis syndrome: preliminary results from a Phase III multicenter trial.* 13th International Symposium on Intensive Care Emergency Medecine. Brussels.

Fisher, C. J. J., Dhainaut, J. F., Opal, S. M., Pribble, J. P., Balk, R. A., Slotman, G. J. *et al.* (1994). Recombinant human interleukin-1 receptor antagonist in the treatment of patients with sepsis syndrome. Results from a randomized, double blind, placebo-controlled trial. *JAMA*, **271**, 1836–43.

Fisher, C., Jr., Agosti, J. M., Opal, S. M., Lowry, S. F., Balk, R. A., Sadoff, J. C *et al.* (1996). Treatment of septic shock with the tumor necrosis factor receptor:Fc fusion protein. The Soluble TNF Receptor Sepsis Study Group. *N Engl J Med*, **334**, 1697–702.

Fraenkel, L., Roubenoff, R., LaValley, M., McAlindon, T., Chaisson, C., Evans, S. *et al.* (1998). The association of peripheral monocyte derived interleukin 1beta (IL- 1beta), IL-1 receptor antagonist, and tumor necrosis factor-alpha with osteoarthritis in the elderly. *J. Rheumatol.*, **25**, 1820–6.

Francis, S. E., Camp, N. J., Dewberry, R. M., Gunn, J., Syrris, P., Carter, N. D. *et al.* (1999). Interleukin-1 receptor antagonist gene polymorphism and coronary artery disease. *Circulation*, **99**, 861–6.

Gabay, C., Smith, M. F., Eidlen, D. and Arend, W. P. (1997). Interleukin 1 receptor antagonist (IL-1ra) is an acute-phase protein. *J. Clin. Invest.*, **99**, 2930–40.

Granowitz, E. V., Santos, A., Poutsiaka, D. D., Cannon, J. G., Wilmore, D. A., Wolff, S. M. *et al.* (1991). Circulating interleukin-1 receptor antagonist levels during experimental endotoxemia in humans. *Lancet*, **338**, 1423–4.

Granowitz, E. V., Clark, B. D., Vannier, E., Callahan, M. V. and Dinarello, C. A. (1992a). Effect of interleukin-1 (IL-1) blockade on cytokine synthesis: I. IL-1 receptor antagonist inhibits IL-1-induced cytokine synthesis and blocks the binding of IL-1 to its type II receptor on human monocytes. *Blood*, **79**, 2356–63.

Granowitz, E. V., Porat, R., Mier, J. W., Pribble, J. P., Stiles, D. M., Bloedow, D. C. *et al.* (1992b). Pharmacokinetics, saftey, and immunomodulatory effects of human recombinant interleukin-1 receptor antagonist in healthy humans. *Cytokine*, **4**, 353–60.

Granowitz, E. V., Porat, R., Mier, J. W., Orencole, S. F., Callahan, M. V., Cannon, J. G. *et al.* (1993). Hematological and immunomodulatory effects of an interleukin-1 receptor antagonist coinfusion during low-dose endotoxemia in healthy humans. *Blood*, **82**, 2985–90.

Greenfeder, S. A., Nunes, P., Kwee, L., Labow, M., Chizzonite, R. A. and Ju, G. (1995). Molecular cloning and characterization of a second subunit of the interleukin-1 receptor complex. *J. Biol. Chem.*, **270**, 13757–65.

Gruetter, M. G., van Oostrum, J., Priestle, J. P., Edelmann, E., Joss, U., Feige, U. *et al.* (1994). A mutational analysis of receptor binding sites of interleukin-1β: differences in binding of human interleukin-1β muteins to human and mouse receptors. *Protein Eng.*, **7**, 663–71.

Guénard, V., Dinarello, C. A., Weston, P. J. and Aebischer, P. (1991). Peripheral nerve regeneration is impeded by interleukin-1 receptor antagonist released from a polymeric guidance channel. *J. Neurosci. Res.*, **29**, 396–400.

Hacker, U. T., Gomolka, M., Keller, E., Eigler, A., Folwaczny, C., Fricke, H. *et al.* (1997). Lack of association betwen an interleukin-1 receptor antagonist gene polymorphism and ulcerative colitis. *GUT*, **40**, 623–7.

Hammerberg, C., Arend, W. P., Fisher, G. J., Chan, L. S., Berger, A. E., Haskill, J. S. *et al.* (1992). Interleukin-1 receptor antagonist in normal and psoriatic epidermis. *J. Clin. Invest.*, **90**, 571–83.

Hirsch, E., Irikura, V. M., Paul, S. M. and Hirsh, D. (1996). Functions of interleukin-1 receptor antagonist in gene knockout and overproducing mice. *Proc. Natl. Acad. Sci. USA*, **93**, 11008–13.

Holmberg, L. A., Seidel, K., Leisenring, W. and Torok-Storb, B. (1994). Aplastic anemia analysis of stromal cell-function in long-term marrow cultures. *Blood*, **84**, 3685–90.

Horai, R., Asano, M., Sudo, K., Kanuka, H., Suzuki, M., Nishihara, M. *et al.* (1998). Production of mice deficient in genes for interleukin (IL)-1α, IL- 1β, IL-1α/β, and IL-1 receptor antagonist shows that IL-1β is crucial in turpentine-induced fever development and glucocorticoid secretion. *J. Exp. Med.*, **187**, 1463–75.

Horai, R., Saijo, S., Tanioka, H., Nakae, S., Sudo, K., Okahara, A., Ikuse, T., Asano, M., and Iwakura, Y. (2000). Development of chronic inflammatory arthropathy resembling rheumatoid arthritis in interleukin 1 receptor antagonist-deficient mice. *J. Exp. Med.* **191**, 313–20.

Huang, Y., Blatt, L. M. and Taylor, M. W. (1995). Type I interferon as an anti-inflammatory agent: inhibition of lipopolysaccharide-induced interleukin-1β and induction of interleukin-1 receptor antagonist. *J. Interferon Cytokine Res.*, **15**, 317–21.

Iizumi, T., Sato, S., Iiyama, T., Hata, R., Amemiya, H., Tomomasa, H. *et al.* (1991). Recombinant human interleukin-1 beta analogue as a regulator of hematopoiesis in patients receiving chemotherapy for urogenital cancers. *Cancer*, **68**, 1520–3.

Jouvenne, P., Vannier, E., Dinarello, C. A. and Miossec, P. (1998). Elevated levels of soluble interleukin-1 receptor type II and interleukin-1 receptor antagonist in patients with chronic arthritis: correlations with markers of inflammation and joint destruction. *Arthritis Rheum.*, **41**, 1083–9.

Katila, H., Hanninen, K. and Hurme, M. (1999). Polymorphisms of the interleukin-1 gene complex in schizophrenia. *Mol. Psychiatry*, **4**, 179–81.

Kitamura, T. and Takaku, F. (1989). A preclinical and Phase I clinical trial of IL-1. *Exp. Med.*, **7**, 170–7.

Knaus, W. A., Harrell, F. E., Fisher, C. J., Wagner, D. P., Opal, S. M., Sadoff, J. C. *et al.* (1993). The clinical evaluation of new drugs for sepsis. *JAMA*, **270**, 1233–41.

Kopp, W. C., Urba, W. J., Rager, H. C., Alvord, W. G., Oppenheim, J. J., Smith, J. W., II *et al.* (1996). Induction of interleukin 1 receptor antagonist after interleukin 1 therapy in patients with cancer. *Clin. Cancer Res.*, **2**, 501–6.

Kristensen, M., Deleuran, B., Eedy, D. J., Feldmann, M., Breathnach, S. M. and Brennan, F. M. (1992). Distribution of interleukin-1 receptor antagonist protein (IRAP), interleukin-1 receptor, and interleukin-1 alpha in normal and psoriatic skin. *Br. J. Dermatol.*, **127**, 305–11.

Ku, G., Thomas, C. E., Akeson, A. L. and Jackson, R. L. (1992). Induction of interleukin-1β expression from human peripheral blood monocyte-derived macrophages by 9-hydroxyoctadecadienoic acid. *J. Biol. Chem.*, **267**, 14183–8.

Kumar, S., McDonnell, P. C., Lehr, R., Tierney, L., Tzimas, M. N., Griswold, D. E., Capper, E. A., Tal-Singer, R., Wells, G. I., Doyle, M. L., and Young, P. R. (2000). Identification and initial characterization of four novel members of the interleukin-1 family. *J. Biol. Chem.* **275**, 10308–14.

Lambriola-Tomkins, E., Chandran, C., Varnell, T. A., Madison, V. S. and Ju, G. (1993). Structure-function analysis of human IL-1α: identification of residues required for binding to the human type I IL-1 receptor. *Protein Eng.*, **6**, 535–9.

Laughlin, M. J., Kirkpatrick, G., Sabiston, N., Peters, W. and Kurtzberg, J. (1993). Hematopoietic recovery following high-dose combined alkylating-agent chemotherapy and autologous bone marrow support in patients in phase I clinical trials of colony stimulating factors: G-CSF, GM-CSF, IL-1, IL-2 and M-CSF. *Ann. Hematol.*, **67**, 267–76.

Lawrence, C. B., Allan, S. M. and Rothwell, N. J. (1998). Interleukin-1beta and the interleukin-1 receptor antagonist act in the striatum to modify excitotoxic brain damage in the rat. *Eur. J. Neurosci.*, **10**, 1188–95.

Lebsack, M. E., Paul, C. C., Bloedow, D. C., Burch, F. X., Sack, M. A., Chase, W. *et al.* (1991). Subcutaneous IL-1 receptor antagonist in patients with rheumatoid arthritis. *Arthr. Rheumatol.*, **34** (suppl), S67.

Loddick, S. A. and Rothwell, N. J. (1996). Neuroprotective effects of human recombinant interleukin-1 receptor antagonist in focal cerebral ischaemia in the rat. *J. Cerebral Blood Flow*, **16**, 932–40.

Lorenzo, J. E., Naprta, A., Rao, Y., Alander, C., Glaccum, M., Widmer, M. *et al.* (1998). Mice lacking the type I interleukin-1 receptor do not lose bone mass after ovariectomy. *Endocrinol.*, **139**, 3022–5.

Lundkvist, J., Sundgren-Andersson, A. K., Tingsborg, S., Ostlund, P., Engfors, C., Alheim, K. *et al.* (1999). Acute-phase responses in transgenic mice with CNS overexpression of IL-1 receptor antagonist. *Am. J. Physiol.*, **276**, R644–51.

Makarov, S. S., Olsen, J. C., Johnston, W. N., Anderle, S. K., Brown, R. R., Baldwin, A. S. *et al.* (1995). Suppression of experimental arthritis by gene transfer of interleukin-1 receptor antagonist cDNA. *Proc. Natl. Acad. Sci. USA*, **92**, 11301–15.

Mandrup-Poulsen, T., Pociot, F., Mølvig, J., Shapiro, L., Nilsson, P., Emdal, T. *et al.* (1994). Monokine antagonism is reduced in patients with insulin-dependent diabetes melitus. *Diabetes*, **43**, 1242–7.

Mandrup-Poulsen, T., Wogensen, L., Jensen, M., Svensson, P., Nilsson, P., Emdal, T. *et al.* (1995). Circulating interleukin-1 receptor antagonist concentrations are increased in adult patients with thermal injury. *Crit. Care Med.*, **23**, 26–33.

Mansfield, J. C., Holden, H., Tarlow, J. K., Di Giovine, F. S., McDowell, T. L., Wilson, A. G. *et al.* (1994). Novel genetic association between ulcerative colitis and the anti-inflammatory cytokine interleukin-1 receptor antagonist. *Gastroenterology*, **106**, 637–42.

Markewitz, A., Faist, E., Lang, S., Endres, S., Fuchs, B. and Reichart, B. (1993). Successful restoration of cell-mediated immune response after cardiopulmonary bypass by immunomodulation. *J. Thorac. Card. Surg.*, **105**, 15–24.

McCall, R. D., Haskill, S., Zimmermann, E. M., Lund, P. K., Thompson, R. C. and Sartor, R. B. (1994). Tissue interleukin 1 and interleukin-1 receptor antagonist expression in enterocolitis in resistant and susceptible rats. *Gastroenterology*, **106**, 960–72.

Mileno, M. D., Margolis, N. H., Clark, B. D., Dinarello, C. A., Burke, J. F. and Gelfand, J. A. (1995). Coagulation of whole blood stimulates interleukin-1β gene expression: absence of gene transcripts in anticoagulated blood. *J. Inf. Dis.*, **172**, 308–11.

Miller, L. C., Lynch, E. A., Isa, S., Logan, J. W., Dinarello, C. A. and Steere, A. C. (1993). Balance of synovial fluid IL-1β and IL-1 receptor antagonist and recovery from Lyme arthritis. *Lancet*, **341**, 146–8.

Mo, J. S., Matsukawa, A., Ohkawara, S. and Yoshinaga, M. (1999). Role and regulation of IL-8 and MCP-1 in LPS-induced uveitis in rabbits. *Exp. Eye Res.*, **68**, 333–40.

Mohankumar, S. M., Mohankumar, P. S. and Quadri, S. K. (1999). Lipopolysaccharide-induced changes in monoamines in specific areas of the brain: blockade by interleukin-1 receptor antagonist. *Brain Res.*, **824**, 232–7.

Murzin, A. G., Lesk, A. M. and Chothia, C. (1992). β-trefoil fold. Patterns of structure and sequence in the Kunitz inhibitors interleukins-1β and 1α and fibroblast growth factors. *J. Mol. Biol.*, **223**, 531–43.

Muzio, M., Polentarutti, N., Sironi, M., Poli, G., De Gioia, L., Introna, M., *et al.* (1995). Cloning and characterization of a new isoform of the interleukin 1 receptor antagonist. *J. Exp. Med.*, **182**, 623–8.

Muzio, M., Polentarutti, N., Facchetti, F., Peri, G., Doni, A., Sironi, M., *et al.* (1999). Characterization of type II intracellular interleukin-1 receptor antagonist (IL-1ra3): a depot IL-1ra. *Eur. J. Immunol.*, **29**, 781–8.

Nemunaitis, J., Appelbaum, F. R., Lilleby, K., Buhles, W. C., Rosenfeld, C., Zeigler, Z. R. *et al.* (1994). Phase I study of recombinant interleukin-1β in patients undergoing autologous bone marrow transplantation for acute myelogenous leukemia. *Blood*, **83**, 3473–9.

Nerad, J. L., Griffiths, J. K., van der Meer, J. W. M., Endres, S., Poutsiaka, D. D., Keusch, G. T. *et al.* (1992). Interleukin-1β (IL-1β), IL-1 receptor antagonist, and TNFα production in whole blood. *J. Leuk. Biol.*, **52**, 687–92.

Nicklin, M. J., Hughes, D. E., Barton, J. L., Ure, J. M., and Duff, G. W. (2000). Arterial inflammation in mice lacking the interleukin 1 receptor antagonist gene. *J. Exp. Med.*, **191**, 303–12.

Norman, J. G., Franz, M. G., Fink, G. S., Messina, J., Fabri, P. J., Gower, W. R. *et al.* (1995a). Decreased mortality of severe acute pancreatitis after proximal cytokine blockade. *Ann. Surg.*, **221**, 625–34.

Norman, J. G., Franz, M. G., Messina, J., Riker, A., Fabri, P. J., Rosemurgy, A. S. *et al.* (1995b). Interleukin-1 receptor antagonist decreases severity of experimental acute pancreatitis. *Surgery*, **117**, 648–55.

Ohno, Y., Fujimoto, M., Nishimura, A. and Aoki, N. (1998). Change of peripheral levels of pituitary hormones and cytokines after injection of interferon (IFN)-beta in patients with chronic hepatitis C. *J. Clin. Endocrinol. Metab.*, **83**, 3681–7.

Pereira, B. J. G., Poutsiaka, D. D., King, A. J., Strom, J. A., Narayan, G., Levey, A. S. *et al.* (1992). *In vitro* production of interleukin-1 receptor antagonist in chronic renal failure, continuous peritoneal disalysis and hemodialysis. *Kidney Int.*, **42**, 1419–24.

Pociot, F., Molvig, J., Wogensen, L., Worsaae, H. and Nerup, J. (1992). A TaqI polymorphism in the human interleukin-1 beta (IL-1 beta) gene correlates with IL-1 beta secretion *in vitro*. *Eur. J. Clin. Invest.*, **22**, 396–402.

Porat, R., Poutsiaka, D. D., Miller, L. C., Granowitz, E. V. and Dinarello, C. A. (1992). Interleukin-1 (IL-1) receptor blockade reduces endotoxin and *Borrelia burgdorferi*-stimulated IL-8 synthesis in human mononuclear cells. *FASEB J*, **6**, 2482–6.

Rambaldi, A., Torcia, M., Bettoni, S., Barbui, T., Vannier, E., Dinarello, C. A. *et al.* (1991). Modulation of cell proliferation and cytokine production in acute myeloblastic leukemia by interleukin-1 receptor antagonist and lack of its expression by leukemic cells. *Blood*, **78**, 3248–53.

Reznikov, L. L., Puren, A. J., Fantuzzi, G., Muhl, H., Shapiro, L., Yoon, D. Y. *et al.* (1998). Spontaneous and inducible cytokine responses in healthy humans receiving a single dose of IFN-alpha2b: increased production of interleukin-1 receptor antagonist and suppression of IL-1-induced IL-8. *J. Interferon Cytokine Res.*, **18**, 897–903.

Rocha, M. F. G., Soares, A. M., Flores, C. A., Steiner, T. S., Lyerly, D. M., Guerrant, R. L. *et al.* (1998). Intestinal secretory factor released by macrophages stimulated with Clostridium difficile toxin A: role of interleukin 1beta. *Infect Immun*, **66**, 4910–6.

Rostoker, G., Rymer, J. C., Bagnard, G., Petit-Phar, M., Griuncelli, M. and Pilatte, Y. (1998). Imbalances in serum proinflammatory cytokines and their soluble receptors: a putative role in the progression of idiopathic IgA nephropathy (IgAN) and Henoch-Schonlein purpura nephritis, and a potential target of immunoglobulin therapy? *Clin. Exp. Immunol.*, **114**, 468–76.

Roubenoff, R., Harris, T. B., Abad, L. W., Wilson, P. W. F., Dallal, G. E. and Dinarello, C. A. (1998). Monocyte cytokine production in an elderly population: effect of age and inflammation. *J. Gerontol.*, **53A**, M20–M26.

Roux-Lombard, P., Modoux, C., Vischer, T., Grassi, J. and Dayer, J.-M. (1992). Inhibitors of inter- leukin 1 activity in synovial fluids and in cultured synovial fluid mononuclear cells. *J. Rheumatol.*, **19**, 517–23.

Schindler, R., Clark, B. D. and Dinarello, C. A. (1990). Dissociation between interleukin-1β mRNA and protein synthesis in human peripheral blood mononuclear cells. *J. Biol. Chem.*, **265**, 10232–7.

Schirò, R., Longoni, D., Rossi, V., Maglia, O., Doni, A., Arsura, M. *et al.* (1993). Supression of juvenile chronic myelogenous leukemia colony growth by interleukin-1 receptor antagonist. *Blood*, **83**, 460–5.

Schreuder, H., Tardif, C., Trump-Kallmeyer, S., Soffientini, A., Sarubbi, E., Akeson, A. *et al.* (1997). A new cytokine-receptor binding mode revealed by the crystal structure of the IL-1 receptor with an antagonist. *Nature*, **386**, 194–200.

Schrijver, H. M., Crusius, J. B., Uitdehaag, B. M., Garcia Gonzalez, M. A., Kostense, P. J., Polman, C. H. *et al.* (1999). Association of interleukin-1beta and interleukin-1 receptor antagonist genes with disease severity in MS. *Neurology*, **52**, 595–9.

Schuld, A., Mullington, J., Hermann, D., Hinze-Selch, D., Fenzel, T., Holsboer, F. *et al.* (1999). Effects of granulocyte colony-stimulating factor on night sleep in humans. *Am. J. Physiol.*, **276**, R1149–R1155.

Smith, D. E., Ranshaw, B. R., Ketchem, R. R., Kubin, M., Garka, K. E., Sims, J. S. (2000). Four new members of the interleukin-1 superfamily. *J. Biol. Chem.*, **275**, 1169–75.

Smith, J. W., Urba, W. J., Curti, B. D., Elwood, L. J., Steis, R. G., Janik, J. E. *et al.* (1992). The toxic and hematologic effects of interleukin-1 alpha administered in a phase I trial to patients with advanced malignancies. *J. Clin. Oncol.*, **10**, 1141–52.

Smith, J. W., Longo, D., Alford, W. G., Janik, J. E., Sharfman, W. H., Gause, B. L. *et al.* (1993). The effects of treatment with interleukin-1α on platelet recovery after high-dose carboplatin. *N. Engl. J. Med.*, **328**, 756–61.

Stokkers, P. C., van Aken, B. E., Basoski, N., Reitsma, P. H., Tytgat, G. N. and van Deventer, S. J. (1998). Five genetic markers in the interleukin 1 family in relation to inflammatory bowel disease. *Gut*, **43**, 33–9.

Tarlow, J. K., Blakemore, A. I. F., Lennard, A., Hughes, H. N., Steinkasserer, A. and Duff, G. W. (1993). Polymorphism in human IL-1 receptor antagonist gene intron-2 is caused by variable numbers of an 86-bp tandem repeat. *Hum. Gen.*, **91**, 403–4.

Tarlow, J. K., Clay, F. E., Cork, M. J., Blakemore, A. I., McDonagh, A. J., Messenger, A. G. *et al.* (1994). Severity of alopecia areata is associated with a polymorphism in the interleukin-1 recep- tor antagonist gene. *J. Invest. Dermatol.*, **103**, 387–90.

Teppo, A. M., Honkanen, E., Ahonen, J. and Gronhagen-Riska, C. (1998). Does increased urinary interleukin-1 receptor antagonist/interleukin-1beta ratio indicate good prognosis in renal trans- plant recipients? *Transplantation*, **66**, 1009–14.

Tewari, A., Buhles, W. C., Jr. and Starnes, H. F., Jr. (1990). Preliminary report: effects of inter- leukin-1 on platelet counts. *Lancet*, **336**, 712–4.

Thea, D. M., Porat, R., Nagimbi, K., Baangi, M., St. Louis, M. E., Kaplan, G *et al.* (1996). Plasma cytokines, plasma cytokine antagonists, and disease progression in African women infected with HIV-1. *Ann. Int. Med.*, **124**, 757–62.

Thomas, C. E., Jackson, R. L., Ohleiler, D. F. and Ku, G. (1994). Multiple lipid oxidation products in low density lipoproteins induce interleukin-1β release from human blood mononuclear cells. *J. Lipid Res.*, **35**, 417–27.

Tilg, H., Mier, J. W., Vogel, W., Aulitzky, W. E., Wiedermann, C. J., Vannier, E. *et al.* (1993). Induction of interleukin-1 receptor antagonist by interferon treatment. *J. Immunol.*, **150**, 4687–92.

Tilg, H., Trehu, E., Atkins, M. B., Dinarello, C. A. and Mier, J. W. (1994). Interleukin-6 (IL-6) as an anti-inflammatory cytokine: Induction of circulating IL-1 receptor antagonist and soluble tumor necrosis factor receptor p55. *Blood*, **83**, 113–8.

Tilg, H., Trehu, E., Shapiro, L., Pape, D., Atkins, M. B., Dinarello, C. A. and Mier, J. W. (1994). Induction of circulating soluble tumour necrosis factor receptor and interleukin 1 receptor antagonist following interleukin-1α infusion in humans. *Cytokine*, **6**, 215–9.

Torcia, M., Lucibello, M., Vannier, E., Fabiani, S., Miliani, A., Guidi, G. *et al.* (1996). Modulation of osteoclast-activating factor activity of multiple myeloma bone marrow cells by different interleukin-1 inhibitors. *Exp. Hematol.*, **24**, 868–74.

van der Poll, T., Bueller, H. R., ten Cate, H., Wortel, C. H., Bauer, K. A., van Deventer, S. J. H. *et al.* (1990). Activation of coagulation after administration of tumor necrosis factor to normal subjects. *New Engl. J. Med.*, **322**, 1622–7.

Vidal-Vanaclocha, F., Amézaga, C., Asumendi, A., Kaplanski, G. and Dinarello, C. A. (1994). Interleukin-1 receptor blockade reduces the number and size of murine B16 melanoma hepatic metastases. *Cancer Res.*, **54**, 2667–72.

Vigers, G. P., Caffes, P., Evans, R. J., Thompson, R. C., Eisenberg, S. P. and Brandhuber, B. J. (1994). X-ray structure of interleukin-1 receptor antagonist at 2.0-A resolution. *J. Biol. Chem.*, **269**, 12874–9.

Vigers, G. P. A., Anderson, L. J., Caffes, P. and Brandhuber, B. J. (1997). Crystal structure of the type I interleukin-1 receptor complexed with interleukin-1β. *Nature*, **386**, 190–4.

Wetzler, M., Kurrzock, R., Lowe, D. G., Kantarjian, H., Gutterman, J. U. and Talpaz, M. (1991). Alteration in bone marrow adherent layer growth factor expression: a novel mechanism of chronic myelogenous leukemia progression. *Blood*, **78**, 2400–6.

Wieczorek, Z., Kluczyk, A., Slon-Usakiewicz, J. J. and Siemion, I. Z. (1996). The search for inhibitors of interleukin-1 based on the sequence of interleukin-1 receptor antagonist. *Biomed. Pept. Proteins Nucleic Acids*, **2**, 123–9.

Yamada, J., Dana, M. R., Zhu, S. N., Alard, P. and Streilein, J. W. (1998). Interleukin 1 receptor antagonist suppresses allosensitization in corneal transplantation. *Arch. Ophthalmol.*, **116**, 1351–7.

Yanofsky, S. D., Baldwin, D. N., Butler, J. H., Holden, F. R., Jacobs, J. W., Balasubramanian, P. *et al.* (1996). High affinity type I interleukin 1 receptor antagonists discovered by screening recombinant peptide libraries. *Proc. Natl. Acad. Sci. USA*, **93**, 7381–6.

Yu, X. Q., Fan, J. M., Nikolic-Paterson, D. J., Yang, N., Mu, W., Pichler, R. *et al.* (1999). IL-1 up-regulates osteopontin expression in experimental crescentic glomerulonephritis in the rat. *Am. J. Pathol.*, **154**, 833–41.

5 Antibodies and soluble receptors

Antibodies and soluble receptors provide a strategy for capturing and blocking cytokines before they interact with their receptors. This strategy is conceptually simple. Interestingly, with the exception of serum therapy against toxins and poisons in a distinct though related area, agonist blockade has not received major attention in classical mainstream pharmacology. With the advent of the cytokine era, this picture has changed dramatically. Antibodies are the single anti-cytokine strategy that has been studied most in one human disease, with consistent results. Thus, in a way, anti-cytokine antibodies, anti-TNF specifically, provide a paradigm for the potential of these novel therapeutic approaches. While the mode of action of antibodies and soluble receptors is intuitively simple, the reality may be more complex. Indeed, antibodies and soluble receptors may have more complex and subtle interactions with the agonist, acting for instance as delivery systems or prolonging the half-life of agonist cytokines. Indeed, the prospect of using these molecules, soluble receptors in particular, as anti-cytokine or growth factor tools has been a powerful force to better understand their biology and has unraveled unsuspected complexities and interactions with agonists.

5.1 Soluble cytokine receptors

Seven transmembrane domain, G protein coupled receptors are not made, nor can they be engineered, as soluble agonist-binding molecules. Therefore, this section is confined to non-chemokine, cytokine receptors. Soluble cytokine receptors should theoretically retain the ligand specificity of the membrane-bound receptors, as well as the affinity, without eliciting any immune response, since they are 'self'. Thus, in theory, they show advantages over antibodies for blocking cytokines. In general, however, a major disadvantage is their fast clearance and short half-life in the circulation. To overcome this, soluble receptors have been coupled with the Fc portion of IgG, which confers a longer half-life—usually of the order of several days. In addition, soluble receptor-Ig fusion proteins are divalent and thus show greater avidity when interacting with transmembrane cytokines, such as membrane-bound TNF, or other membrane-associated cytokines. The generation of soluble receptors is part of the cytokines' homeostatic mechanisms. Therefore, understanding the pathophysiology of soluble cytokine receptors is fundamental to their therapeutic exploitation.

Soluble receptors leave the cells producing them and can be active in the cellular micro-environment or in body fluids (Fernandez-Botran *et al.*, 1996; Heaney and Golde,

1996). The discovery that membrane-bound receptors are released in body fluids has changed our understanding of ligand–receptor interactions, as well as the mode of action of hormones and cytokines. Ligand concentrations can be modified by soluble receptors, by down-regulation of the number of membrane-bound receptors released, and they may compete with membrane-bound receptors for the ligands, thus reducing the number of free active ligands. Soluble receptors can also render cells in tissues able to respond to ligands for which they express an incomplete set of receptor molecules.

5.1.1 Mechanisms of generation

Soluble receptors are produced by expression of an alternative mRNA splice, which generates an appropriate transcript encoding a soluble isoform, by proteolytic cleavage or by the action of phospholipase C (Table 5.1). This enzyme is active on GPI linked receptors and is only involved as far as we know—to date—in the release of the soluble ciliary neurotrophic factor (CNTF) receptor.

Alternative splicing yields different soluble isoforms of cytokine receptors through different mechanisms. The simplest and most common one involves exclusion of the exon encoding the transmembrane portion of the receptor, and is exemplified by the GM-CSF receptor α chain. A second mechanism involves inclusion in the mature mRNA transcript of a 'soluble exon', which causes the protein chain to terminate before the transmembrane exon. Thus, under these conditions, the membrane-bound isoforms are actually the result of alternative splicing. This is the mechanism of generation of soluble receptors for IL-4, IL-5, and leukemia inhibitory factor (LIF).

The first cytokine receptor for which differential splicing was shown to generate membrane-bound and soluble forms was the mouse IL-4 receptor. The mRNA encoding the

Table 5.1 Mechanisms of generation of soluble cytokine receptors

Proteolytic cleavage	TNF, RI, and II
	IL-1 RII
	IL-2Rα
	IL-6Rα
	M-CSFR(fms)
	c-kit
Alternative splicing	(IL-1RII)
	IL-1RAcP
	IL-4Rα
	IL-5Rα
	(IL-6Rα)
	IL-7R
	IL-9R
	GM-CSFRα
	LIF-R
	IFNα/βR
	c-kit
	gp130
Cleavage/GPI linked	CNTFRα

The parenthesis for IL-1RII and IL-6Rα indicated that, while an alternative spliced RNA has been demonstrated, available *in vitro* information suggests a major role for proteolytic shedding. The soluble form of c-kit originates from proteolytic cleavage of an automatively spliced form.

soluble version of the IL-4 receptor contains a 114-bp insertion upstream of the transmembrane domain, which resulted in extra six amino acids and premature termination. The resulting soluble receptor lacks the transmembrane and cytoplasmic domains. For the IL-7 receptor, deletion of the sequences encoding the transmembrane domain alters the translational reading frame, resulting in 27 new amino acids and premature termination. Alternative splicing regulates the generation of mRNA encoding soluble forms of various cytokine receptors, including those for IL-5, IL-6, IL-1 type II, interferon-α/β, and GM-CSF. Differential splicing generates a soluble version of the IL-1 receptor accessory protein (IL-1RAcP), which can compete with membrane bound IL-1RacP and block the formation of signaling complexes (Jensen *et al.*, 2000). Incompletely spliced IL-1RI transcripts are generated in monocytes exposed to endotoxin (Penton-Rol *et al.*, 1999). Their functional significance has not been established.

Proteolytic cleavage is involved in the generation of soluble forms of the TNF receptors p55 (type I) and p75 (type II), of the IL-1 type II decoy receptor, and the IL-2 receptor α chain. The IL-6 receptor α chain can be released by proteolysis of the membrane-bound isoform or by alternative splicing. How much these two mechanisms contribute to the soluble IL-6 receptor found in biological fluids under normal and pathological conditions is unknown. The soluble form of c-kit is generated both by proteolytic cleavage and alternative splicing. Expression of the membrane-bound and soluble isoforms of cytokine receptors can be differentially regulated, at least in the case of IL-4.

Release of the type II IL-1 decoy receptor has been extensively investigated (Fig. 5.1). Anti-inflammatory agents (glucocorticoid hormones, IL-4, IL-13) enhance expression of the type II decoy receptor and consequently its release. In monocytes exposed to dexamethasone, the number of surface receptors increased from 3×10^3/cell to $\approx 12 \times 10^3$ over a period of 24 h and over the same time $\approx 20 \times 10^3$ receptors are released. Thus, under these conditions, augmented release is associated with, and dependent on, increased expression of the membrane-bound isoforms, and is gene expression- and protein synthesis-dependent.

A second rapid pathway of regulation of type II receptor release is shared with the TNF receptors. Chemo-attractants and agents that mimic elements in the signal transduction pathway of G-protein coupled receptors (phorbol esters, calcium ionophores), as well as

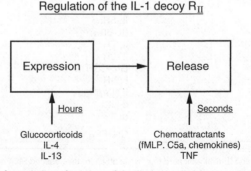

Regulation of the IL-1 decoy R$_{II}$

Fig. 5.1 Pathways of regulation of release of the IL-1 type II decoy receptor.

TNF but not other pro- or anti-inflammatory cytokines, cause rapid release of the type II decoy receptor and of the TNF receptors (Orlando *et al.*, 1997 and references therein).

The enzyme systems involved in regulating the shedding of cytokine receptors have not been molecularly identified. For the TNF and IL-1 type II decoy receptors, spontaneous release is to some extent dependent on enzymes belonging to the serine protease group. However, recent findings with inhibitors strongly suggest that matrix metalloproteinases play a major role in activating the release of type II IL-1 and IL-6 and TNF receptors (Orlando *et al.*, 1997). At least for some proteolytically-released receptors (e.g. the TNF receptor), the metalloproteinase involved is the TNFα converting enzyme (TACE).

TNF causes rapid shedding of the p55 and p75 receptor and of the type II IL-1 decoy receptor. Work with specific blocking antibodies suggests that proteolytic cleavage of the p75 receptor is induced by TNF binding to the p55 receptor.

A novel IL 18 binding protein (IL 18BP), although not a true receptor but rather a decoy one, has been described (Novick *et al.*, 1999). It is constitutively expressed and secreted, binds IL 18, acts as a natural inhibitor of IL 18 as well as of LPS-induced IFNγ and suppresses the Th1 response. Four human and two mouse isoforms of IL 18BP exist each resulting from mRNA splicing and found in various cDNA libraries. Of these, human IL 18BP isoform 'a' exhibited the greatest affinity for IL 18 (Kim *et al.*, 2000).

IL-12 is a peculiar cytokine, in that it consists of two covalently linked chains (p40 and p35), one of which is structurally similar to the IL-6 receptor α chain. Homodimers of the p40 act as IL-12 receptor antagonists by binding the receptor β1 chain, not the signal transducing β2 chain. However, in the case of human IL-12, the p40 homodimer shows lower affinity for the receptor than the heterodimeric agonist cytokine.

5.1.2 Antagonistic effects

Virtually all soluble cytokine receptors, even those with much lower affinities than the membrane receptors, inhibit the binding and biological activity of cytokines *in vitro*. The exception to this rule are the soluble versions of the IL-6, IL-11 and CNTF receptors, generated by proteolytic cleavage or by differential splicing, which bind the soluble cytokine and interact with the signal transducing gp130 molecule (transignaling, see Fig. 1.6). Thus, under most circumstances, interaction of a soluble cytokine receptor with its agonist prevents it binding to a functional membrane receptor and hence blocks subsequent signaling and responses. Soluble cytokine receptors block cytokines competitively. Therefore, the inhibitory effects depend on the concentrations of soluble receptors and agonistic/antagonistic cytokines (e.g. IL-1 and IL-1ra) as well as their relative affinities.

In certain receptors, the affinities of the membrane-bound forms are orders of magnitude higher than those of the soluble versions. A typical example is the IL-2 receptor α-chain. The soluble IL-2 receptor α chain, like its membrane-bound form alone, binds IL-2 with an affinity approximately 10^3 times lower than that of the functional membrane-bound IL-2 receptor, which includes the ß and γ subunits associated with the α chain (Kd 100 nM versus 10 pM). Thus, in spite of the fact that the soluble version of the α chain of the IL-2 receptor can block IL-2 *in vitro*, high concentrations are needed for inhibition. A similar situation applies to the GM-CSF receptor α chain. In contrast, for a series of cytokines, the soluble receptor has comparable affinity to the membrane-bound receptor. These include the IL-4 receptor, the two TNF receptors and the human IL-1 type II decoy receptor.

5.1.3 Pro-cytokine function of soluble receptors

As discussed above, with the exception of the soluble IL-6/IL-11/CNTF receptor α chains, which presents the agonist to gp130, soluble cytokine receptors can act as competitive inhibitors of the relevant ligands. However, under certain conditions soluble cytokine receptors act as cytokine carrier proteins and potentiate the activity of their agonists *in vivo*.

Different mechanisms underlie these seemingly paradoxical effects of soluble cytokine receptors. A first general mechanism of potentiation of agonist activity by soluble receptors is ligand stabilization. For instance, soluble TNF receptors reportedly increase the *in vitro* biological half-life of TNF. The *in vivo* relevance of the *in vitro* decay of TNF is a matter of speculation. Perhaps more directly related to *in vivo* conditions is the observation that soluble IL-4 receptors reduce the susceptibility of IL-4 to degradation by proteolytic enzymes both *in vitro* and *in vivo*. Prolongation of biological half-life is a first general mechanism whereby soluble cytokine receptors potentiate the action of cytokines.

A second general mechanism through which soluble receptors can exert pro-cytokine activity is by affecting the pharmacokinetic behavior of agonists *in vivo*. For instance, TNFα and IL-4 soluble cytokine receptors cause a dose-dependent increase in the half-life of their ligands and a concomitant decrease in blood clearance and elimination in the urine. Cytokine receptors share this 'carrier' effect with monoclonal antibodies. Monoclonal antibodies against certain cytokines including IL-1, IL-3, IL-6, and IL-7, potentiate the activity of cytokines *in vivo*.

In conclusion, soluble cytokine receptors can have divergent effects on the bioactivity of cytokines. Their *in vivo* function can be represented with the image of a balance: on the one hand, these receptors can inhibit cytokine binding activity; and, on the other hand, they can increase stability and prolong the *in vivo* half-life. The concentration of the agonist, as well as the availability of membrane receptors on target cells, dictates the final biological outcome of this balance. The general concept that soluble cytokine receptors can have dual influence on cytokine function has obvious implications for the design of studies in humans.

5.1.4 Soluble cytokine receptors in human diseases

A variety of signals regulate the production of soluble cytokine receptors by affecting the differential splicing of RNA, by generally regulating receptor expression, or by influencing the shedding of the membrane-bound receptor. Soluble cytokine receptor levels in the blood and in biological fluids are, threrefore, profoundly modified by a variety of pathological and physiological states. A detailed discussion of the soluble cytokine receptors in pathophysiology is beyond the scope of this chapter. However, to the extent that these receptors are considered in the context of anti-cytokine strategies, their presence in pathological conditions requiring pharmacological intervention needs to be carefully considered. Table 5.2 summarizes pathological conditions in which elevated levels of soluble IL-1, TNF, IL-2, and IL-6 receptors have been detected and provides indications as to the clinical significance of these measurements. Thus, the use of soluble cytokine receptors as drugs falls within a context of already high levels. While the actual *in vivo* relevance of these high levels—agonistic or antagonistic—has not been elucidated, increasing the concentrations by exogenous administration should shift the balance towards the antagonistic, anti-cytokine action of soluble receptors.

Table 5.2   Soluble cytokine receptors in human diseases

Receptor	Pathology	Disease	Elevated	Related to disease course
sIL-2Rα	Hematologic malignancy	Adult T cell leukemia, Hairy cell leukemia,CML, T-ALL, T-CLL, lymphomas, myeloma	+	+
	Solid tumors	GI, breast, lung, gynecological melanoma	+	–
	Autoimmune/ Inflammatory	Graves', RA, scleroderma, Wegener, SLE	+	+
	Infections	Tubercolosis, HIV, leishmania	+	+
		Diverse	+	–
	Transplantation	Diverse organs	+	±
sIL-1 RII	Hematologic malignancy	Hairy cell leukemia	+	–
	Infections	Sepsis	+	–
	Autoimmune	RA	+	–
	Other	Major surgery	+	–
sIL-6R	Hematological malignancy	Multiple myeloma	+	–
	Autoimmune	RA, IBD, interstitial lung diseases	+	–
		Juvenile RA	decreased	–
	Infection	Sepsis	decreased	–
		Cerebral malaria	+	+
sTNFR (I and II)	Infection	Sepsis, HIV	+	+
		TB, malaria, CMV, endocarditis	+	–
	Autoimmune	Juvenile RA, SLE	+	–
	Transplantation	Kidney	+	–
	Other	Myocardial infarction	+	–

Abbreviations: RA, rheumatoid arthritis; TB, tuberculosis; CMV, cytomegalovirus; IBD, inflammatory bowel disease; SLE, systemic lupus erythematosus, GI, gastrointestinal; CML, chronic myeloid leukemia; ALL, acute

5.1.5   Viral cytokine receptors as a paradigm

Viruses provide a paradigm for the *in vivo* capacity of cytokine receptors to modulate the function of cytokines. Several viruses, particularly the poxvirus family, 'capture' cytokine receptors and use them to subvert host immune responses (Smith, 1996). The viral 'piracy' of cytokines and their receptors is widespread, and includes the presence in the virus genome of genes encoding immunosuppressive cytokines (IL-10, Epstein-Barr virus), soluble cytokine receptors and cytokine-binding molecules, and transmembrane cytokine receptors. The latter include members of the seven transmembrane domain, G protein-coupled, chemokine receptors, such as US28 in the case of cytomegalovirus.

Table 5.3 summarizes soluble cytokine receptors encoded by viruses. These include interferon receptors, TNF receptors, and IL-1 receptors. The soluble IL-1 receptor

Table 5.3   Selected viral cytokine receptors

Protein	Virus	Specificity
B15R+	Vaccinia	IL-1β, not IL-1α and IL-1ra
T2	Shape papilloma	TNFα and β
TNFR	Myxoma	TNFα and β (rabbit)
B28R	Vaccinia	TNFα and β
crmB	Cowpox	TNFα and β
G2R/G4R	Variola	TNFα and β
M-T7	Myxoma	IFNγ, chemokines
B8R	Vaccinia	IFNγ
B18R+	Vaccinia	IFNα/β
US28	CMV	CC chemokines ≠
ECRF3	Herpes Virus Saimiri	CC chemokines (CXCR2 like)≠
KSV-GPCR	KSV/HHV8	CC chemokines °≠

+ Released and membrane bound
≠ Membrane bound, signal transducing
° Constitutively active as a proliferation inducing receptor.

encoded by pox viruses is more related structurally and functionally, to the type II decoy receptor than to the type I signal transducing receptor.

Work with viruses that produce, or do not produce, soluble IL-1 receptors has provided strong evidence for the actual *in vivo* involvement of IL-1 in the pathogenesis of fever. Thus, while soluble cytokine receptors may subserve different functions, including presentation of the agonist to signal-transducing moieties and prolongation of agonist half-ife, experiments conducted by 'Mother Nature' with viruses suggest that, at least for certain cytokines, such as IL-1, TNF, and interferon, soluble cytokine receptors constitute a mechanism of negative regulation of the action of cytokines.

5.2 Soluble cytokine receptors as pharmacological agents

From a pharmacological perspective, soluble cytokine receptors can either function as such, or represent targets for agents that up-regulate their production. Cytokines with anti-inflammatory activity, such as IL-4 and IL-13, augment expression and release of the type II IL-1 decoy receptor. The prototypic immunosuppressive/anti-inflammatory agents, glucocorticoid hormones, exert a similar activity. Augmented production of soluble type II IL-1 receptor is likely to contribute to the anti-inflammatory activity of these agents (Colotta *et al.*, 1993; Re *et al.*, 1994).

Modulation of soluble cytokine receptors production may be an unwanted action of cytokine-targeted therapeutic strategies. For instance, inhibitors of matrix metalloproteases inhibit release of TNF and thus may act as anti-TNF agents. However, these same agents inhibit the shedding of TNF receptors, as well as that of other cytokines' receptors (IL-1 and IL-6). Thus, inhibition of production of soluble cytokine receptors may limit the action of matrix metalloprotease inhibitors, which block TNF processing.

Soluble cytokine receptors are attractive therapeutic agents with a potential to inhibit cytokine activity. When compared to anti-cytokine monoclonal antibodies, soluble cytokine receptors have comparable or higher affinity for the agonist and are not recognized as nonself by the immune system.

The major problem related to the use of soluble cytokine receptors as drugs is their relatively short half-life *in vivo*. The estimated half-lives for soluble receptors of IL-4, IL-1 (RI) and IFNγ after i.v. injection is 1–3 h, 6 h, and 3 h, respectively. The half-lives of monoclonal antibodies are usually orders of magnitude greater. Constructing fusion proteins between soluble receptors and the Fc portion of an immunoglobulin has circumvented this intrinsic limitation of soluble cytokine receptors. The advantage of these hybrid receptor molecules is an increased half-life, similar to that of antibodies. Moreover, the dimeric nature of hybrid receptor constructs in principle confers a greater avidity for membrane bound agonists such as membrane 26kD TNF, which is biologically active, or, multimeric soluble agonists.

Soluble cytokine receptors can act as 'carriers' for cytokines by stabilizing the agonist and protecting it from proteolytic degradation (see above). This property of soluble cytokine receptors could be exploited to enhance the activity of exogenously administered cytokines. However, establishing the 'right' potentiating dose of soluble cytokine receptors has prevented utilization of this property. Thus, at this time, the carrier function of soluble cytokine receptors represents only a potential negative consequence of insufficient dosing of soluble cytokine receptors.

5.2.1 Soluble TNF receptors

Once again, TNF provides the most interesting example of how a soluble receptor can act as an inhibitor (Eigler *et al.*, 1997). In 1988–90, various groups had found that human urine is rich in TNF-inhibitory proteins (Lantz *et al.*, 1990). Working on several hundred liters of urine, this inhibitor was purified and sequenced, and demonstrated to act by binding the TNF molecule (Engelmann *et al.*, 1989). It was thus termed TNF-binding protein (TBP). Then, it was found that these inhibitors were in fact soluble forms of the two TNF receptors (p55 and p75) (Engelmann *et al.*, 1990; Seckinger *et al.*, 1990).

Soluble p55 (type I) receptors, as well as IgG1 chimeric type I and type II receptors, have been developed as anti-inflammatory/immunosuppressive agents. Fusion proteins combining extracellular TNF receptors with Ig heavy chain sequences have been constructed, the main goal being to achieve longer *in vivo* half-life. In addition, these fusion proteins also have higher binding affinity for TNF under equilibrium conditions when compared to monomeric receptors and cellular TNF receptors, possibly because of interaction of two receptors moieties with the same soluble TNF complex. The binding affinities of the TNF receptor type I and type II are similar in magnitude, but their binding kinetics differ with the type II receptor exchanging TNF at a faster rate. On this basis it was suggested that RI fusion proteins have better TNF neutralizing activity and less pronounced carrier 'activity'.

All the various forms of soluble TNF receptors studied have shown anti-inflammatory/immunosuppressive activity in a variety of preclinical models of local and systemic inflammation. Interestingly enough, under certain conditions, TNF blockade results in worsening of the clinical picture, an effect related to the protective action exerted by TNF on certain districts. Soluble TNF receptors were reported to be protective in some of the animal models, where anti-TNF antibodies are protective, including endotoxic shock

(Lesslauer *et al.*, 1991; Bertini *et al.*, 1993) and experimental autoimmune encephalomyelitis (Baker *et al.*, 1994; Selmaj *et al.*, 1995).

TNF receptor fusion proteins are undergoing clinical evaluation in inflammatory conditions. TNF receptor-Fc fusion proteins have been evaluated in sepsis patients (e.g. Zenaide *et al.*, 1995; Fisher *et al.*, 1996; Shaw Warren, 1997). By and large, in spite of some promising results in phase II studies, a variety of biotechnological strategies have not shown convincing efficacy in sepsis. In a study of 141 patients treated randomly with placebo or TNFRI fusion protein, no reduction in mortality was observed and actually at higher doses, anti-TNF treatment was associated with increased mortality (Fisher *et al.*, 1996). In contrast, in a recent 498-patient phase II study, a fusion protein of TNFRI and the Fc portion of IgG1 resulted in a substantial reduction of mortality in the prospectively defined severe sepsis patient group. It was speculated that the pharmacokinetics and pharmacodynamic properties of the two fusion proteins may underlie this difference. Previous inconsistent results with other approaches, as well as the heterogeneity of the septic population, cautions against an over-optimistic interpretation of the results. The role of cytokines and cytokine blockade in septic shock is discussed in Chapter 13. While the two TNF receptor fusion proteins have yielded divergent results in septic shock, anti-TNF strategies including soluble TNF receptors, (e.g. Moreland *et al.*, 1997) have yielded concordant beneficial results in rheumatoid arthritis (see below, Section 5.4). In particular, in patients with persistent active disease, the combination of a TNFRII (p75, etanercept) Fc fusion protein with methotrexate proved safe, well tolerated and better than methotrexate alone (Weinblatt *et al.*, 1999; Pisetsky, 2000). Etanercept was also active in juvenile rheumatoid arthritis as second line therapy (Lovell *et al*,. 2000)

5.2.2 Soluble IL-1 receptors

Although several lines of evidence indicate that the type II decoy receptor is a major negative pathway of regulation of the IL-1 system (see Chapter 1), efforts aimed at exploiting soluble IL-1 receptors therapeutically have been focused mainly on the type I receptor. Chimeric IL-1RI has been shown to have anti-inflammatory activity in a variety of experimental models, including experimental autoimmune encephalomyelitis, lung inflammation, and ocular inflammation. Moreover, this molecule has also been shown to prolong the survival of cardiac allografts. In humans, soluble IL-1RI has been shown to reduce the clinical manifestations of late-phase allergic reactions following subcutaneous inoculation of allergen. At the time of writing, we are not aware of further developments using sIL-1RI. Based on current understanding of ligand recognition, affinity, and physiological function, one would expect that the type II soluble receptor would be a better candidate than IL-1RI for inhibiting IL-1 activity (Colotta *et al.*, 1994). In fact, soluble IL-1RI binds IL-1ra as efficiently as IL-1ß, the main form of IL-1 present in the circulation. The IL-1ra is produced in large excess, compared to IL-1ß, under a variety of pathological conditions. Hence, soluble IL-1RI, by interfering with this physiological pathway of negative regulation of IL-1, would be self-defeating. In contrast, the type II receptor, whose only function to date is to block IL-1, binds IL-1ß with much higher affinity and with more favorable on and off rates than the receptor antagonist (Ghetta *et al.*, 1994; van Deuren *et al.*, 1997). As expected on the basis of these binding characteristics, while soluble IL-1RI interferes with the anti-IL-1 action of IL-1ra, soluble IL-1RII and IL-1ra have additive or synergistic anti-IL-1 activity *in vitro*.

5.2.3 Soluble IL-4 and IFNγ receptors

The therapeutic potential of soluble IL-4 receptor has been demonstrated in a variety of preclinical models, including allogeneic transplantation, IgE production, and cutaneous leishmaniasis. In particular, soluble IL-4 receptor was shown to inhibit predominantly Th2 responses with a subsequent shift to Th1 responses (Fernandez-Botran *et al.*, 1996).

Therapy with soluble IFNγ receptor has been shown to have significant potential for the treatment of autoimmune diseases and for the prevention of acute and chronic graft versus host disease in murine models.

The Th1/Th2 paradigm (see Chapter 1) provides an interesting perspective for the exploitation of soluble IL-4 and IFNγ receptors. Given the central role that IL-4 and IFNγ play in Th2 and Th1 responses, respectively, soluble receptors for these cytokines could represent useful tools to orient immunity, rather than acting as mere suppressants of immune reactions.

5.3 Antibodies

Since the pioneering work of Kitasano and von Behring at the end of the nineteenth century with anti-diphtheria toxin antiserum, antibodies have represented a classic tool to block the action of exogenous and endogenous toxins. Studies in which monoclonal or polyclonal antisera have been used to dissect the role of cytokines in pathology in animals have provided an obvious preclinical rational for therapeutic attempts in humans. The major theoretical advantage of antibodies over, for instance, natural soluble receptors, to block the action of cytokines, is the long half-life in body fluids of these molecules. A major stumbling block, on the other hand, is represented by the fact that antibody molecules act as antigen for the immune system and thus generate the production of endogenous antibodies against these molecules.

Various forms of engineering have been used to minimize the antigenicity of antibody molecules, including the construction of chimeric molecules consisting of human Ig constant regions, coupled with mouse Fv regions or more extensive humanization. In the latter case, the genetic sequences of complementarity determining regions of mouse immunoglobulin chains are transplanted into a human immunoglobulin gene context. The resulting antibodies contain largely (about 95%) human sequences, with only a small proportion (5%) of murine sequences. While engineered, humanized antibodies or hybrid or human antibodies dominate the field and will do so even more in the future, one should not forget that classic antisera have been invaluable to prove the *in vivo* potential of anti-TNF antibodies in humans, in a condition (Jarisch-Herxmeier reaction) where a single treatment was required (see below). In general, the antibody-based approach has been invaluable because it has provided the first unequivocal evidence that in a human disease, rheumatoid arthritis, blocking inflammatory cytokines, TNF in particular, results in unequivocal clinical responses. Consequently, the antibody approach has given a strong momentum to the whole field of anti-cytokine strategies. Here we will discuss anti-cytokine antibodies that have been studied in human disorders or that are undergoing

Table 5.4   Animal models where anti-TNF antibodies are protective

Endotoxin shock	Bleomycin- or silica-induced lung fibrosis
Septic shock	Experimental autoimmune encephalomyelitis
Cerebral malaria	Cerebral ischemia
Bacterial meningitis	Arthritis
Drug-induced gastric ulcer	

clinical evaluation. Emphasis will be on anti-TNF antibodies, as these are the anti-cytokine strategy most extensively investigated in humans.

5.3.1 Anti-TNFα

As early as in 1985 (only one year after TNF cloning was published (Pennica *et al.*, 1984)) Beutler, Milsark and Cerami reported that anti-TNF antibodies protected mice against endotoxic shock (Beutler *et al.*, 1985). Anti-TNF antibodies have been extensively investigated in a wide array of preclinical pathological conditions (Table 5.4) and represent the individual anti-cytokine strategy that has undergone most extensive evaluation in humans. Technical (better antibodies were generated against mouse TNF than, for instance, mouse IL-1) and historical reasons account for the wider experience in blocking TNF, rather than other cytokines, with antibodies. Antibody preparations used in humans include chimeric (human IgG1/mouseFv) monoclonal antibody, F(ab')2 fragments, humanized monoclonal antibodies, as well as old-fashioned (sheep) antiserum.

Septic shock

Septic shock is the first human pathological condition in which anti-cytokine strategies have been studied (Abraham *et al.*, 1995, 1998; Cohen and Carlet, 1996; Grau and Maennel, 1997). Clinical evaluation of blocking TNF was based on a wealth of results in preclinical models, which indicated that TNF plays a central role in septic shock.

The comments already made on the lack of consistent beneficial results of anti-cytokine strategies in septic shock (see Chapter 3 and this chapter, soluble cytokine receptors) also apply to anti-TNF antibodies. The issue of cytokines and septic shock is discussed in Chapter 13.

Rheumatoid arthritis

Rheumatoid arthritis is the single human disease that has been most extensively studied in terms of anti-cytokine strategies. Interestingly, different strategies (antibodies, soluble receptors) aimed at blocking the same cytokine, TNF, or different cytokines (IL-1, IL-6) have concomitantly indicated that anti-cytokine therapy has a potential to affect disease in rheumatoid arthritis. Thus, studies in rheumatoid arthritis have served to establish proof of the principle that blocking inflammatory cytokines can be beneficial in human pathology.

Pathogenesis and anti-TNF antibody therapy

Rheumatoid arthritis is a chronic inflammatory autoimmune disease, which involves multiple joints and affects approximately 1% of the population, with three-fold higher inci-

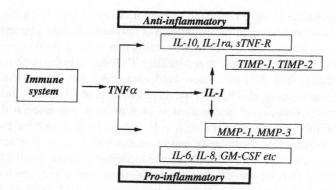

Fig. 5.2 Central role of TNF in the pathogenesis of rheumatoid arthritis. (Reproduced with permission from Feldmann *et al.*, 1997.)

dence among women than men. Rheumatoid arthritis has severe cumulative disabling effects and in severe forms shows mortality rates comparable to low-grade lymphomas. Animal models, including the classical collagen-induced arthritis and recently developed transgenic mice, have been invaluable to delineate the pathogenesis of this autoimmune disease and potential therapeutic strategies (Feldmann *et al.*, 1996; Ivashkiv, 1996; Feldmann *et al.*1997; Firestein and Zvaifler, 1997). As diagrammatically illustrated in Fig. 5.2, one consequence of the ill-understood autoimmune reaction is that inflammatory cytokines are produced. There is indication that TNF represents the primary initiator of the cytokine cascade as indicated, for instance, by blocking of the production of other mediators, such as IL-1, as a consequence of TNF inhibition. The subsequent pathogenesis of cytokine damage of the joint can be summarized with the image of a balance (Fig. 5.3). In rheumatoid synovium the balance between pro- and anti-inflammatory molecules is shifted in favor of pro-inflammatory mediators (TNF, IL-1 and possibly IL-6) (Feldmann *et al.*, 1996). It should be emphasized that even in this cascade model of the pathogenesis of rheumatoid arthritis, with TNF on the top, other molecules such as IL-1, IL-6, or chemokines play a central role. For instance, there is evidence that in TNF transgenic mice, blocking IL-1 with IL-1ra results in inhibition of disease, particularly of bone erosions.

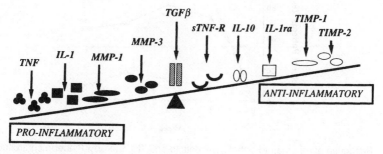

Fig. 5.3 Pro- versus anti-inflammatory cytokines in rheumatoid arthritis. (Reproduced with permission from Feldmann *et al.*, 1997.)

Based on preclinical *in vitro* results and experiments conducted in preclinical rodent models, a series of pioneering clinical studies was initiated using the chimeric cA2 anti-TNFα monoclonal antibody. It was clearly established in these, as well as in studies with humanized anti-TNFα antibodies, that blocking TNF has clinical activity in human rheumatoid arthritis (Fig. 5.4; for review Feldmann *et al.*, 1997). A discussion of the actual clinical results obtained is beyond the scope of this book devoted to the pharmacology of cytokines. As discussed below, clinical improvement was associated to reduced serum levels of inflammatory markers, such as C reactive protein, reduced production of inflammatory cytokines, of chemokines, and of adhesion molecules. This action of anti-TNF therapy on molecules involved in leukocyte recruitment may explain why the clinical benefits lasted beyond the presence of measurable anti-TNFα antibodies in the circulation. However, benefits were transient indicating that TNF production is not the *primum movens* of this autoimmune disease, as one would indeed expect. Moreover, once again, a substantial proportion of patients receiving anti-TNF antibodies developed an anti-murine antibody response. These initial efforts using anti-TNF chimeric antibodies were followed by trials which used soluble TNF receptors, humanized anti-TNFα antibodies, the IL-1ra. In general, an impressive amount of converging results indicate that blocking TNF or other pro-inflammatory cytokines has potential as a therapeutic target in human rheumatoid arthritis (Pisetsky, 2000).

The most common causes of death in rheumatoid arthritis are cardiovascular and cerebrovascular disease. It will be of interest to assess whether anti-TNF therapy reduces vascular deaths, given the role attributed to inflammatory mediators in the pathogenesis of vascular disorders (see Chapter 9).

In the perspective of anti-murine antibody response, it is of interest that in preclinical models, synergism was observed between anti-CD4 antibodies and anti-TNF antibodies with a concomitant reduction in the production of anti-antibodies. Whether these observations in preclinical models are useful in the perspective of a better use of antibodies in the human disease remains to be elucidated.

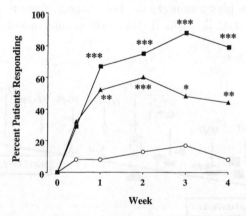

Fig. 5.4 Response of rheumatoid arthritis patients to anti-TNF therapy. Placebo controlled trial: ○ placebo; ▲ 1 mg/kg cA2; ■ 10 mg/kg cA2. (Reproduced with permission from Feldmann *et al.*, 1997.)

Antibody and TNF levels

A considerable amount of information has accumulated on the pharmacokinetics of anti-TNF antibodies. For instance, cA2 serum concentrations were found to increase with the dose of cA2 administered, maximum levels observed after infusion being predictable, based on the distribution of the total dose within the vascular space. Measurable levels of cA2 were present in the serum at 8 weeks after treatment with 10 or 20 mg/kg. The maximal concentration was 277 μg/ml and the area under the curve (μg/ml/h) was 54.775 after a 10 mg/kg dose. The median volume of distribution ranged in various studies between $\approx$ 4000 and 5000 for the same dose and the terminal half-life from 219 to 240 h. When TNF was measured in the circulation, the surprising observation was that immunoreactive cytokine levels were increased after antibody administration. However, this molecule was biologically inactive upon neutralization by antibody.

Mechanism of action

The rationale for treating rheumatoid arthritis patients with anti-TNF antibodies rested in the dominant role played by this cytokine in the cascade, as discussed above. Therefore, it would be logical to assume that this is in fact the major mechanism of action of anti-TNF therapy in this disease. Indeed, evidence was obtained that production of downstream mediators, including various cytokines and adhesion molecules, as well as acute-phase reactants (C-reactive protein), is dramatically inhibited after anti-TNF therapy. Inhibition of IL-6 production may account, for instance, for blocking of acute-phase reactant production in the liver. Moreover, since IL-6 may play a positive role in local inflammation by amplifying chemokine production (Romano *et al.*, 1997), blocking this mediator may also contribute to therapeutic activity. Inhibition of IL-6 production following cA2 administration may account for, or contribute to, the reduction in thrombocytosis typical of rheumatoid arthritis. Anemia is commonly observed in active rheumatoid arthritis, and anti-TNF therapy was found beneficial in restoring erythrocyte counts. This may reflect the action of TNF in directly suppressing erythroid development.

Anti-TNF treatment was shown to result in inhibition of chemokine production and adhesion molecule expression, as assessed *in situ*, as well as systemically by measuring soluble forms of endothelial adhesion molecules. It is likely that the blocking of leukocyte recruitment may represent a major target for the anti-inflammatory action of TNF blockade under these conditions. This may explain why clinical benefit is also observed at times when anti-TNF antibody is no longer detectable in the circulation. Anti-TNF antibodies also result in decreased levels of matrix metalloproteinases, responsible for tissue destruction, and of vascular endothelial growth factor (VEGF,) presumably a crucial determinant of angiogenesis, which is associated with pannus formation.

While inhibition of TNF and secondary blockade of mediators involved, for instance, in leukocyte recruitment is likely to play a central role in the anti-inflammatory action of anti-TNF antibodies, intriguing observations point to more subtle actions of this therapeutic strategy. In studies conducted in Japan, it was found that the cA2 hybrid antibody increased serum levels of IL-10 in 4/6 patients tested (Ohshima *et al.*, 1996). Since IL-10 is a potent immunosuppressive and anti-inflammatory cytokine with therapeutic potential in human diseases, this may contribute to the mechanism of action of cA2.

cA2 also recognizes and binds with high affinity the 26 kD monomeric transmembrane form of TNFα. The cA2 hybrid molecule is an IgG1 isotype, capable of mediating antibody-dependent cellular cytotoxicity and complement-dependent cytotoxicity. Therefore, this reagent could deplete cells bearing membrane TNF. It was in fact found that granulocyte and monocyte counts fall after cA2 administration, whereas lymphocyte number tends to increase. While these changes in counts may reflect alterations in distribution between circulating and marginating pools, one could also speculate that cA2 is indeed cytotoxic for activated myelomonocytic cells (Lalani *et al.*, 1997). It is of interest that the other anti-TNFα molecule with activity in rheumatoid arthritis (Zhang *et al.*, 1997), CDP571, consists of the hypervariable regions of a mouse anti-TNFα monoclonal antibody grafted on human IgG4, and does not trigger ADCC. It has been suggested that while CDP571 and cA2 are equally effective in controlling the early acute phase response in rheumatoid arthritis, cA2 is more effective in reducing joint counts and other clinical endpoints of disease activity. It is evident that elucidation of the actual mechanisms of action of anti-TNFα antibodies in rheumatoid arthritis has profound implications for the design of more effective therapeutic strategies.

Potential side-effects

No obvious major alteration in susceptibility to infectious agents or evidence of immunosuppression was seen in anti-TNF-treated patients. Administration of monoclonal antibodies to humans is frequently associated with the formation of human anti-mouse antibody (HAMA). Chimerization reduces the incidence of HAMA, but anti-idiotype or anti-variable region antibodies are expected and do occur. The frequency of HAMA after administration of cA2 varies considerably from study to study ranging form < 5% to 25–30%. It would be logical to expect that the presence in a molecule of a lower proportion of mouse sequences is associated with a lower incidence of HAMA. However, at present there is no unequivocal evidence that humanized antibodies are less effective in eliciting HAMA production than hybrid antibodies. In 7 of 69 cA2-treated patients, anti-double stranded DNA antibodies were observed and in one patient, anti-TNF may have precipitated a Lupus-like syndrome (Feldman *et al.* 1997).

Serious infections and the sepsis have been reported after marketing of soluble TNFRII (etanercept). These reports call for cautious monitoring of patients developing infections.

Inflammatory bowel disease

Crohn's disease

Any portion of the gastro-intestinal tract can be affected by Crohn's disease, an inflammatory disorder characterized by granulomatous lesions and by the presence of substantial amounts of TNFα. Following a single-patient study, a number of studies have investigated the potential of anti-TNFα antibodies in this disease. There is unequivocal evidence for therapeutic activity of anti-TNF antibodies in Crohn's disease (van Dullemen *et al.*, 1995; Rutgeerts *et al.*, 1997; Stack *et al.*, 1997; Targan *et al.*, 1997; Bell and Kamm, 2000). For instance, in a recently reported study, the effect of humanized CDP571 antibody was investigated in a randomized protocol (van Dullemen *et al.*, 1995; Stack *et al.*, 1996, 1997). Results confirmed the potential of anti-TNF therapy as assessed by scores for disease activity and colonoscopy.

One of the anti-TNF antibody preparations (infliximab) has been licensed in USA and Europe (Bell and Kamm, 2000).

Ulcerative cholitis

Ulcerative cholitis affects the mucosa of the large bowel. Again, while the etiology of the disease is not fully understood, there is evidence that TNF may play a role in this disorder. Steroid refractory ulcerative cholitis was investigated for treatment with anti-TNF monoclonal antibodies (hybrid cA2 and humanized CDP571). As for Crohn's disease, encouraging results were obtained though patient numbers are still small and call for a cautious approach (Bell and Kamm, 2000).

Jarisch-Herxheimer reaction

The Jarisch-Herxheimer reaction is a systemic inflammatory syndrome, which was first described after treatment of secondary syphilis with chemotherapy. This reaction has been described in a variety of bacterial infections, including brucellosis, leptospirosis, Lyme disease, and relapsing fevers. The clinical and pathophysiologic features of the Jarisch-Herxheimer reactions are similar to those that follow exposure to endotoxin, and thus resemble septic shock syndrome or systemic inflammatory response syndrome. The fatality rate of this reaction is approximately 5% and is associated with increased cytokine production, in particular TNFα. Most likely, bacterial products released as a consequence of anti-microbial cytotoxic therapy, activate mononuclear phagocytes, endothelial cells, and other cells, to release pro-inflammatory cytokines, which mediate this reaction. Anti-TNFα therapy was studied in patients undergoing anti-microbial treatment for louse-borne relapsing fever due to *Borrelia recurrentis* infections. In a randomized, double blind, placebo-controlled trial of 49 patients given sheep anti-TNF Fab immediately before intramuscular injection of penicillin, anti-TNFα antibody was found effective in suppressing the Jarisch-Herxheimer reaction (Fekade *et al.*, 1996).

5.3.2 Anti-IL-6

There have been reports that anti-IL-6 monoclonal antibodies have beneficial effects in rheumatoid arthritis (reviewed in Feldman *et al.*, 1997). Since IL-6 inhibits IL-1 and TNF production *in vitro* and *in vivo*, results were somewhat surprising and were interpreted in the light of a role of IL-6 in sustaining lymphocyte autoreactivity. However, recent results obtained with IL-6 knock-out mice and anti-IL-6 reagents, indicate that this cytokine plays an unsuspected positive role as an amplification loop for local inflammation. In particular there is evidence that IL-6, in concert with soluble IL-6 receptor, induces chemokine production *in vitro* and *in vivo* and augments ICAM-1 expression in endothelial cells (Romano *et al.*, 1997). This observation on the dual role of IL-6 in the regulation of inflammation may explain the early therapeutic efficacy observed with anti-IL-6 monoclonal antibodies in rheumatoid arthritis.

The results obtained with sIL-6R point out a common feature of the IL-6 family of cytokines (IL-6, IL-11, and CNTF), where addition of the specific cytokine binding receptor (IL-6R, IL-11R, and CNTFRα) in the soluble form can bind the cytokine and the signal transduction protein gp130 thus triggering an activation signal (Taga *et al.*, 1989; Davis *et al.*, 1993; Karow *et al.*, 1996). In these cases, administration of soluble receptor may not be inhibitory but may even induce responsiveness to the cytokine in cells that normally do not respond to it (see Chapter 1). In fact, while the signal transduction protein is almost ubiquitously distributed, IL-6R, IL-11R, and CNTFRα are not.

5.3.3 Anti-IL-5

IL-5 is a crucial mediator of Th2 reactions. In particular, evidence in preclinical models indicates that IL-5 plays a central role in the regulation of eosinophil production and recruitment. Accordingly, there is also evidence that IL-5 plays a central role in allergic inflammation such as asthma (Chand *et al.*, 1992; Danzig and Cuss, 1997), a disease that is assuming the proportion of an epidemic. A humanized anti-IL-5 antibody is at present undergoing initial clinical evaluation.

5.4 Problems associated with the use of soluble receptors and antibodies

The use of soluble receptors and antibodies poses, in some cases, a peculiar problem. In fact, these molecules often have relatively long circulating half-life, compared to the generally very short ones of the cytokine they bind. Thus, they may have the effect of stabilizing the circulating levels of cytokines (reviewed in Klein and Brailly, 1995). While the cytokine bound to the antibody or the receptor is inactive, it may be slowly released and the inhibitor may thus act as a reservoir (the term 'chaperone' has also been used for this effect; Sehgal, 1996).

For instance, in the case of IL-6, some antibodies that effectively neutralize its activity *in vitro*, increase its levels when administered *in vivo* to mice or baboons (Mihara *et al.*, 1991; May *et al.*, 1993; Ndubuisi *et al.*, 1998). Prolongation of pharmacokinetic half-life of the respective cytokine was also reported with IL-3, IL-4, and IL-7 (Finkelman *et al.*, 1993; Jones and Ziltener, 1993). Administration of soluble TNF receptor to mice actually prolongs the kinetics of serum TNF bioactivity due to endogenous TNF (induced by LPS injection) or exogenously administered TNF (Ghezzi *et al.*, 1994), and evidence that soluble TNF receptor could prolong the kinetics of endogenous TNF produced was also reported with soluble TNF receptor-IgG fusion proteins in models of gram-negative sepsis in mice (Evans *et al.*, 1994). It should be noted, however, that in this case the neutralizing properties of the soluble receptors prevail over the stabilizing ones, as a protective effect against LPS or TNF lethality, was observed in animal models despite this 'carrier' property (Mohler *et al.*, 1993).

The stabilizing effect is not only observed *in vivo*, due to the prolonged plasma half-life of the cytokine, but also *in vitro*. TNF for instance, is bioactive as a trimer. *In vitro* it spontaneously deoligomerizes over long incubation periods, particularly at low concentrations (Aderka *et al.*, 1992). It was reported that soluble TNF receptors stabilize the TNF trimer and thus increase TNF activity recovered after several days of incubation (Aderka *et al.*, 1992). It is important to note that this effect is not observed when a short-time TNF activity is studied (such as the standard 24-h cytotoxicity assay) but in assays requiring long-term incubations (such as the stimulation of cell growth over a 7-day period (Aderka *et al.*, 1992)). This stabilizing effect on the bioactivity of low concentrations of TNF is observed at lower receptor/TNF molar ratios (about 1:1), and the inhibitory effect of sTNFR prevails when concentrations are increased to a receptor/TNF ratio of 10:1 or higher (Aderka *et al.*, 1992; Ghezzi *et al.*, 1994). Also in mice, injection of TNF complexed with a soluble receptor at receptor/agonist molar ratios of 0.01:1–1:1, induced much higher IL-6 levels than TNF alone, and a clear inhibitory effect was observed only at molar ratios higher than 5:1 (Ghezzi *et al.*, 1994).

These observations stress the importance of evaluating the balance between the neutralizing activity of the inhibitor (i.e. its affinity for the cytokine) and its stabilizing effect. Various factors must be taken into consideration, such as the plasma half-life of the cytokine and of the inhibitory molecule, as well as kinetics of binding and release of the cytokine from the inhibitor (e.g. Evans *et al.*, 1994).

5.4.1 Other cytokine-binding peptides

Screening of a phage displayed random peptide library has led to the identification of small (15-amino acid) peptides that inhibit TNF activity. Although the sequences of these peptides are not present in TNFR, they have been shown to act by binding TNF, and this approach is worth mentioning because it can represent an alternative strategy for molecular drug design of cytokine antagonists (Chirinos-Rojas *et al.*, 1998).

References

Abraham, E., Wunderink, R., Silverman, H. *et al.* (1995). Efficacy and safety of monoclonal antibody to human tumor necrosis factor alpha in patients with sepsis syndrome. A randomized, controlled, double-blind, multicenter clinical trial. TNF-alpha MAb Sepsis Study Group. *JAMA*, **273**, 934–41.

Abraham, E., Anzueto, A., Gutierrez, G. *et al.* (1998). Double-blind randomised controlled trial of monoclonal antibody to human tumor necrosis factor in treatment of septic shock. *Lancet*, **351**, 929–33.

Aderka, D., Engelmann, H., Maor, Y. *et al.* (1992). Stabilization of the bioactivity of tumor necrosis factor by its soluble receptors. *J. Exp. Med.*, **175**, 323–9.

Baker, D., Butler, D., Scallon, B. J. *et al.* (1994). Control of established experimental allergic encephalomyelitis by inhibition of tumor necrosis factor (TNF) activity within the central nervous system using monoclonal antibodies and TNF receptor-immunoglobulin fusion proteins. *Eur. J. Immunol.*, **24**, 2040–8.

Bell, S., and Kamm, M. A. (2000). Antibodies to tumour necrosis factor a as treatment for Crohn's disease. *Lancet*, **355**, 858–60.

Bertini, R., Delgado, R., Faggioni, R. *et al.* (1993). Urinary TNF-binding protein (TNF soluble receptor) protects mice against the lethal effect of TNF and endotoxic shock. *Eur. Cytokine Netw.*, **4**, 39–42.

Beutler, B., Milsark, I. W., and Cerami, A. C. (1985). Passive immunization against cachectin/tumor necrosis factor protects against lethal effect of endotoxin. *Science*, **229**, 869–71.

Chand, N., Harrison, J. E., Rooney, S. *et al.* (1992). Anti-IL-5 monoclonal antibody inhibits allergic late phase bronchial eosinophilia in guinea pigs: a therapeutic approach. *Eur. J. Pharmacol.*, **211**, 121–3.

Chirinos-Rojas, C., Steward, M. W., Partidos, C. D. (1998). A peptidomimetic antagonist of TNF-α-mediated cytotoxicity identified from a phage-displayed random peptide library. *J. Immunol.*, **161**, 5621–6.

Cohen, J. and Carlet, J. (1996). INTERSEPT: an international, multicenter, placebo-controlled trial of monoclonal antibody to human tumor necrosis factor-alpha in patients with sepsis. International Sepsis Trial Study Group. *Crit. Care. Med.*, **24**, 1431–40.

Colotta, F., Re, F., Muzio, M. *et al.* (1993). Interleukin-1 type II receptor: a decoy target for IL-1 that is regulated by IL-4. *Science*, **261**, 472–5.

Colotta, F., Dower, S. K., Sims, J. E., and Mantovani, A. (1994). The type II 'decoy' receptor: novel regulatory pathway for interleukin-1. *Immunol. Today.*, **15**, 562–6.

Danzig, M. and Cuss, F. (1997). Inhibition of interleukin-5 with a monoclonal antibody attenuates allergic inflammation. *Allergy*, **52**, 787–94.

Davis, S., Aldrich, T. H., Nancy, I. *et al.* (1993). Released form of CNTF receptor α component as a soluble mediator of CNTF responses. *Science*, **259**, 1736–9.

Eigler, A., Sinha, B., Hartmann, G., and Endres, S. (1997). Taming TNF: strategies to restrain this proinflammatory cytokine. *Immunol. Today.*, **18**, 487–92.

Engelmann, H., Aderka, D., Rubinstein, M. *et al.* (1989). A tumor necrosis factor-binding protein purified to homogeneity from human urine protects cells from tumor necrosis factor toxicity. *J. Biol. Chem.*, **264**, 11974.

Engelmann, H., Novick, D., and Wallach, D. (1990). Two tumor necrosis factor-binding protein purified from human urine. Evidence for immunological cross-reactivity with cell surface tumor necrosis factor receptors. *J. Biol. Chem.*, **265**, 1531–6.

Evans, T. J., Moyes, D., Carpenter, A. *et al.* (1994). Protective effect of 55- but not 75-kD soluble tumor necrosis factor receptor-immunoglobulin G fusion proteins in an animal model of Gram-negative sepsis. *J. Exp. Med.*, **180**, 2173–9.

Fekade, D., Knox, K., Hussein, K. *et al.* (1996). Prevention of jarisch-herxheimer reactions by treatment with antibodies against tumor necrosis factor α. *New Engl. J. Med.*, **335**, 311–5.

Feldmann, M., Brennan, F. M., and Maini, R. N. (1996). Rheumatoid Arthritis. *Cell*, **85**, 307–10.

Feldmann, M., Elliott, M. J., Woody, J. N., and Maini, R. N. (1997) Anti-tumor necrosis factor-alfa therapy of rheumatoid arthritis. In *Adv. Immunol.* (ed. F. J. Dixon), Vol 64, pp. 283–350. Academic Press, San Diego.

Fernandez-Botran, R., Chilton, P. M., and Ma, Y. (1996). Soluble cytokine receptors: their roles in immunoregulation, disease, and therapy. In *Adv. Immunol.* (ed. F. J. Dixon), Vol 63. pp. 269–336. Academic Press, San Diego.

Finkelman, F. D., Madden, K. B., Morris, S. C. *et al.* (1993). Anti-cytokine antibodies as carrier proteins. Prolongation of *in vivo* effects of exogenous cytokines by injection of cytokine-anti-cytokine antibody complexes. *J. Immunol.*, **151**, 1235–44.

Firestein, G. S. and Zvaifler, N. J. (1997). Anticytokine therapy in rheumatoid arthritis. *New Engl. J. Med.*, **337**, 195–7.

Fisher, C. J., Agosti, J. M., Opal, S. M. *et al.* (1996). Treatment of septic shock with the tumor necrosis factor receptor: Fc fusion protein. *New Engl. J. Med.*, **334**, 1697–1702.

Ghezzi, P., Benigni, F., Gascon, M. P., and Ythier, A. (1994). sTNFR-p55 both neutralizes and sta-bilizes TNF (abstract presented at the 2nd International Cytokine Conference, Banff, Canada, October 1–5, 1994). *Cytokine*, **6**, 553.

Grau, G. E. and Maennel, D. N. (1997). TNF inhibition and sepsis. Sounding a cautionary note. *Nature Med.*, **3**, 1193–5.

Heaney, M. L. and Golde, D. V. (1996). Soluble cytokine receptors. *Blood*, **87**, 847–57.

Ivashkiv, L. B. (1996) Cytokine expression and cell activation in inflammatory arthritis. In *Adv. Immunol.* (ed. F. J. Dixon), Vol 63, pp. 337–374. Academic Press, San Diego.

Jensen, L. E., Muzio, M., Mantovani, A., Whitehead, A. S. (2000). Interleukin-1 signalling cascade in liver cells and the involvement of a soluble form of the interleukin-1 accessory protein. *J. Immunol.*, in press.

Jones, A. T. and Ziltener, H. J. (1993). Enhancement of the biologic effects of interleukin-3 *in vivo* by anti- interleukin-3 antibodies. *Blood*, **82**, 1133–41.

Karow, J., Hudson, K. R., Hall, M. A. *et al.* (1996). Mediation of interleukin-11-dependent biologi-cal responses by a soluble form of the interleukin-11 receptor. *Biochem. J.*, **318**, 489–95.

Kim, S-H., Eisenstein, M., Reznikov, L. *et al.* (2000). Structural requirements of six naturally occurring isoforms of the interleukin-18 binding protein to inhibit interleukin-18. *Proc. Natl. Acad. Sci. USA*, **97**, 1190–5.

Klein, B. and Brailly, H. (1995). Cytokine-binding proteins: stimulating antagonists. *Immunol.Today*, **16**, 216–20.

Lalani, A. S., Graham, K., Mossman, K. *et al.* (1997). The purified myxoma virus gamma inter-feron receptor homolog M-T7 interacts with the heparin-binding domains of chemokines. *J. Virol.*, **71**, 4356–63.

Lantz, M., Grullberg, U., Nilsson, E., and Olsson, K. (1990). Characterization *in vitro* of a human tumor necrosis factor-binding protein. A soluble form of a tumor necrosis factor receptor. *J. Clin. Invest.*, **81**, 1396.

Lesslauer, W., Tabuchi, H., Gentz, R. *et al.* (1991). Recombinant soluble tumor necrosis factor recep-tor proteins protect mice from lipopolysaccharide-induced lethality. *Eur. J. Immunol.*, **21**, 2883–6.

Lovell, D. J., Giannini, E. H., Reiff, A. *et al.* (2000). Etanercept in children with polyarticular juve-nile rheumatoid arthritis. *New Engl. J. Med.*, **342**, 763–9.

May, L. T., Neta, R., Moldawer, L. L. *et al.* (1993). Antibodies chaperone circulating IL-6. Paradoxical effects of anti-IL-6 'neutralizing' antibodies *in vivo*. *J. Immunol.*, **151**, 3225–36.

Mihara, M., Koishihara, Y., Fukui, H. *et al.* (1991). Murine anti-human IL-6 monoclonal antibody prolongs the half-life in circulating blood and thus prolongs the bioactivity of human IL-6 in mice. *Immunology*, **74**, 55–9.

Mohler, K. M., Torrance, D. S., Smith, C. A. *et al.* (1993). Soluble tumor necrosis factor (TNF) receptors are effective therapeutic agents in lethal endotoxemia and function simultaneously as both TNF carriers and TNF antagonists. *J. Immunol.*, **151**, 1548–61.

Moreland, L. W., Baumgartner, S. W., Schiff, M. H. *et al.* (1997). Treatment of rheumatoid arthritis with a recombinant human tumor necrosis factor receptor (p75)-Fc fusion protein. *New Engl. J. Med.*, **337**, 141–7.

Ndubuisi, M. I., Patel, K., Rayanade, R. J. *et al.* (1998). Distinct classes of chaperoned IL-6 in human blood: differential immunological and biological availability. *J. Immunol.*, **160**, 494–501.

Novick, D., Kim, S-H., Fantuzzi, G. *et al*, (1999). Interleukin-18 binding protein: a novel modulator of the Th1 cytokine response. *Immunity*, **10**, 127–36.

Ohshima, S., Saeki, Y., Mima, T. *et al.* (1996). Possible mechanism for the long-term efficacy of anti-TNFalfa antibody (cA2) therapy in RA. *Arthritis Rheum.*, **39**, S242 (abstract).

Orlando, S., Sironi, M., Bianchi, G. *et al.* (1997). Role of the metalloproteases in the release of the IL-1 type II decoy receptor. *J. Biol. Chem.*, **272**, 31764–9.

Pennica, D., Nedwin, G. E., Hayflick, J. S. *et al.* (1984). Human tumor necrosis factor: precurtsor structure, expression and homology to lymphotoxin. *Nature*, **312**, 724–7.

Penton-Rol G., Orlando S., Polentarutti N. *et al.* (1999). Bacterial lipopolysaccharide causes rapid shedding, followed by inhibition of mRNA expression, of the IL-1 type II receptor, with concomitant up-regulation of the type I receptor and induction of incompletely spliced transcripts. *J. Immunol.*, **162**, 2931–8.

Pisetsky, D. S. (2000). Tumor necrosis factor blockers in rheumatoid arthritis. *New Engl. J. Med.*, **342**, 810–11.

Re, F., Muzio, M., De Rossi, M. *et al.* (1994). The type II 'receptor' as a decoy target for interleukin 1 in polymorphonuclear leukocytes: characterization of induction by dexamethasone and ligand binding properties of the released decoy receptor. *J. Exp. Med.*, **79**, 739–43.

Romano, M., Sironi, M., Toniatti, C. *et al.* (1997). Role of IL-6 and its soluble receptor in induction of chemokines and leukocyte recruitment. *Immunity*, **6**, 315–25.

Rutgeerts, P., D'Haens, G., and van Deventer, S. J. H. (1997). Retreatment with anti-TNF-α chimeric antibody (cA2) effectively maintains cA2-induced remission in Crohn's disease. *Gastroenterology*, **112** (supplement), A1078 (abstract).

Seckinger, P., Zhang, J.-H., Hauptmann, B., and Dayer, J.-M. (1990). Characterizatio of a tumor necrosis factor α (TNF-α) inhibitor: evidence of immunological cross-reactivity with the TNF receptor. *Proc. Natl. Acad. Sci.USA*, **87**, 5188–92.

Sehgal, P. B. (1996). Interleukin-6-type cytokines *in vivo*: regulated bioavailability. *Proc. Soc. Exp. Biol. Med.*, **213**, 238–47.

Selmaj, K., Papierz, W., Glabinski, A., and Kohno, T. (1995). Prevention of chronic relapsing experimental autoimmune encephalomyelitis by soluble tumor necrosis factor receptor I. *J. Neuroimmunol.*, **56**, 135–41.

Shaw Warren, H. (1997). Strategies for the treatment of sepsis. *New Engl. J. Med.*, **336**, 952–3.

Smith, G. L. (1996). Virus proteins that bind cytokines,chemokines or interferons. *Curr. Opin. Immunol.*, **8**, 467–71.

Stack, W., Mann, S., Roy, A. *et al.* (1996). The effects of CDP571, an engineered human IgG4 anti-TNFalfa antibody in Crohn's disease. *Gastroenterology*, **110**, A284 (abstract).

Stack, W. A., Mann, S. D., Roy, A. J. *et al.* (1997). Randomised controlled trial of CDP571 antibody to tumour necrosis factor-α in Crohn's disease. *Lancet*, **349**, 521–4.

Taga, T., Hibi, M., Hirata, Y. *et al.* (1989). Interleukin-6 triggers the association of its receptor with a possible signal transducer, gp130. *Cell*, **58**, 573–81.

Targan, S. R., Hanauer, S. B., van Deventer, S. J. *et al.* (1997). A short-term study of chimeric monoclonal antibody cA2 to tumor necrosis factor alpha for Crohn's disease. Crohn's Disease cA2 Study Group. *New Engl. J. Med.*, **337**, 1029–35.

van Deuren, M., van der Ven-Jongekrijg, J., Vannier, E. *et al.* (1997). The pattern of Interleukin-1β (IL-1β) and its modulating agents IL-1 receptor antagonist and IL-1 soluble receptor type II in acute meningococcal infections. *Blood*, **90**, 1101–8.

van Dullemen, H. M., van Deventer, S. J., Hommes, D. W., Bijl, H. A., Jansen, J., Tytgat, G. N. *et al.* (1995). Treatment of Crohn's disease with anti-tumor necrosis factor chimeric monoclonal antibody (cA2). *Gastroenterology*, **109**, 129–35.

Weinblatt, M. E., Kremer, J. M., Bankhurst, A. D. *et al.* (1999). A trial of etanercept, a recombinant tumor necrosis factor receptor: fc fusion protein, in patients with rheumatoid arthritis receiving methotrexate. *New Engl. J. Med.,* **340**, 253–9.

Zenaide, M., Quezado, N., Banks, S. M., and Natanson, C. (1995). New strategies for combatting sepsis: the magic bullets missed the mark...but the search continues. *Tibtech,* **13**, 56–63.

Zhang, C., Baumgartner, R. A., Yamada, K., and Beaven, M. A. (1997). Mitogen-activated protein (MAP) kinase regulates production of tumor necrosis factor-alpha and release of arachidonic acid in mast cells—indications of communication between p38 and p42 MAP kinases. *J. Biol. Chem.,* **272**, 13397–402.

6 Anti-inflammatory and immunosuppressive cytokines

The action of cytokines is under the control of several negative regulation circuits. These include glucocorticoid hormones (see Fig. 1.3, Chapter 1 and Chapter 2), soluble cytokine receptors (see Chapter 5), and anti-inflammatory/immunosuppressive cytokines. In a schematic view, these include IL-10, transforming growth factor β (TGFβ), IL-4, and IL-13. (IL-1ra, a specific IL-1 antagonist, is discussed in Chapter 4). None of these molecules has a purely negative action on immunocompetent cells. For instance, B cell growth, differentiation, and function is promoted by these molecules and IL-4 and IL-13 stimulate the differentiation of dendritic cells. However, there is no question that the most obvious role of IL-10 and TGFβ is to inhibit inflammatory responses and immunity, as vividly illustrated in gene targeted mice. In contrast, IL-4 and IL-13 fulfill more complex functions in specific immunity, IL-4 being a major determinant of Th2 differentiation and a T cell growth factor. TGFβ has a broad spectrum of action, which includes virtually all cell types, whereas IL-10 is restricted to cells of hematopoietic origin. It is, therefore, hardly surprising that the therapeutic potential of IL-10 in humans is under increasing scrutiny (for review see: Mosmann, 1994; Bromberg, 1995; de Vries, 1995; Geissler, 1996).

6.1 IL-10

IL-10 was initially discovered as a murine Th2 cell product, which inhibited cytokine synthesis by Th1 cells in the mouse (Mosmann, 1994; de Vries, 1995). Subsequent work, however, has shown that human IL-10 is not a typical Th2 cell product in that it is also produced by CD4$^+$ Th0 and Th1 cells, and a variety of other cell types including CD8+ T cells, B cells, monocytes/macrophages, keratinocytes, and tumor lines such as lymphomas, certain melanomas, ovarian, and colon carcinomas. Two herpes viruses have acquired an IL-10-like gene. Epstein-Barr virus (EBV) and equine herpes virus (EHV) encode a functional IL-10 homologue. The EBV cytokine, encoded by the open reading frame BCRF1, has IL-10 activity on both mouse and human cells. The homology with IL-10 of BCRF1 is higher at the protein level (84%) than the DNA (71%), suggesting that the sequence has been conserved for functional reasons. These two viruses have a two-fold advantage in encoding a functional IL-10-related cytokine. On the one hand, viral IL-10 inhibits the synthesis of macrophage and T cell cytokines that would otherwise contribute to antiviral activity. On the other hand, IL-10 stimulates B cell proliferation, which would be beneficial since EBV infects B cells. The human IL-10 gene maps on chromosome 1 and encodes a protein consisting of 160 amino acids with a predicted molecular size of 18.5 kD. IL-10 is in fact a homodimer with a molecular weight of 37 kD.

6.1.1 Receptor and signal transduction

The human and mouse IL-10 receptors have been cloned. The human IL-10 receptor gene is on chromosome 11. It is expressed in a restricted fashion, mainly on hematopoietic cells and cell lines. It is structurally related to interferon receptors. The signaling in response to IL-10 has been studied to a limited extent. Using the mouse IL-10 receptor, it has been shown that IL-10 activation leads to tyrosine phosphorylation of jak-1 and tic-2 but not of jak-2 and jak-3. In addition, IL-10 completely inhibits p56 lyn tyrosine kinase activation and all subsequent events in this pathway leading to ras activation, as observed in monocytes exposed to LPS. IL-10 induces factors that belong to the p91 family of proteins. These molecules bind to interferon γ-responsive promoter elements. This pathway, therefore, provides a molecular basis for IL-10's ability to inhibit IFNγ-mediated macrophage activation.

6.1.2 Biological activity

Macrophages are a major target for the suppressive action of IL-10 (Table 6.1). IL-10 inhibits different facets of the activation of macrophages as well as ontogenetically and functionally related cells, such as granulocytes and dendritic cells. IL-10 inhibits the production of inflammatory cytokines (TNFα, IL-1, IL-6, and IL-12), besides various chemokines and colony-stimulating factors. This suppressive action is observed irrespective of the stimulus (LPS or IFNγ). It decreases macrophage or dendritic cell functions that

Table 6.1   Effects of IL-10

Cells	Function	Effect
Monocytes/macrophages	IL-1, TNF, IL-6, IL-12, CSF, chemokines	Inhibition
	NO synthase	Inhibition
	Class II	Inhibition
	Differentiation to mature macrophages	Stimulation
	IL-1ra	Stimulation
	Antigen uptake	Stimulation
	CCR2, CCR5 (chemokine receptors)	Stimulation
	CXCR4 (chemokine receptor)	Inhibition
Dendritic cells	Differentiation	Inhibition
	Maturation	Inhibition
	Antigen presentation	Inhibition
Neutrophils/eosinophils	Cytokines	Inhibition
T cells (Th1)	Proliferation, cytokines	Inhibition
B cells	Proliferation	Promotion
	Ig production	Promotion
Mast cells	Differentiation from precursors (+IL-3 and IL-4)	Promotion

are related to antigen presentation and T cell differentiation, such as class II major histo-compatibility complex (MHC) expression and IL-12 production. IFNγ-induced synthesis of nitric oxide, a major pathway of resistance against intracellular parasites, is blocked by IL-10, which also inhibits cytokine production in LPS-stimulated neutrophils and eosinophils. Most importantly, it inhibits the differentiation of monocytes to dendritic cells induced by GM-CSF and IL-4 or IL-13. Concomitantly, IL-10 promotes the differentiation of monocytes to mature macrophages. Interestingly, IL-10 stimulates the endocytic activity of macrophages and dendritic cells, in terms of both fluid phase macropynocytosis and mannose receptor-mediated uptake. This stimulation results in antigen uptake and clearance from the extracellular fluid, with blocked presentation (Allavena *et al.,* 1998).

IL-10 suppresses a variety of T-cell responses. The action on T cells is at least partly mediated by inhibition of accessory cell function, including class II MHC antigen expression, IL-1 and IL-12 production. However, IL-10 also directly inhibits growth and cytokine production in T cells.

IL-10 exerts stimulatory effects on B cells *in vivo*. It augments MHC class II expression in mouse B cells and promotes their survival. In human B cells, IL-10 promotes the proliferation induced by anti-CD40 and differentiation into plasma cells. IL-10 and IL-2 are synergistic in stimulating the proliferation of normal B cells and immunoglobulin secretion, possibly because of up-regulation of IL-2 receptors. IL-10 co-stimulates mast cell growth in the presence of IL-3 and IL-4.

IL-10's inhibition of cytokine production by phagocytes is not completely non-selective. For instance, it inhibits the production of primary proinflammatory cytokines such as IL-1, but augments that of IL-1ra.

During macrophage activation, production of IL-10 is a relatively late event, occurring after peak induction of the pro-inflammatory cytokines and chemokines. This is consistent with the view that IL-10 is a negative pathway of regulation of cytokine production in phagocytes and dendritic cells. IL-10 production itself is under the control of other cytokines. For instance, IFNγ suppresses IL-10 production by activated mononuclear phagocytes. Also, IL-10 inhibits IL-10 mRNA expression, an important autoregulatory feedback loop.

6.1.3 IL-10 in preclinical models

IL-10 has potential as an anti-inflammatory/immunosuppressive agent in a variety of conditions ranging from T-cell-mediated autoimmune diseases, such as type I diabetes and multiple sclerosis, to transplant rejection. Because IL-10 inhibits secretion of pro-inflammatory cytokines and up-regulates IL-1ra expression, it is a candidate anti-inflammatory agent for the treatment of sepsis, rheumatoid arthritis, and psoriasis. The development of IL-10-deficient knock-out mice has provided a strong preclinical background for evaluation in humans (Rennick *et al.,* 1995). IL-10 gene targeted mice have normal development of hematopoietic cells, including lymphocytes, and normal antibody responses. However, under conventional conditions, they presented growth retardation and anemia. Moreover—and most important—they suffered from severe chronic inflammatory bowel disease. When they were kept in a pathogen-free environment, the disease was milder.

These results indicate that under normal conditions IL-10 plays a central role in controlling the development of chronic inflammatory responses, which, in its absence, cause a chronic inflammatory disorder localized in the gut as a result of uncontrolled inflammatory cytokine induction by enteric microorganisms. As expected, in knock-out mice treated with IL-10, the inflammatory bowel disease improved. IL-10 also offered a potential in the treatment of inflammatory bowel disease in an immunodeficient mouse model based on the transfer of CD4 memory T cells. IL-10 protected the mice from colitis. These results indicate that IL-10 is potentially useful for the treatment of inflammatory bowel disease (Crohn's disease and ulcerative colitis) in humans.

IL-10 prevents mice from dying after administration of microbial toxins. IL-10 given before, or shortly after (30 min), LPS prevents septic shock in mice. In this model, death depends largely on pro-inflammatory cytokines, primarily TNFα, secreted by macrophages. IL-10 also protected mice against lethal shock induced by the superantigen staphylococcal enterotoxin B (SEB). Unlike LPS-induced shock, the SEB reaction depends on TNFα produced by activated T cells. Thus, IL-10 prevents lethal shock caused by bacterial toxins which act by inducing TNF in macrophages and T cells.

IL-10 appears to be a proliferation factor for B-cell lymphoma in AIDS, Burkitt's lymphoma, and myeloma. IL-10 produced by tumor cells or by tumor-associated macrophages may be a tool to subvert host immune responses by malignancies (see Chapter 10). More interestingly, from the point of view of direct therapeutic application, IL-10 inhibits the growth of chronic myeloid leukemia cells, acting by blocking endogenous production of GM-CSF.

6.1.4 IL-10 in humans

Phase I studies in healthy human volunteers investigated the pharmacokinetics and immunomodulatory capacity of IL-10 (Chernoff *et al.,* 1995; Huhn *et al.,* 1996; Pajkrt *et al.,* 1997a). IL-10 was administered as a single intravenous injection at doses from 0.1 to 100 μg/kg. IL-10 was well tolerated with no adverse effects at doses as high as 25 mg/kg. Adverse reactions consisted of mild to moderate flu-like symptoms, mainly at the highest dose. Interestingly, considering that IL-10 stimulates the growth of activated B cells and immunoglobulin production, serum Ig levels were not modified in IL-10-treated volunteers.

As expected, IL-10 inhibited production of pro-inflammatory cytokines in mononuclear cells stimulated *in vitro* with LPS—even at low doses, though it affected the numbers of circulating myeloid and lymphoid elements. A single i.v. injection of IL-10 caused a transient, dose-dependent decrease in circulating neutrophils and monocytes, with a concomitant increase in lymphocytes. The mechanism of this unexpected action is unknown. The finding that IL-10 up-regulates the expression of certain chemokine receptors in monocytes (Sozzani *et al.,* 1998) may provide an explanation. The half-life of IL-10 in the terminal phase was 2.3–3.7 h, a range usually observed for cytokines. The capacity to produce inflammatory cytokines after IL-10 in volunteers was still reduced 48 h after treatment.

In a placebo-controlled cross-over study in healthy human volunteers, the effect of IL-10 on the changes in coagulation or fibrinolysis caused by LPS *in vivo* were studied. IL-10 (25 μg/kg) was given 2 min before LPS challenge. It potently modulated the fibrinolytic system and inhibited procoagulant functions during endotoxemia in humans. IL-10 is under investigation in human inflammatory diseases, such as Crohn's disease and rheumatoid arthritis, at the time of writing (Pajkrt *et al.,* 1997a, 1997b). Schreiber *et al.* (1995) reported that topical IL-10 treatment of three steroid-resistant patients with ulcerative colitis resulted in beneficial effects and inhibition of inflammatory cytokine production. Repeated i.v. administration to patients with Crohn's disease had beneficial effects and was well tolerated (van Deventer *et al.*, 1997). Encouraging results, correlated with changes in immune parameters, were observed in a phase II study in psoriasis (Asadullah *et al.*, 1998).

6.2 Transforming Growth Factor-β (TGFβ)

The family of TGFβ includes more than 20 related polypeptides fundamental in the regulation of cell growth, differentiation, migration, and organ construction. Some members of the family dictate the body plan during embryogenesis and others regulate the formation of cartilage, bone, and sexual organs, promote repair, and have immune and endocrine activity. The distinct factors that constitute the family can be grouped in clusters based on sequence similarity. Classically, TGFβ-related molecules have been divided into four families: TGFβ; the activin/inhibins; Mullerian inhibiting substances; and decapentaplegic-related factors, including bone morphogenic proteins. Discovery of new molecules and activity has shown that the TGFβ family is in fact a continuum whose clusters can be identified as shown in Fig. 6.1. Among these molecules, TGFβ has potent actions on immunocompetent and inflammatory cells. The most extensively studied isoform is TGFβ-1, though receptor usage suggests that other TGFβ-1-related molecules should have similar activites (Massagué *et al.*, 1994; Wahl, 1994).

6.2.1 Structure

The biologically active forms of TGFβ and related molecules are disulphide-linked dimers containing subunits of approximately 110 amino acids. Subunits are synthesized as the C-terminal portion of a long precursor. A peptidase cleaves the active domain, which may remain non-covalently associated with the propeptide, forming a latent complex unable to bind the receptor but which can be activated in the extracellular medium. Members of the family show sequence similarity in the active domain, where the most conserved feature is the spacing of seven cysteines. TGFβ-2 has been crystallized. Six of the cysteines form a structure known as the cysteine knot. The seventh is involved in homodimer formation.

6.2.2 Receptors

Classically, the main components of TGFβ receptors were identified as type I (53 kD), type II (70–85 kD) and type III (200–400 kD) (Serra and Moses, 1996; Heldin *et al.*, 1997). The type III receptor is in fact a proteoglycan that binds TGFβ and presents it to the signalling type I and type II receptors, without having any signalling function itself. The type I and type II receptors are serine/threonine kinase receptors. The TGFβ receptors autophosphorylate on serine and threonine and signal as a heteromeric complex. TGFβ1 first binds TβRII, then TβRI is recruited into the complex. Studies on *Drosophila* and *Caenorhabtidis elegans* have been invaluable in showing how signals are transduced from serine/threonine kinase receptors to the nucleus, with identification of the Mad and Sma genes. Vertebrate homologues of Mad and Sma have been designated SMAD; there are at

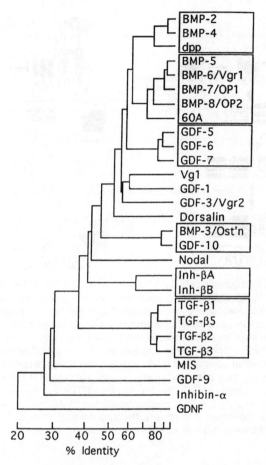

Fig. 6.1 The TGFβ family. The family includes distinct molecules that can be grouped in clusters. 60A and dpp are from *Drosophila* and Vg1 is from *Xenopus*. (Reprinted from Massagué *et al.* (1994), p. 172, with permission from Elsevier Science.)

least nine. After activation of the receptors, SMAD from hetero-oligomeric complexes translocate to the nucleus and regulate transcription of target genes (Fig. 6.2). Interestingly, inhibitory SMAD bind receptors and prevent phosphorylation and signaling.

6.2.3 Activity

TGFβ affects cells of different ontogenetic origin, including fibroblasts, epithelial cells, and hematopoietic elements. TGFβ potently inhibits the growth of many cells. Inhibition of lymphoid cell proliferation is a major mechanism responsible for the immunosuppressive activity of this molecule. In spite of the fact that TGFβ is antiproliferative, under certain conditions it can promote growth during development, and tissue repair.

A variety of cell types, including macrophages, produce TGFβ. A major source of TGFβ-1 are platelets, which store these molecules in the α-granules. Upon stimulation, platelets deliver TGFβ-1 to wounded tissues and thus stimulate healing. TGFβ-1 is very

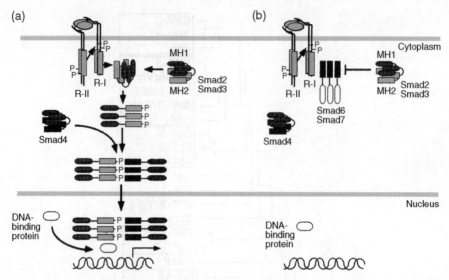

Fig. 6.2 Agonistic and antagonistic SMAD proteins in TGFβ signalling. (a) A hypothetical signal transduction pathway for TGFβ. TGFβ binding leads to the assembly of a heterotetrameric receptor complex in which the type II receptor phosphorylates and activates the type I receptor. Pathway-restricted SMADs (Smad2 and Smad3), which may be anchored in the cytoplasm in homotrimeric forms, are phosphorylated, leading to heteromerization with the common-mediator Smad4. The hetero-oligomeric complex is then translocated to the nucleus, where it binds DNA directly or complexed with other component(s) and affects transcription of specific genes. It is not known whether the hetero-oligomer between Smad2, Smad3, and Smad4 is a hexamer or has another stoichiometry. (b) Inhibitory SMADs (Smad6 and Smad7) bind to the receptors and prevent the phosphorylation and signalling activity of pathway-restricted SMAD. It is not know whether inhibitory SMADs occur as monomers or multimers. (Reprinted with permission from Heldin *et al.*, *Nature* **390**, 465, 1997. Macmillan Magazines Ltd.)

likely a major determinant of formation and accumulation of fibrotic tissue in disorders of the kidney, liver, and lung. TGFβ stimulates tissue growth directly or by stimulating chemotaxis and production of extracellular components, cell adhesion receptors, and mitogenic cytokines.

The biological activity of TGFβ on inflammatory cells is to some extent contradictory. TGFβ is chemotactic for a variety of leukocyte populations, including macrophages and neutrophils, and local administration of the molecule elicits a leukocyte infiltrate (Wahl, 1994). In addition, it seems to induce cytokine production and to augment adhesion. However, TGFβ has potent anti-inflammatory action on many cells. For instance, it inhibits the expression of adhesion molecules and adhesion in leukocyte/endothelial cell interactions. It inhibits cytokine production in endothelial cells and the expression of NO synthase. While local TGFβ is mainly pro-inflammatory, systemic TGFβ appears to be predominantly anti-inflammatory (Wahl, 1994).

TGFβ-1 knock-out mice have provided strong evidence that the main function of TGFβ-1 is anti-inflammatory/immunosuppressive. Perhaps surprisingly, TGFβ-1 gene-targeted mice are normal at birth and for 2–3 weeks thereafter. Subsequently they succumb to an inflammatory condition consisting of widespread leukocyte adhesion to endothelium and infiltration into vital organs, which eventually leads to organ failure, cachexia, and death. This apparently straightforward model of genetic manipulation is in fact complicated by the fact that maternal TGFβ-1 is transferred to the offspring. Maternal TGFβ-1, an endocrine source of this molecule, is sufficient for embryogenesis and birth of the knock-outs. It may also be a confounding factor for the subsequent development of the inflammatory conditions.

TGFβ-1 thus appears to act mainly as an anti-inflammatory/immunosuppressive cytokine produced by a variety of cells, notably platelets and macrophages. The finding that this molecule interacts with, and affects, virtually all cells of the body, modifying fundamental functions such as matrix deposition and proliferation, is a major limitation for its therapeutic exploitation. On the other hand, TGFβ antagonism may be of interest in diseases such as scarring or fibrotic diseases of parenchymal tissues (lungs, liver, kidney), where tissue overgrowth is a major pathogenetic mechanism.

6.3 IL-4 and IL-13

IL-4 and IL-13 have complex immunoregulatory properties encompassing virtually all leukocyte populations (de Vries and Zurawski, 1995). IL-4 plays a central role in orienting immunity towards type II responses (see Chapter 1). As part of their significance in the orientation of immunity towards eosinophil-mast cell-basophil-mediated resistance, IL-4 and IL-13 inhibit the pro-inflammatory functions of macrophages. This is why we discuss them in this chapter on anti-inflammatory/immunosuppressive cytokines.

6.3.1 Molecular properties of IL-4 and IL-13

The IL-4 and IL-13 genes are located on human chromosome 5q31, in the same region as IL-5, IL-3, and GM-CSF (Table 6.2). The homology between these two proteins is only 30% but their tertiary structures are similar, both being α-helical proteins consisting of four antiparallel α-helixes.

6.3.2 Receptors, signal transduction, and activity

IL-4 and IL-13 share receptor proteins and have overlapping spectra of action (Table 6.3 and Figs 6.3 and 6.4). IL-4 is a cytokine that utilizes the common γ chain, shared by other cytokine receptors (IL-2, IL-7, IL-9, IL-15). This chain interacts with the tyrosine

Table 6.2 **Molecular properties of IL-4 and IL-13**

	IL-4	IL-13
Chromosome (human)	5q31	5q31
Protein	4 antiparallel α helixes	4 antiparallel α helixes
Producers	T cells (Th2) mastocytes/basophils	T cells, B cells mastocytes/basophils
Kinetics of production	Early and transient	Early and sustained
Antagonism	IL-4.Y124D	IL-4.Y124D

Table 6.3   Cellular targets of IL-4 and IL-13 (human)

Cells	IL-4	IL-13
Phagocytes (Mø, PMN)	↓ NO, IL-1, TNF, IL-6, G, GM-CSF, IL-12 ↑ IL-1ra, decoy IL-1RII, MDC	↓ NO, IL-1, TNF, IL-6, G, GM-CSF, IL-12 ↑ IL-1ra, decoy IL-1RII, MDC
Dendritic cells	↑ Differentiation (+GM-CSF)	↑ Differentiation (+GM-CSF)
T cells	Growth, cytokine production	No effect
B cells[a]	Growth, IgE, IgG4	Growth, IgE, IgG4
Endothelial cells	↑ VCAM-1, MCP-1 eotaxin, ↓ E selectin	↑ VCAM-1, MCP-1 eotaxin, ↓ E selectin
Mesothelial cells	↑ VCAM-1, MCP-1	↑ VCAM-1, MCP-1

[a] IL-13 has no effect on mouse B cells.

kinase Jak-3 and activates Stat-6. The IL-4 binding moiety is a 240 kD molecule (IL-4Rα). A third chain, IL-13Rα, is subsequently recruited into the complex. IL-13 primarily binds IL-13Rα1 and does not interact with common γ chain containing IL-4 receptor complexes. A second high-affinity IL-13 chain (α2) has been cloned but its functions is not yet clear (Fig. 6.3).

As summarized in Fig. 6.4, the spectra of action of IL-4 and IL-13 overlap, with some important distinguishing features. IL-4 is a T-cell growth factor and a mediator of Th2 differentiation and function. IL-13 is not active on T-cells. IL-4 is also a B-cell growth factor and a switch factor to IgE and IgG4, consistently with a central role in Th2 immunity. Human IL-13 has similar activity on B cells, but the mouse molecule is inactive at this level.

IL-4 and IL-13 both have functions related to the regulation of leukocyte traffick in type II responses. They induce VCAM-1 in endothelial and mesothelial cells and inhibit E selectin expression. Eosinophils and basophils have the VCAM-1 counter-receptor

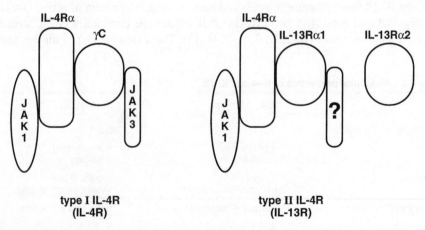

Fig. 6.3   The IL-4 and IL-13 receptors. The function of the IL-13 α2 chain is not known.

PRODUCTION   ACTION

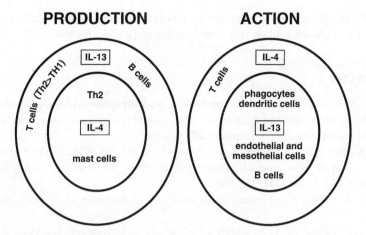

Fig. 6.4 A diagrammatic representation of the spectrum of action and production of IL-4 and IL-13.

VLA-4. In addition, IL-4 (and presumably IL-13) induces the endothelium to produce eotaxin, a chemokine that attracts eosinophils and basophils (Mantovani *et al.*, 1997). Both molecules promote the differentiation of monocytes to dendritic cells (Piemonti *et al.*, 1995). Moreover, they inhibit various macrophage and neutrophil functions related to inflammation, including cytokine production. These molecules inhibit chemokine (e.g. MCP-1) production in monocytes but induce or co-stimulate production of the same mediators in endothelial cells (Mantovani *et al.*, 1997). IL-4 and IL-13 induce production of the chemokine MDC which amplifies Th2 cell recruitment (Mantovani *et al.*, 2000).

IL-4 and IL-13 have complex effects on components of the IL-1 system. They inhibit agonist production, up-regulate expression of intracellular and soluble IL-1 receptor antagonists, and augment production and release of the IL-1 type II decoy receptor (see Chapter 1).

6.3.3 Production

IL-4 and IL-13 are produced by cells of the basophil/mast cell lineage and by T cells. Polarized Th2 cells and cytotoxic T cells with a type II phenotype are characterized by IL-4 and IL-13 production. At least in humans, Th1 cells too produce some IL-13, though less. B cells produce IL-13 but not IL-4. By and large IL-13 is produced in larger amounts and release is more sustained than IL-4 (Fig. 6.4).

6.3.4 Selective receptor agonists and antagonists

Replacement of the tyrosine residue at position 124 of human IL-4 with an aspartic acid, results in a molecule that binds the IL-4 receptor and has no agonist activity. The antagonist, IL-4Y124D, acts against both IL-4 and IL-13. At 50–100-fold excess concentration, it inhibits IL-4 or IL-13 driven IgE synthesis. Interestingly, hIL-4Y124D also inhibits IgE synthesis in SCID mice transplanted with human hematopoietic cells (de Vries and Zurawski, 1995). IL-4R121E binds receptors containing the γc chain (class I) but not IL-13 Rα containing receptors (class II). Accordingly, this mutein has no activity on endothelial cells but retains activity for immunocompetent cells (Shanafelt *et al.*, 1998). A soluble IL-4R chimeric Ig protein is undergoing clinical evaluation.

References

Allavena, P., Piemonti, L., Longoni, D., Bernasconi, S., Stoppacciaro, A., Ruco, L., *et al.* (1998). Interleukin-10 prevents the differentation of monocytes to dendritic cells but promotes their maturation to macrophages. *Eur. J. Immunol.*, **28**, 359–69.

Asadullah, K., Sterry, W., Stephanek, K., Jasulaitis, D., Audring, H., Volk, H. D., *et al.* (1998). IL-10 is a key cytokine in psoriasis. Proof of principle by IL-10 therapy: a new therapeutic approach. *J. Clin. Invest.*, **101**, 783–94.

Bromberg, J. S. (1995). IL-10 immunosuppression in transplantation. *Curr. Opin. Immunol.*, **7**, 639–43.

Chernoff, A. E., Granowitz, E. V., Shapiro, L., Vannier, E., Lonnemann, G., Angel, J. B., *et al.* (1995). A randomized, controlled trial of IL-10 in humans. *J. Immunol.*, **154**, 5492–9.

de Vries, J. E. (1995). Immunosuppressive and anti-inflammatory properties of interleukin-10. *Ann. Med.*, **27**, 537–41.

de Vries, J. E. and Zurawski, G. (1995). Immunoregulatory properties of IL-13: its potential role in atopic disease. *Int. Arch. Allergy. Immunol.*, **106**, 175–9.

Geissler, K. (1996). Current status of clinical development of interleukin-10. *Curr. Opin. Hematol.*, **3**, 203–8.

Heldin, C-H., Miyazono, K., and ten Dijke, P. (1997). TGF-β signalling from cell membrane to nucleus through SMAD proteins. *Nature*, **390**, 465–71.

Huhn, R. D., Radwanski, E., O'Connell, S. M., Sturgill, M. G., Clarke, L., Cody, R. P., *et al.* (1996). Pharmacokinetics and immunomodulatory properties of intravenously administered recombinant human interleukin 10 in healthy volunteers. *Blood*, **87**, 699–705.

Mantovani, A., Bussolino, F., and Introna, M. (1997). Cytokine regulation of endothelial cell function: from molecular level to the bed side. *Immunol. Today*, **18**, 231–9.

Mantovani A., Gray, P. A., Van Damme J., Sozzani, S. (2000). Macrophage derived chemokine. *J. Leukoc. Biol.*, in press.

Massagué, J., Attisano, L., and Wrana, J. L. (1994). The TGF-beta family and its composite receptors. *Trends Cell Biol.*, **4**, 172–8.

Mosmann, T. R. (1994). Properties and functions of interleukin-10. *Adv. Immunol.*, **56**, 1–26.

Pajkrt, D., Camoglio, L., Tiel-van Buul, M. C. M., de Bruin, K., Cutler, D. L., Affrime, M. B., *et al.* (1997a). Attenuation of proinflammatory response by recombinant human IL-10 in human endotoxemia. *J. Immunol.*, **158**, 3971–7.

Pajkrt, D., van der Poll, T., Levi, M., Cutler, D. L., Affrime, M. B., van den Ende, A., *et al.* (1997b). Interleukin-10 inhibits activation of coagulation and fibrinolysis during human endotoxemia. *Blood*, **89**, 2701–5.

Piemonti, L., Bernasconi, S., Luini, W., Trobonjaca, Z., Minty, A., Allavena, P., *et al.* (1995). IL-13 supports differentiation of dendritic cells from circulating precursors in concert with GM-CSF. *Eur. Cytokine Netw.*, **6**, 245–52.

Rennick, D., Davidson, N., and Berg, D. (1995). Interleukin-10 gene knock-out mice: a model of chronic inflammation. *Clin. Immunol. Immunopathol.*, **76**, 174–8.

Schreiber, S., Heinig, T., Thiele, H. G., and Raedler, A. (1995). Immunoregulatory role of interleukin 10 in patients with inflammatory bowel disease. *Gastroenterology*, **108**, 1434–44.

Serra, R. and Moses, H. L. (1996). Tumor suppressor genes in the TGF-β signaling pathway. *Nature Med.*, **2**, 390–1.

Shanafelt, A. B., Forte, C. A., Kasper, J. J., Sanchez-Pescador, L., Wetzel, M., Gundel, R., and Greve, J. M. (1998). An immune cell-selective interleukin-4 agonist. *Proc. Natl. Acad. Sci. USA*, **95**, 9454–8.

Sozzani, S., Ghezzi, S., Iannolo, G., Luini, W., Borsatti, A., Polentarutti, N., *et al.* (1998). Interleukin-10 increases CCR5 expression and HIV infection in human monocytes. *J. Exp. Med.*, **187**, 439–44.

van Deventer, S. J., Elson, C. O., and Fedorak, R. N. (1997). Multiple doses of intravenous interleukin 10 in steroid-refractory Crohn's disease. Crohn's Disease Study Group. *Gastroenterology*, **113**, 383–9.

Wahl, S. M. (1994). Transforming growth factor beta: the good, the bad, and the ugly. *J. Exp. Med.*, **180**, 1587–90.

7 Pharmacology of chemokines

Chemokines are a group of small cytokines whose eponimous function is to attract leukocytes. A brief overview of some of their general features is given in Chapter 1 and the reader is referred to recent reviews (Rollins, 1997; Baggiolini, 1998; Mantovani et al., 1998; Mantovani, 1999) for a more detailed analysis of the molecular and biological properties of this class of cytokines.

Chemokines are involved in a wide range of pathophysiological processes, including inflammation/allergy, immunity, angiogenesis, atherosclerosis, hemopoiesis, brain ontogeny, and viral infections. The recognition that chemokine receptors are a port of entry for HIV has given a strong stimulus to the development of chemokine-targeted agents. Pharmacology of chemokines is now an area of intense efforts and high expectations.

Classic pharmacology is largely founded on analysis of ligands interacting with seven transmembrane domain receptors. Chemokine receptors belong to this class of serpentine receptors. These features distinguishing them from other cytokines justify dealing with the emerging field of chemokine pharmacology in a chapter of its own.

7.1 Synthesis inhibitors

Classic immunosuppressive and anti-inflammatory drugs are potent inhibitors of the production of certain chemokines, such as IL-8 and Monocyte Chemotactic Protein-1 (MCP-1). Active molecules include glucocorticoid hormones, FK506, cyclosporin A (Poon et al., 1991; Zipfel et al., 1991; Mukaida et al., 1992. 1994; Wertheim et al., 1993; Loetscher et al., 1994; Sozzani et al., 1996) (see Table 7.1). The identification of 5' regulatory sequences has provided a means of defining some of the molecular targets. Given the promiscuity of transcription factors, such as NF-kB, it is still not clear whether this approach will eventually lead to the development of selective anti-chemokine agents.

Table 7.1   Some inhibitors of chemokine synthesis

Agent	Chemokine	Selectivity
Glucocorticoid hormones	IL-8, MCP-1, etc.	No
Cyclosporin-A, FK506	IL-8, MCP-1, etc.	No
Bindarit	MCP-1	Some
Statins	MCP-1	No

Chemokine production was also inhibited by various agents that inhibit cytokine production, such as MAP kinase inhibitors, PDEIV inhibitors, PPARγ agonists, etc. (see Chapter 2). Lipoxin A4 and aspirin-triggered lipoxins, inhibited the TNF-stimulated production of macrophage inflammatory protein-2 (MIP-2) and blocked leukocyte recruitment (Hachicha *et al.*, 1999).

The compound 2-methyl-2[[1-(phenylmethyl)-1H-indazol-3yl]methoxy] propanoic acid (Bindarit) was recently found to inhibit chemokine production in a relatively specific way, though at high concentrations (Sironi *et al.*, 1999). Bindarit inhibited MCP-1 production in human monocytes, with no effect on production of IL-8, RANTES and MIP-1α. Bindarit also blocked synthesis of TNF to some extent, but not of IL-1 or IL-6. Although recent results indicate that it inhibits p38 MAP kinase, the molecular mechanisms responsible for selectivity have not been defined.

Agents that affect cholesterol metabolism can affect MCP-1 production. Lovastatin and Mevastatin (two inhibitors of cholesterol which block 3-hydroxy-3-methylglutaryl coenzyme A (HMG-CoA) reductase), inhibit MCP-1 production in mononuclear phagocytes and smooth muscle cells (Romano *et al.*, 2000). The effect of Lovastatin was reversed by the addition of mevalonate, as expected considering its activity on HMG-CoA. Given the fundamental role of MCP-1 in the pathogenesis of atherosclerosis (see Chapter 9), it is tempting to speculate that inhibition of chemokine synthesis, in addition to cholesterol lowering, is in fact a major part of these agents' activity in the prevention of acute myocardial infarction.

7.2 Processing

Naturally occurring post-traslationally modified forms of both CXC and CC families have been identified. IL-8 has long been known to occur in isoforms that differ by the extension of the N-terminal region. A number of proteases, including thrombin, are reported to be responsible for these truncations. Neutrophil activating protein-2 (NAP-2) is generated by proteolytic cleavage of its precursor platelet basic protein. This process results in the generation of intermediates, such as connective tissue activating peptide and ß-thromboglobulin. Only NAP-2 is a potent chemoattractant for neutrophils. Isoforms of the human ELR+ CXC chemokine granulocyte chemotactic protein-2 (GCP-2) show no difference in chemotactic activity.

Post-translational modification at the N-terminus affects dramatically the activity of CC chemokines (see below). A natural isoform of MCP-2, MCP-2(6–76), has been identified. This molecule is biologically inactive and can block the chemotactic activity of MCP-2, as well as that of MCP-1, MCP-3, and RANTES (Proost *et al.*, 1998).

Dipeptidyl-peptidase IV/CD26, has recently been shown to process a variety of chemokines. CD26 has unique specificity compared to other exopeptidase. It cleaves dipetides at the N-terminus with a penultimate Pro, or Ala residues (Van Damme, 1999). CD26, which is expressed on a variety of cell types including epithelial and endothelial cells, has been shown to process the N-terminus of a number of chemokines, such as RANTES, GCP-2, and stromal cell derived factor 1 (SDF-1). Processing of RANTES by CD26 resulted in an antagonist for chemotaxis with enhanced antiviral activity against macrophage tropic HIV strains. In contrast, both the chemotactic activity and the antiviral activity of SDF1 were reduced following truncation by CD26. CD26 also processes the CC chemokine macrophage derived chemokine (MDC). It originates first a 3–69 and then a 5–69 MDC with reduced capacity to interact with its cognate receptor CCR4.

These results suggest that extracellular processing of chemokines by proteases may be an important way to tune the activity and function of the chemokine system in different physiological and pathological conditions. Whether inhibitors of certain proteolytic enzymes, such as CD26-dipeptidyl peptidase IV, can represent a valuable strategy to modulate the action of key chemokines remains to be elucidated (Proost *et al.,* 1998, 1999; Shioda *et al.,* 1998; Van Damme *et al.,* 1999).

7.3 Modulation of receptor expression

The spectrum of action of chemokines is largely dictated by the expression of appropriate receptors in different cell populations. Activation or deactivation of leukocytes is associated with profound changes in receptor expression. A systematic effort to clarify this has been made in monocytes and dendritic cells (Sica *et al.,* 1997; Penton-Rol *et al.,* 1998; Sozzani *et al.,* 1998a, 1998b). Primary pro-inflammatory signals, such as bacterial endotoxin, IL-1, TNF, and IFNγ, cause rapid selective down-regulation of certain chemokine receptors (CCR2 in particular). This may serve as a mechanism to keep mononuclear phagocytes at sites of inflammation and infection, and to focus their action. Reciprocally, certain anti-inflammatory signals, such as IL-10 and glucocorticoid hormones, up-regulate chemokine receptors in monocytes, particularly CCR2 and CCR5 (Sozzani *et al.,* 1998b). These changes are relevant for the susceptibility of monocytes to HIV infection and may explain the rapid disappearance of monocytes that follows acute glucocorticoid treatment (Penton-Rol *et al.,* 1999).

Thus, pro- and anti-inflammatory signals have reciprocal and divergent effects on agonist production or receptor expression in mononuclear phagocytes and dendritic cells. Regulation of receptor expression was mediated by rapid changes in the stability of mRNA transcripts. Therefore, transcript stability might be a target for selectively regulating chemokine receptor expression.

7.4 Antagonists

7.4.1 Viral chemokines and chemokine-binding proteins

Viruses interact with the chemokine system using different strategies, including the expression of viral serpentine homologues, chemokine ligands, and secreted chemokine-binding proteins (Lalani and McFadden, 1997; Wells and Schwartz, 1997). The latter two are involved in the viruses' strategy to block or divert the host-immune response. As such they provide a paradigm for intervention on the chemokine system.

Table 7.2 summarizes the properties of selected viral molecules related to the chemokine system. vMIP-II is a product of human Herpes virus 8 (HHV8), which is involved in the pathogenesis of Kaposi's sarcoma and body-cavity lymphoma. vMIP-II interacts with various chemokine receptors, notably with the HIV co-receptors CCR5 and CXCR4. No agonist activity was detected on these receptors (Boshoff *et al.,* 1997; Kledal *et al.,* 1997). This viral chemokine also interacts with CCR3 and CCR8, and agonist

Table 7.2   Selected viral molecules affecting the chemokine system*

Class	Virus	Molecule	Agonist/receptor recognized
Viral receptors	CMV	US28	Various CC
	HHV8	GPCR[1]	Various CC and CXC[1]
Viral chemokines	HHV8	vMIPI, II, III	CCR5, CCR3, CCR8, CCR4
	Molluscum contagiosum	MC148R	CCR1[2]
Viral chemokine binding proteins	Myxoma	Type I/T7/IFNγR family	Various, heparin binding domain
		Type II/T1/35kD	CC, not CXC

* Selected examples of different classes are given.
[1] The GPCR receptor is constitutively active. Most ligands (e.g. gro) do not affect signaling, whereas IP10 and SDF1 inhibit (inverse agonists).
[2] Based on inhibition of MIP-1α chemotaxis. However, it inhibits hematopoietic precursors as MIP-1α does.

activity has been reported on cells expressing these receptors (Boshoff *et al.*, 1997; Sozzani *et al.*, 1998c). vMIP-II is an attractant for Th2 cells, which express CCR3 and CCR8 (Sozzani *et al.*, 1998c). The HHV8-encoded chemokine vMIP-III reportedly recognizes CCR4, a receptor also preferentially expressed on Th2 cells (Bonecchi *et al.*, 1998; Stine *et al.*, 2000). Preferential attraction of Th2 cells was also recently reported for vMIP-I, which is a functional agonist for CCR8 (Endres *et al.*, 1999). These molecules may thus be a component of the viral strategy to subvert immunity, by orienting responses towards an ineffective Th2 pattern (Fig. 7.1).

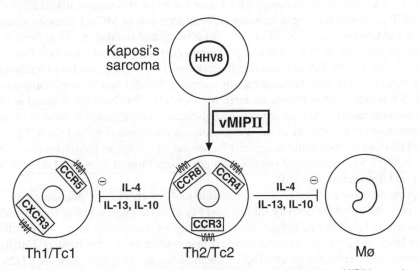

Fig. 7.1   Th2 attraction as a strategy to subvert effective antiviral immunity. vMIPII is a molecule that diverts immunity from effective Th1 responses to an ineffective Th2-dominated pattern. Similar activity is shown by vMIP-I and vMIP-III which interact with CCR3 and CCR4, respectively.

The MC14841 and MC148R2 chemokines encoded by *Molluscum contagiosum* types I and II (a pox virus pathogenic in humans) are structurally related to MIP-1ß and MCP-1, with a deletion in the first five aminoacids (Krathwohl *et al.*, 1997). As discussed below, this part of the molecule is essential for the activity of MCP-1. Thus, the *Molluscum contagiosum* chemokines have no chemotactic activity and block monocyte chemotaxis in response to MIP-1α, presumably by blocking CCR1. Intriguingly, *Molluscum contagiosum* chemokines inhibited the proliferation of human hematopoietic precursors more effectively than MIP-1α. This implies that these viral chemokines have agonist activity on as yet undefined receptor(s).

7.4.2 Peptides

The development of peptide antagonists for chemokines was based initially on selective deletion or substitution of NH_2-terminal residues or by scanning mutagenesis. These studies identified the fundamental role of the ELR (Glu–Leu–Arg) motif just before the CXC in IL-8. IL-8 provided the first chemokine antagonist (Baggiolini and Moser, 1997). An IL-8 analogue in which truncation had resulted in N-terminal arginine (RIL-8) was not active on neutrophils but had considerable affinity for the receptor and blocked biological activity. Substitution within the ELR also yielded antagonists such as (AAR)IL-8. Similar approaches on the backbone of other CXC chemokines, such as gro-α, were followed to generate antagonists. In general, the N-terminal modification appears to result in the generation of antagonists for some but not all receptors. For instance, no peptide antagonist generated in this way has been reported for CXCR3.

Loetscher *et al.* in 1998 found that N-terminal peptides of SDF-1 are weak agonist for CXCR4 and that the analogue 1–9 peptide with a P2G substitution, when dimerized, has antagonist properties.

NH_2 terminal truncation or modification also resulted in the generation of potent antagonists for CC chemokine receptors. This is true for molecules such as RANTES, MCP-1, and MCP-3. Removal of eight residues at the N-terminus of MCP-1 gives an antagonist (Gong and Clarklewis, 1995). MCP-1(9–76) is of special interest, as it has been used in models of diseases such as arthritis, with appreciable therapeutic results (Gong *et al.*, 1997). Expression of RANTES in *E.coli*, gave Met-RANTES, a functional antagonist or weak partial agonist for chemo-attractant receptors. Similar results were obtained when MCP-3 was expressed in *Pychia pastoris*. Met-RANTES has been investigated *in vivo* in experimental models, such as arthritis and glomerulonephritis, and in models of airway inflammation (Plater-Zyberk *et al.*, 1997). Aminoxypentane modified RANTES (AOP-RANTES) was an even better antagonist for several CC receptors (Simmons *et al.*, 1997). AOP-RANTES is internalized but does not elicit signal transduction, and the receptor is prevented from being recycled.

Peptide antagonists have proved a valuable tool for chemokine pharmacology. They have provided structure–activity information essential for understanding ligand–receptor interactions. In addition, before the availability of knock-out mice, they validated chemokines as targets for pharmacological intervention in disease models. Finally, the discovery of N-terminal processing of chemokines by enzymes such as CD26 (see above), suggests that the generation of peptide antagonists may offer a strategy for fine tuning the chemokine system.

7.4.3 Small antagonists

Efforts have been made to develop small antagonists directed against HIV fusion co-receptors, particularly those most frequently used: CXCR4 and CCR5. Three classes of small chemicals that antagonize CXCR4 ligands (Fig. 7.2) have been identified (Doranz *et al.*, 1997; Murakami *et al.*, 1997; Schols *et al.*, 1997): AMD3100, a bicyclam with competitive inhibitory activity for SDF1; a molecule isolated from *Limulus polyphemus* (Polyphemusin II); a peptide identified originally as an anti-HIV molecule and subsequently as a CXCR4 antagonist (ALX40-4C).

In terms of simple chemicals, evidence has been presented at meetings, or in the patent literature, of the development of antagonists both against CXC and CC receptors. To date, only two, SB225002 and TAK-779, have surfaced in a peer-reviewed paper (White *et al.*, 1998; Baba *et al.*, 1999). SB225002 (Fig. 7.3) is a urea-based inhibitor of CXCR2 with activity in the nanomolar range and considerable selectivity for CXCR2. TAK-779 antag-

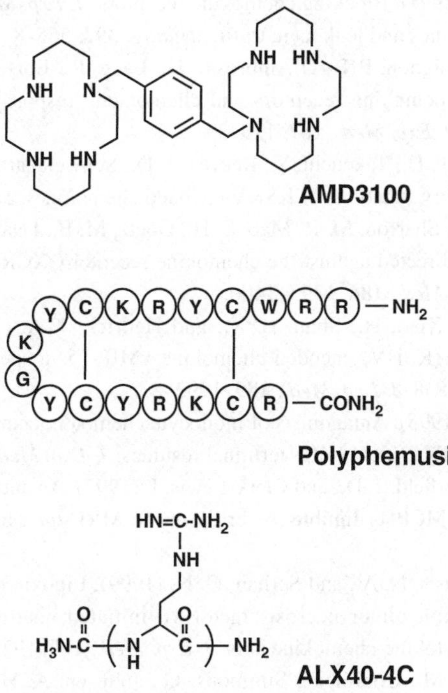

AMD3100

Polyphemusin II

ALX40-4C

Fig. 7.2 Small-molecular-weight CXCR4 antagonists.

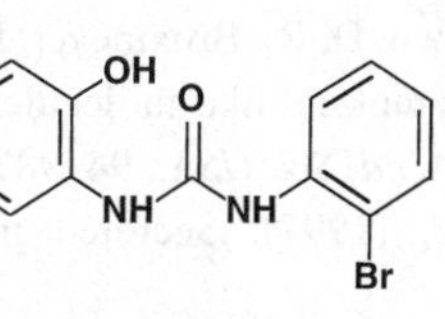

SB 225002

Fig. 7.3 A chemical antagonist for CXCR2.

onized CCR5, to a lesser extent CCR2B, and had no activity on CCR1, CCR3, CCR4 (Baba *et al.*, 1999). These first reports will most likely be followed by others describing chemokine-receptor antagonists based on different molecular scaffolds.

The recent identification of small molecules mimicking G-CSF and erythropoietin range (Tian *et al.*, 1998; Qureshi *et al.*, 1999)) has raised the possibility of a new era of small, simple chemical pharmacology of cytokines. This may even be more true for chemokines given the serpentine nature of their receptors.

References

Baba, M., Nishimura, O., Kanzaki, N., Okamoto, M., Sawada, H., Iizawa, Y. *et al.* (1999). A small-molecule, nonpeptide CCR5 antagonist with highly potent and selective anti-HIV-1 activity. *Proc. Natl. Acad. Sci. USA*, **96**, 5698–703.

Baggiolini, M. and Moser, B. (1997). Blocking chemokine receptors. *J. Exp. Med.*, **186**, 1189–91.

Baggiolini, M. (1998). Chemokines and leukocyte traffic. *Nature*, **392**, 565–8.

Bonecchi, R., Bianchi, G., Bordignon, P. P., D'Ambrosio, D., Lang, R., Borsatti, A. *et al.* (1998). Differential expression of chemokine receptors and chemotactic responsiveness of type 1 T helper cells (Th1) and Th2. *J. Exp. Med.*, **187**, 129–34.

Boshoff, C., Endo, Y., Collins, P. D., Takeuchi, Y., Reeves, J. D., Schweickart, V. L. *et al.* (1997). Angiogenic and HIV-inhibitory functions of KSHV-encoded chemokines. *Science*, **278**, 290–4.

Doranz, B. J., GrovitFerbas, K., Sharron, M. P., Mao, S. H., Goetz, M. B., Daar, E. S. *et al.* (1997). A small-molecule inhibitor directed against the chemokine receptor CXCR4 prevents its use as an HIV-1 coreceptor. *J. Exp. Med.*, **186**, 1395–1400.

Endres, M. J., Garlisi, C. G., Xiao, H., Shan, L. X., and Hedrick, J. A. (1999).The Kaposi's sarcoma-related herpesvirus (KSHV)-encoded chemokine vMIP-I is a specific agonist for the CC chemokine receptor (CCR)8. *J. Exp. Med.*, **189**, 1993–8.

Gong, J. H. and Clarklewis, I. (1995). Antagonists of monocyte chemoattractant protein 1 identified by modification of functionally critical NH2- terminal residues. *J. Exp. Med.*, **181**, 631–40.

Gong, J. H., Ratkay, L. G., Waterfield, J. D., and Clark-Lewis, I. (1997). An antagonist of Monocyte Chemoattractant Protein-1 (MCP-1) Inhibits Arthritis in the MRL-*lpr* Mouse Model. *J. Exp. Med.*, **186**, 131–7.

Hachicha, M., Pouliot, M., Petasis, N. A., and Serhan, C. N. (1999). Lipoxin (LX)A4 and aspirin-triggered 15-epi-LXA4 inhibit tumor necrosis factor 1α-initiated neutrophil responses and trafficking: regulators of a cytokine-chemokine axis. *J. Exp. Med.*, **189**, 1923–9.

Kledal, T. N., Rosenkilde, M. M., Coulin, F., Simmons, G., Johnsen, A. H., Alouani, S. *et al.* (1997). A broad-spectrum chemokine antagonist encoded by Kaposi's sarcoma- associated herpesvirus. *Science*, **277**, 1656–9.

Krathwohl, M. D., Hromas, R., Brown, D. R., Broxmeyer, H. E., and Fife, K. H. (1997). Functional characterization of the C-C chemokine-like molecules encoded by molluscum contagiosum virus types 1 and 2. *Proc. Natl. Acad. Sci. USA.*, **94**, 9875–80.

Lalani, A. S. and McFadden, G. (1997). Secreted poxvirus chemokine binding proteins. *J. Leukocyte. Biol.*, **62**, 570–6.

Loetscher, P., Dewald, B., Baggiolini, M., and Seitz, M. (1994). Monocyte chemoattractant protein 1 and interleukin 8 production by rheumatoid synoviocytes. Effects of anti-rheumatic drugs. *Cytokine*, **6**, 162–70.

Loetscher, P., Gong, J. H., Dewald, B., Baggiolini, M., and Clark-Lewis, I. (1998). N-terminal peptides of stromal cell-derived factor-1 with CXC chemokine receptor 4 agonist and antagonist activities. *J. Biol. Chem.*, **273**, 22279–83.

Mantovani, A. (1999). The chemokine system: redundancy for robust outputs. *Immunol. Today*, **20**, 254–7.

Mantovani, A., Allavena, P., Vecchi, A., and Sozzani, S. (1998). Chemokines and chemokine receptors during activation and deactivation of monocytes and dendritic cells and in amplification of Th1 versus Th2 responses. *Int. J. Clin. Lab. Res.*, **28**, 77–82.

Mukaida, N., Gussella, G. L., Kasahara, T., Ko, Y., Zachariae, C. O., Kawai, T. *et al.* (1992). Molecular analysis of the inhibition of interleukin-8 production by dexamethasone in a human fibrosarcoma cell line. *Immunology*, **75**, 674–9.

Mukaida, N., Morita, M., Ishikawa, Y., Rice, N., Okamoto, S., Kasahara, T. *et al.* (1994). Novel mechanism of glucocorticoid-mediated gene repression. Nuclear factor-kappa B is target for glucocorticoid-mediated interleukin 8 gene repression. *J. Biol. Chem.*, **269**, 13289–95.

Murakami, T., Nakajima, T., Koyanagi, N., Tachibana, K., Fujii, N., Tamamura, H. *et al.* (1997). A small molecule CXCR4 inhibitor that blocks T cell line-tropic HIV-1 infection. *J. Exp. Med.*, **186**, 1389–93.

Penton-Rol, G., Polentarutti, N., Luini, W., Borsatti, A., Mancinelli, R., Sica, A. *et al.* (1998). Selective inhibition of expression of the chemokine receptor CCR2 in human monocytes by IFN-γ. *J. Immunol.*, **160**, 3869–73.

Penton-Rol G., Cota, M., Polentarutti, N., Luini, W., Borsatti, A., Sica, A. *et al.* (1999). Up-regulation of CCR2 chemokine receptor expression and increased susceptibility to the multitropic HIV strain 89,6 in monocytes exposed to glucocorticoid hormones. *J. Immunol.*, **163**, 3524–9.

Plater-Zyberk, C., Hoogewerf, A. J., Proudfoot, A. E. I., Power, C. A., and Wells, T. N. C. (1997). Effect of a CC chemokine receptor antagonist on collagen induced arthritis in DBA/1 mice. *Immunol. Lett.*, **57**, 117–20.

Poon, M., Megyesi, J., Green, R. S., Zhang, H., Rollins, B. J., Safirstein, R. *et al.* (1991). *In vivo* and *in vitro* inhibition of JE gene expression by glucocorticoids. *J. Biol. Chem.*, **266**, 22375–9.

Proost, P., Struyf, S., Couvreur, M., Lenaerts, J-P., Conings, R., Menten, P. *et al.* (1998). Posttranslational modifications affect the activity of the human monocyte chemotactic proteins MCP-1 and MCP-2: identification of MCP-2(6–76) as a natural chemokine inhibitor. *J. Immunol.*, **160**, 4034–41.

Proost, P., Struyf, S., Schols, D., Opdenakker, G., Sozzani, S., Allavena, P. *et al.* (1999). Truncation of macrophage-derived chemokine by CD26/dipeptidyl-peptidase IV beyond its predicted cleavage site affect chemotactic activity and CC chemokine receptor 4 interaction. *J. Biol. Chem.*, **274**, 3988–99.

Qureshi, S. A., Kim, R. M., Konteatis, Z., Biazzo, D. E., Motamedi, H., Rodrigues, R. *et al.* (1999). Mimicry of erythropoietin by a nonpeptide molecule. *Proc. Natl. Acad. Sci. USA.*, **96**, 12156–61.

Rollins, B. J. (1997). Chemokines. *Blood*, **90**, 909–28.

Romano, M., Diomede, L., Sironi, M., Massimiliano, L., Sottocorno, M., Polentarutti, N. *et al.* (2000) Inihibition of monocyte chemotactic protein-1 synthesis by statins. *Lab. Invest.* (In press.)

Schols, D., Struyf, S., Vandamme, J., Este, J. A., Henson, G., and DeClercq, E. (1997). Inhibition of T-tropic HIV strains by selective antagonization of the chemokine receptor CXCR4. *J. Exp. Med.*, **186**, 1383–8.

Shioda, T., Kato, H., Ohnishi, Y., Tashiro, K., Ikegawa, M., Nakayama, E. E. *et al.* (1998). Anti-HIV-1 and chemotactic activities of human stromal cell-derived factor 1 alpha (SDF-1 alpha) and SDF-1 beta are abolished by CD26/dipeptidyl peptidase IV-mediated cleavage. *Proc. Natl. Acad. Sci. USA.*, **95**, 6331–6.

Sica, A., Saccani, A., Borsatti, A., Power, C. A., Wells, T. N. C., Luini, W. *et al.* (1997). Bacterial lipopolysaccharide rapidly inhibits expression of C-C chemokine receptors in human monocytes. *J. Exp. Med.*, **185**, 969–74.

Simmons, G., Clapham, P. R., Picard, L., Offord, R. E., Rosenkilde, M. M., Schwartz, T. W. *et al.* (1997). Potent HIV inhibition of HIV infectivity in macrophages and lymphocytes by a novel CCR5 antagonist. *Science*, **276**, 276–9.

Sironi, M., Guglielmotti, A., Polentarutti, N., Fioretti, F., Milanese, C., Romano, M. *et al.* (1999). A small synthetic molecule able to selectively inhibit the production of the CC chemokine monocyte chemotactic protein-1. *Eur Cytokine Netw.*, **10**, 437–41.

Sozzani, S., Allavena, P., Proost, P., Van Damme, J., and Mantovani, A. (1996) Chemokines as targets for pharmacological intervention. In *Progress in Drug Research* (ed. E. Jucker), pp. 53–80 Birkhaüser Verlag, Basel.

Sozzani, S., Allavena, P., D'Amico, G., Luini, W., Bianchi, G., Kataura, M. *et al.* (1998a). Cutting edge: Differential regulation of chemokine receptors during dendritic cell maturation: a model for their trafficking properties. *J. Immunol.*, **161**, 1083–6.

Sozzani, S., Ghezzi, S., Iannolo, G., Luini, W., Borsatti, A., Polentarutti, N. *et al.* (1998b). Interleukin-10 increases CCR5 expression and HIV infection in human monocytes. *J. Exp. Med.*, **187**, 439–44.

Sozzani, S., Luini, W., Bianchi, G., Allavena, P., Wells, T. N. C., Napolitano, M. *et al.* (1998c). The viral chemokine macrophage inflammatory protein-II is a selective Th2 chemoattractant. *Blood*, **92**, 4036–9.

Stine, J. T., Wood, C., Hill, M., Epp, A., Raport, C., Schweickart, V. *et al.* (2000). The KSHV-encoded CC chemokine vMIP-III is a CCR4 agonist, stimulates angiogenesis, and selectively chemoattracts TH2 cells. *Blood*, **951**, 1151–7.

Tian, S. S., Lamb, P., King, A. G., Miller, S. G., Kessler, L., Luengo J. I. *et al.* (1998). A small, non-peptidyl mimic of granulocyte-colony-stimulating factor. *Science*, **281**, 257–259.

Van Damme, J., Struyf, S., Wuyts, A., Van Coilie, E., Menten, P., Schols, D., Sozzani, S., De Meester, I., and Proost, P. (1999). The role of CD26/DPP IV in chemokine processing. In *Chemokines* (ed. A. Mantovani.), Karger, Basel, pp. 42–56.

Wells, T. N. C. and Schwartz, T. W. (1997). Plagiarism of the host immune system: lessons about chemokine immunology from viruses. *Curr. Opin. Biotechnol.*, **8**, 741–8.

Wertheim, W. A., Kunkel, S. L., Standiford, T. J., Burdick, M. D., Becker, F. S., Wilke, C. A. *et al.* (1993). Regulation of neutrophil-derived IL-8: the role of prostaglandin E2, dexamethasone, and IL-4. *J. Immunol.*, **151**, 2166–75.

White, J. R., Lee, J. M., Young, P. R., Hertzberg, R. P., Jurewicz, A. J., Chaikin, M. A. *et al.* (1998). Identification of a potent, selective non-peptide CXCR2 antagonist that inhibits interleukin-8-induced neutrophil migration. *J. Biol. Chem.*, **273**, 10095–8.

Zipfel, P. F., Bialonski, A., and Skerka, C. (1991). Induction of members of the IL-8/NAP-1 gene family in human T lymphocytes is suppressed by cyclosporin A. *Biochem. Biophys. Res. Commun.*, **181**, 179–83.

Part II

Pharmacology in a context

8 Nervous system

The production of cytokines and the presence of cytokine receptors in the brain is well documented and is summarized in Table 8.1. Among the central effects of cytokines, fever was probably the first activity demonstrated to be mediated by IL-1. Since then, when purified recombinant cytokines became available, new physiological actions of cytokines on the brain were described. Table 8.2 outlines the most important central activities of cytokines on the brain. In addition, cytokines cause glial proliferation (Fattori

Table 8.1   Cytokine and cytokine receptors expression in the brain

Cytokine	Neurons	Astrocytes	Oligodendrocytes	Microglia
IL-1	C/R	C/R	C/R	C
IL-2	C/R		R	R
IL-3	C/R	C/R	R	R
IL-4		R	R	R
IL-5		C		C/R
IL-6	C/R	C/R		C/R
IL-7		R	R	R
IL-8	R	C/R		R
IL-9		R		
IL-10		C/R		C/R
IL-11		C		
IL-12				C
IL-15		C		C
TNF	R	C/R	R	C/R
IFN-gamma		C/R		R
TGF-beta		C/R	C/R	C/R
GM-CSF	R	C/R	R	R
M-CSF		C	R	C/R

C, Cytokine; R, Receptor.
Modified from Sternberg *et al.* (1989) *The Journal of Clinical Investigations*, **100**, 2643, by copyright permission of The American Society for Clinical Investigation.

Table 8.2   Central effects of cytokines

Fever	(IL-1, TNF, IL-6, IL-8, MIP-1,CNTF)
Sleepiness	(IL-1, TNF)
Anorexia	(IL-1, TNF, IL-6)
HPAA activation	IL-1, TNF, IL-6 and other gp130-user cytokines

HPAA, hypothalamus–pituitary–adrenal axis.

Table 8.3   Cytokines in CNS diseases

Meningitis (bacterial)[a]	IL-1, TNF
Cerebral malaria[a]	TNF
Multiple sclerosis/EAE[a, b]	TNF, IL-1, IL-12, IL-18
Alzheimer disease	IL-1, TNF, IL-6
Cerebral ischemia[a]	IL-1, TNF
AIDS dementia	TNF
Myasthenia gravis[a]	IL-12
Stroke[a]	TNF

[a] Diseases where inhibition of cytokines is protective in animal models.
[b] EAE, experimental autoimmune encephalomyelitis.

et al., 1995), induction of adhesion molecules, and β-amyloid and other acute-phase proteins in the central nervous system (CNS) (Vandenabeele and Fiers, 1991). Excitotoxic amino acids induce the synthesis of TNF and IL-1 (Minami *et al.*, 1991). Conversely, TNF potentiates glutamate neurotoxicity in human fetal brain cell cultures (Chao and Hu, 1994).

As a result, a pathogenic effect of cytokines, particularly TNF, IL-6, and IL-1, was proposed in some diseases of the CNS that have an inflammatory component. A list of these diseases is shown in Table 8.3. Various pharmacological approaches have been used to inhibit cytokine production in the CNS as a consequence of the identification of IL-1 or TNF in these diseases. Pentoxifylline, an inhibitor of TNF production, has been shown to be active in animal models of bacterial meningitis and EAE (Saez-Llorens *et al.*, 1990; Nataf *et al.*, 1993; Okuda *et al.*, 1996). It also inhibits, at least in part, LPS fever (Goldbach *et al.*, 1997).

As TNF has been implicated in cancer-associated cachexia and/or anorexia (Stovroff *et al.*, 1988; Sherry *et al.*, 1989; Tracey *et al.*, 1990; Gelin *et al.*, 1991), pentoxifylline was also studied in a randomized, double blind, placebo-controlled trial on 70 patients with cancer cachexia/anorexia but was ineffective (Goldberg *et al.*, 1995). One possible interpretation for these results is that other cytokines may be important in cancer cachexia/anorexia. In fact, IL-6 was proposed to trigger cancer cachexia (Hack *et al.*, 1996). Using an experimental model, where human tumor cells were transplanted into nude mice, it was found that with some tumor cells a much stronger cachectic/anorectic action was observed when the cells were implanted into the brain than in the paw. This was associated with a strong IL-6 production from the host, rather than from the tumor. In one of these models of brain tumors, administration of anti-IL-6 receptor antibodies had a protective effect (Ghezzi, unpublished). In this respect, the importance of IL-6 is also supported by a study in patients with lymphoma, where administration of an anti-IL-6 monoclonal antibody had a clear effect on cancer cachexia (Emilie *et al.*, 1994).

8.1   Effects of cytokines on the brain

8.1.1   Fever

As we have mentioned above, IL-1 was the first cytokine to be identified as an endogenous pyrogen. Other cytokines are pyrogenic, although on a weight basis IL-1 is the most potent. Pyrogenic cytokines include TNF (Dinarello *et al.*, 1986), IL-6 (Dinarello *et al.*, 1991), IL-8 (Zampronio *et al.*, 1994), MIP-1α (Davatelis *et al.*, 1989) and CNTF (Shapiro *et al.*, 1993).

Obviously, the demonstration of a direct pyrogenic effect does not necessarily mean that a cytokine is an endogenous pyrogen. This would only be confirmed if that cytokine was detected (in the brain or in the periphery) during fever and, more conclusively, if fever is inhibited by antibodies or specific inhibitors.

To date, this has only been reported for IL-1 (Long *et al.*, 1990a) and IL-6 (Rothwell *et al.*, 1991). Rothwell *et al.* showed that intracerebroventricular injection of anti-IL-6 antibody inhibited the pyrogenic response to IL-1 and LPS (Rothwell *et al.*, 1991), indicating that even IL-1 fever may be partially mediated by IL-6. The latter is a much less potent pyrogen than IL-1, but as noted by Shapiro *et al.* (Shapiro *et al.*, 1993), IL-6 levels in humans with infection or following experimental endotoxin fever are 100–1000-times those of IL-1. However, in evaluating the relative roles of cytokines in fever, one has to consider their being part of a complex network, and studies with IL-6-deficient mice have shown that central IL-6 is necessary for fever response to LPS or IL-1 (Chai *et al.*, 1996).

A biphasic fever was reported with TNF, a first peak due to the direct effect of TNF was followed by a second one due to IL-1 induction by TNF (Dinarello *et al.*, 1986). The role of TNF as an endogenous pyrogen is controversial; it was reported that anti-TNF antibodies enhanced rather than inhibited LPS- or stress-induced fever, and it was suggested that TNF acts as an endogenous antipyretic (Long *et al.*, 1990a, 1990b). It should be noted that these data were obtained in rats and contrast a previous report that anti-TNF reduced LPS fever in rabbits (Nagai *et al.*, 1988). It is also interesting to note that, unlike IL-1, IL-6 is pyrogenic but not somnogenic (Opp *et al.*, 1989).

8.1.2 Anorexia

Anorexia is a component of the acute-phase response to acute and chronic inflammatory, infectious, and invasive diseases. Centrally or peripherally administered, IL-1 or TNF (like LPS) induces anorexia (Plata-Salaman *et al.*, 1988; Bodnar *et al.*, 1989; Hellerstein *et al.*, 1989; Plata-Salaman, 1991; Masotto *et al.*, 1992). It has been suggested that this is a central effect, and local application (*in vivo* and *in vitro*) of IL-1 affects the activity of glucose-responsive neurons in the hypothalamus by a prostaglandin-dependent mechanism (Kuriyama *et al.*, 1990). Anorexia can be viewed as one aspect of a series of changes in the metabolism and induction of catabolic hormones, including cortisol, glucagon, and catecholamines, resulting in weight loss, catabolism of vital proteins and lipid stores, and lean tissue wasting (Tracey and Cerami, 1992).

Anorexia induced by IL-1 is associated with conditioned taste aversion and it was suggested to be secondary to the toxicity of this cytokine, which would result in a 'sickness behavior', although this was based only on evidence that the dose–response curves of IL-1 for these effects are similar (Tazi *et al.*, 1988). Induction of taste aversion was also reported for TNF (Bernstein *et al.*, 1991). The role of gp130-user cytokines in anorexia is more complex. Chronic administration of IL-6 (at doses up to 0.4 mg/kg, i.p. for 5 days) did not change food intake in mice, whereas CNTF markedly reduced food intake (Fantuzzi *et al.*, 1995a; Gloaguen *et al.*, 1997). However, anti-IL-6 antibodies partially inhibited the decrease in food intake associated with turpentine-induced inflammation (Oldenburg *et al.*, 1993).

Several lines of evidence suggest that cytokines, particularly TNF, might mediate cancer cachexia; implantation of tumor cells genetically engineered to produce TNF induces anorexia and cachexia in mice (Oliff *et al.*, 1987; Tracey *et al.*, 1990), thus TNF might be a mediator of cancer-associated cachexia and anorexia. In fact, anti-TNF antibodies attenuate anorexia in various experimental tumor models (Stovroff *et al.*, 1988; Sherry *et al.*, 1989).

8.2 Cytokine-mediated diseases of the CNS

8.2.1 Infections

In some parasitic and bacterial infections, such as meningitis and cerebral malaria, IL-1, IL-6, IL-8, or TNF have been detected and antibodies against TNF or IL-1 are protective (Grau *et al.*, 1987; Saukkonen *et al.*, 1990). Meningitis also provides an interesting example of pharmacological intervention aimed at inhibiting the production of inflammatory cytokines. In fact, unlike most cytokine-mediated diseases, this is one of the few cases when the time of production of cytokines can be foreseen. In bacterial meningitis, human and animal studies, mainly by McCracken's group, have shown that release of LPS, which triggers the cytokine cascade, is a result of the bacterial lysis induced by antibiotic therapy (Grau *et al.*, 1987, Mustafa *et al.*, 1989a, 1989b, 1990). In this case, the release of cytokines can be inhibited by administering DEX with antibiotics (Odio *et al.*, 1991) and this is now common practice. Therefore, this might thus be a pathology in which inhibitors of IL-1 and TNF synthesis can be tested. For instance, pentoxifylline is protective in animal models of bacterial meningitis (Saez-Llorens *et al.*, 1990).

8.2.2 AIDS dementia

TNF, IL-1, and IL-6 have been detected in the CSF of AIDS patients and this was suggested to have a role in AIDS dementia (Gallo *et al.*, 1989; Grimaldi *et al.*, 1991). The observation that intracerebroventricular injection of the viral envelope protein gp120, which is also neurotoxic (for a review on gp120 neurotoxicity see Brenneman *et al.*, 1993), induces brain IL-1 in rats (Sundar *et al.*, 1991) suggests a mechanism for this effect. One hypothesis is that cytokines might act by increasing the synthesis of toxic tryptophan metabolites (see 2.2.3).

8.2.3 Alzheimer's disease

In vitro, IL-1 and IL-6 can activate β-amyloid gene expression (Donnelly *et al.*, 1990; Vandenabeele and Fiers, 1991), raising the possibility that amyloidogenesis associated with Alzheimer's disease might be due to an IL-1/IL-6-driven acute-phase reponse in the brain (Vandenabeele and Fiers, 1991). Conversely, β-amyloid activates cytokine production (Meda *et al.*, 1995). Due to the lack of animal models, the hypothesis of a role of cytokines, although sound, has not been experimentally demonstrated. However, this hypothesis is supported by the fact that IL-1 and IL-6 have been detected in brains from patients with Alzheimer's disease (Griffin *et al.*, 1989; Wood *et al.*, 1993). Another neurodegenerative disease where TNF and IL-1 gene expression is enhanced is scrapie, a transmissible subacute spongiform encephalopathy (Campbell *et al.*, 1994).

8.2.4 Cerebral ischemia

Various lines of evidence suggest that TNF and IL-1 are implicated in cerebral ischemia (Barone *et al.*, 1999). Cytokines are induced *in vivo* by excitotoxins (Minami *et al.*, 1991) and TNF is detected in ischemic brain regions of rats after middle cerebral artery occlusion (Meistrell III *et al.*, 1997; Bertorelli *et al.*, 1998). TNF was also reported to synergize with glutamate in inducing neurotoxicity in human fetal brain cell cultures (Chao and Hu, 1994). Strong evidence in favor of a pathogenic role of TNF also comes from papers showing that administration of anti-TNF antibodies is protective in these models (Meistrell III *et al.*, 1997). It should be noted, however, that a study with gene targeted mice lacking both TNFR p55 and p75 indicated that they are more susceptible to excitotoxic and ischemic brain damage (Bruce *et al.*, 1996). Thus, TNF may also have protective effects, although the mechanisms for this still have to be elucidated. It is possible that this is related to the protective effect of IL-1/TNF against oxidative stress that was well characterized in pulmonary toxicology. In the same models, like in NMDA receptor-mediated neurotoxicity, IL-1Ra is protective, indicating that IL-1 is a mediator of excitotoxic and ischemic neuronal damage (Relton and Rothwell, 1992; Rothwell *et al.*, 1997).

8.2.5 Experimental allergic encephalomyelitis (EAE)/multiple sclerosis (MS)

EAE is an autoimmune demyelinating disease with an important inflammatory component that is considered an animal model of MS (Raine, 1994). Induction of cytokines in this disease has been well studied (Brosnan *et al.*, 1995; Olsson, 1995; Woodroofe, 1995). In acute models of EAE, three phases have been identified (Issazadeh *et al.*, 1995; Olsson, 1995). In a first phase, the appearance of the first inflammatory cells coincides with production of lymphotoxin and IL-12. Then an acute phase of the disease follows, accompanied by production of IFN-γ and TNF. TGF-β and IL-10 are induced during the recovery phase. Further support for the role of pro-inflammatory cytokines comes from the detection of TNF and IL-1 in MS patients (Hofman *et al.*, 1989; Hauser *et al.*, 1990; Sharief and Hentges, 1991; Rieckmann *et al.*, 1995).

The first cytokine to be implicated was TNF, since in 1990 Ruddle *et al.* reported that anti-TNF antibodies had a protective effect in EAE (Ruddle *et al.*, 1990). Similarly, a protective effect of soluble TNFR was reported (Selmaj and Raine, 1995). The importance of TNF as a pharmacological target in EAE was confirmed by the protective effect of various inhibitors of its production, including pentoxifylline (Nataf *et al.*, 1993; Rott *et al.*, 1993; Okuda *et al.*, 1996) or rolipram (Sommer *et al.*, 1995). As mentioned in Chapter 2, these agents act by increasing cAMP levels. Studies in TNF-deficient mice suggest that TNF is not required for the progression of MBP-induced EAE, but accelerates the onset of disease (Kassiotis *et al.*, 1999).

Administration of IL-13 or IL-10, known inhibitors of TNF production, is also protective in rat EAE (Cash *et al.*, 1994; Rott *et al.*, 1994). Along the same line, retinoids improve the clinical course of chronic relapsing EAE, and this correlates with development of Th2 cells and production of IL-4 (Racke *et al.*, 1995). A drastic anti-cytokine approach, such as that consisting of the elimination of macrophages by treatment with liposomes containing dichloromethylene diphosphonate (Cl$_2$MDP), also suppresses the expression of EAE (Huitinga *et al.*, 1990). Furthermore, administration of glucocorticoids suppresses the development of the disease and a role for endogenous glucocorticoids in regulating the susceptibility to EAE (MacPhee *et al.*, 1989; Mason, 1991) will be discussed below. Also inhibition of IL-12 is protective (Leonard *et al.*, 1995), and this cytokine is currently considered an important pharmacological target in MS (Adorini *et al.*, 1996; Gately *et al.*, 1998). Experiments with IL-12-deficient mice have also demonstrated the role of this cytokine in a model of experimental autoimmune myasthenia gravis (Moiola *et al.*, 1998).

Targeting IFNs has given controversial results; in particular, a protective effect of the administration of IFN-γ was reported in rats (Voorthuis *et al.*, 1990), and neutralization of endogenous IFN-γ led to exacerbation of the disease (Lublin *et al.*, 1993; Duong *et al.*, 1992, 1994). However, in MS patients administration of IFN-γ led to exacerbation of the disease (Panitch *et al.*, 1987), while, IFN-β is beneficial in patients (The IFN-β Multiple Sclerosis Study Group and the University of British Columbia MS/MRI Analysis Group). In animal models, however, IFN-β has a protective or aggravating effect depending on the length of treatment (Ruuls *et al.*, 1996). The mechanism of action of IFN-β is far from being defined. It might act by inhibiting production of cytokines implicated in MS, such as IL-12 and IFN-γ (Cousens *et al.*, 1997), or up-regulating IL-10 (Rudick *et al.*, 1996), but inhibition of migration of T-cells might also be important (Leppert *et al.*, 1996). Some reports also suggest a possible protective effect of IL-6. In fact, IL-6 is induced during EAE (Gijbels *et al.*, 1990). Administration of rIL-6 to mice suppresses demyelination induced by Theiler's murine encephalomyelitis virus (Rodriguez *et al.*, 1994), and anti-IL-6 antibodies that paradoxically increase the levels of bioactive IL-6 protect against EAE (Gijbels *et al.*, 1995). This could be explained by the reported inhibitory effect of IL-6 on TNF production (Aderka *et al.*, 1989; Fattori *et al.*, 1994), but one should not forget that IL-6 was originally described as an IFN-β (Zilberstein *et al.*, 1986). Indeed, IL-6 gene targeted mice are resistant to the development of EAE (Mendel *et al.*, 1998; Okuda *et al.*, 1998; Samoilova *et al.*, 1998).

It should be pointed out that data obtained from experiments using transgenic mice are not the ultimate demonstration of a role of a cytokine in autoimmunity, and these data should be considered critically (Steinman, 1997).

8.2.6 Stress

While stress has a glucocorticoid-mediated inhibitory effect on cytokine production (see below), stimulatory effects were also reported. Immobilization stress and other forms of 'psychological' stress, like open-field stress or conditioned aversion, also induce brain IL-1 mRNA and serum IL-6 (LeMay *et al.*, 1990; Zhou *et al.*, 1993). The mechanisms of these effects have not yet been defined but they may involve the stimulation of IL-6 production by adrenaline or ACTH (Van Gool *et al.*, 1990; DeRijk *et al.*, 1994). Stress also induces hyperthermia, which is enhanced by anti-TNF antibodies, suggesting that TNF might counterbalance the effect of IL-6 (Long *et al.*, 1990b).

8.3 Cytokine production in the CNS

Shortly after the cloning of IL-1, it was reported that the normal human brain contains immunoreactive IL-1β, particularly in hypothalamic neurons (Breder *et al.*, 1988), as does rat brain (Bandtlow *et al.*, 1990), which also expresses IL-1ra (Gatti and Bartfai, 1993). Widespread TNF immunoreactivity was detected in murine brain (Breder *et al.*, 1993, 1994). *In situ* hybridization studies have confirmed the presence of IL-6 mRNA in normal rat brain (Schobitz *et al.*, 1992) and IL-6 can be induced in the brain following intracerebroventricular injection of LPS (Di Santo *et al.*, 1996, 1997). In patients with meningitis IL-6 was often detected in cerebrospinal fluid (CSF) even when it was undetectable in serum (Houssiau *et al.*, 1988; Leist *et al.*, 1988; Rusconi *et al.*, 1991) suggesting that the brain was the actual source of IL-6.

Rat hypothalamus and hippocampus also express mRNA for a neutrophil chemoattractant CXC chemokine, IL-8 (Licinio and Wong, 1992). Brain expression of various chemokine receptors was reported (Horuk *et al.*, 1997). Reportedly, the brain parenchyma is refractory to leukocyte infiltration induced by injection of recombinant IL-8 (Andersson *et al.*, 1992). However, there was a report of neurological disease in transgenic mice expressing the chemokine N51/KC in oligodendrocytes (Tani *et al.*, 1996). Overexpression of IL-6 in the brain also leads to astrocytosis and gliosis (Fattori *et al.*, 1995) and subsequent augmentation of the production of other cytokines such as IL-1 and TNF (Di Santo *et al.*, 1996). MCP-1 is produced in the brain following infection, brain trauma or during EAE (Glabinski *et al.*, 1995. 1996; Berman *et al.*, 1996; Bernasconi *et al.*, 1996) and MIP-1 is also elevated in EAE (Karpus *et al.*, 1995).

Regarding the cell sources of cytokines in the brain, a large number of studies have documented production of TNF, IL-1 or IL-6 by endothelial, glial or astrocytic cells in the CNS (Riccardi-Castagnoli *et al.*, 1990; Fabry *et al.*, 1993; Sébire *et al.*, 1993; Tada *et al.*, 1993). Others have pointed out production of IL-1 or TNF by neurons(Breder *et al.*, 1988). In particular, Gahring *et al.* (Gahring *et al.*, 1996) found constitutive TNF alpha immunoreactivity in normal, unstimulated brain in glial and microglial-like cells but it was predominant in neuronal-like cells. It is likely that the TNF-producing cells in the CNS may differ with the disease. While in EAE, which has a strong inflammatory component, TNF is produced mainly by glial cells (Renno *et al.*, 1995), in excitotoxic and ischemic brain injury a neuronal TNF production was reported (Liu *et al.*, 1994; Bruce *et al.*, 1996).

8.4 Cytokine receptors in the brain

There are reports that IL-1Ra inhibits IL-1-induced fever, anorexia, activation of the HPAA, and induction of sleep, thus indicating that these effects are likely to be receptor-mediated (Opp and Krueger, 1991). Not only does IL-1Ra inhibit the central effects of directly administered IL-1 (Opp and Krueger, 1991) but it also prevents LPS-induced fever (Smith and Kluger, 1992), thus confirming a role for IL-1 as an endogenous mediator. IL-1Ra does not discriminate IL-1RI from IL-1RII but a monoclonal antibody to mouse IL-1RI prevents some of the effects of IL-1, even of mild inflammatory stimuli like turpentine, indicating that IL-1RI might be involved in the neuroendocrine response to inflammation (Rivier *et al.*, 1989). Studies with receptor type selective deletion mutants of IL-1-beta supported the concept that IL-1RI is involved in hypothalamus-pituitary-adrenal axis activation by IL-1 (Van Dam *et al.*, 1998). More conclusive results have been obtained with IL-1RI-deficient mice (reviewed in: Alheim and Bartfai, 1998).

Studies with IL-1 receptor accessory protein (IL-1RAcP)-deficient mice have shown that febrile response to IL-1 involves the IL-1RAcp (Zetterstrom *et al.*, 1998). One paper reported that a monoclonal antibody claimed to neutralize mouse IL-1RII inhibited IL-1 fever in rats (Luheshi *et al.*, 1993). However, that particular monoclonal antibody had never been conclusively shown to recognize an IL-1 receptor, and a recent report by Immunex has in fact shown that it recognized an MHC class II antigen instead (Gayle *et al.*, 1994).

Two types of TNF receptors (TNFR) have also been identified in brain by various techniques: TNFRI (or p55) and TNFRII (p75). Studies using knock-out mice or specific anti-p55 or anti-p75 agonist antibodies have suggested that p55 has the major role in one central action of TNF (Benigni *et al.*, 1996). With respect to the role of TNFR in the CNS, there was a report showing that administration of small fragments of TNF alpha to rabbits reproduced the sleep-inducing, pyrogenic and anorectic actions of TNF (Kapas *et al.*, 1992). This suggested the existence of biologically active regions in the TNF molecule and a mechanism different from the widely accepted receptor clustering by TNF trimers (Engelmann *et al.*, 1990; Beutler and van Huffel, 1994).

8.5 Second messengers of cytokine action in the brain

8.5.1 Prostaglandins

The role of prostaglandins in fever is supported by many studies, which report that IL-1, IL-6, and TNF induce prostaglandin production (particularly PGE_2) in a variety of cells, including hypothalamic explants, and the pyrogenic activity of these cytokines is inhibited by cyclooxygenase inhibitors (Wolfe and Coceani, 1979; Dinarello *et al.*, 1986, 1988, 1991; Sirko *et al.*, 1989). There seems to be a certain degree of specificity in the action of some cytokines on prostaglandin synthesis. IL-1 induces PGE_2 synthesis both in the brain (as detected from CSF levels) and in peripheral blood mononuclear cells *in vitro*, whereas IL-6 induces PGE_2 in the brain but not in peripheral blood mononuclear cells (Dinarello *et al.*, 1991).

MIP-1 and IL-8 seem to be exceptions to the generalization that fever is mediated by PGE_2. Their pyrogenic activity is independent of prostaglandins and not inhibited by cyclo-oxygenase inhibitors (Davatelis *et al.*, 1989; Zampronio *et al.*, 1994), although fever induced by IL-8 is inhibited by glucocorticoids (Zampronio *et al.*, 1994). This indicates that prostaglandin-independent mechanisms may be involved in the pyrogenicity of some cytokines.

Prostaglandins (or other arachidonic acid oxygenation products) are involved in other activities of IL-1 or TNF. For example, ibuprofen antagonizes IL-1-induced anorexia (Hellerstein *et al.*, 1989) and CRH release (Lyson and McCann, 1992).

8.5.2 Nitric oxide

NO has a great importance as a neuronal messenger by activating soluble guanylate cyclase and thus mediating increased cGMP formation in response to stimulation of the NMDA receptor in the brain (Schuman and Madison, 1994). Intracerebroventricular injection of an NO synthase inhibitor reduces the IL-1-induced increase of non-rapid eye movement sleep suggesting possible mediation by NO; however, such treatment had no effect on IL-1 fever (Kapas *et al.*, 1994). A role for NO has also been suggested in activation of the HPAA by cytokines, since NO synthase inhibitors blocked IL-2-induced CRH release and IL-1-induced CRH and ACTH release by rat hypothalamic and pituitary cells (Brunetti *et al.*, 1993; Karanth *et al.*, 1993). NO may also be neuroprotective as shown by studies with iNOS-deficient mice in traumatic brain injury (Sinz *et al.*, 1999).

8.6 Effect of psychotropic drugs on cytokine production

Several drugs acting on the CNS, such as psychotropic drugs or neurotrasmitter receptor antagonists have been reported to affect cytokine production. Although, as it will be clear later, these agents do not necessarily do so through a central action, these drugs have been included in this chapter as these effects might be of interest in the development of drugs for the therapy of cytokine-mediated diseases of the CNS. The first psychotropic drug that was reported to inhibit cytokine production is actually the oldest anti-psychotic agent, chlorpromazine (CPZ). As early as 1954 Chedid reported that CPZ had a protective action against bacterial endotoxin (Chédid, 1954) and soon after that other groups investigated this effect (Abernathy *et al.*, 1957). When it became clear that TNF was the major mediator of endotoxic shock, the possibility that CPZ might exert its protective effect on this target was considered. It was found that administration of CPZ to mice or guinea-pigs protected these animals from endotoxic shock and completely inhibited the appearance of LPS-induced serum TNF levels (Gadina *et al.*, 1991). CPZ only inhibited the production of TNF and IL-1, but did not affect that of IL-6 (Mengozzi *et al.*, 1994). Interestingly, the production of IL-10 was up-regulated by CPZ (Mengozzi *et al.*, 1994; Tarazona *et al.*, 1995). As CPZ passes the blood–brain barrier, it is also a potent inhibitor of brain TNF production (Mengozzi *et al.*, 1994).

The inhibitory effect of CPZ on TNF production was not mediated by endogenous glucocorticoids, as inhibition was also observed in adrenalectomized mice (Gadina *et al.*, 1991). Furthermore, CPZ was able to inhibit TNF production by monocytes *in vitro* (Zinetti *et al.*, 1995). Various attempts were made to correlate the inhibition of TNF production with one of the many pharmacological activities of CPZ. In fact, CPZ is a histamine receptor antagonist, serotonin (5-HT) receptor antagonist, adrenoceptor antagonist, dopamine receptor antagonist, phospholipase A_2 inhibitor (Baldessarini, 1985; Vadas *et al.*, 1986), and antioxidant (Slater, 1968; Jeding *et al.*, 1995). Some of these activities might explain its inhibition of TNF production and, in fact, other α-blockers (both α_1 and α_2, including prazosin, idazoxan and phenoxybenzamine), antiserotoninergic (including methysergide, metergoline and the catecholamine depletor, reserpine), and antihistaminic (chlorpheniramine, promethazine) drugs were the most potent inhibitors of TNF production, while the β-blocker, L-propranolol, and antidopaminergic (fluphenazine, haloperidol) or anticholinergic (scopolamine) drugs were also active, although to a lesser extent (Bertini *et al.*, 1993).

However, a study with various newly-synthesized analogues of CPZ that were devoid of these pharmacological actions indicated that none of these activities was essential for the inhibition of TNF production (Ghezzi *et al.*, 1996). Actually, this study concluded that probably CPZ acted as an antioxidant (Ghezzi *et al.*, 1996). Also, as some of these derivatives were quaternary ammonium salt that did not cross the blood–brain barrier, it was concluded that the effect of CPZ on TNF production *in vivo* did not take place through a central action (Ghezzi *et al.*, 1996).

Although these studies might indicate an usefulness of CPZ in septic shock, it should be pointed out that CPZ has a potent hypotensive action (Ghezzi *et al.*, 1996), which makes its use in shock patients problematic. This probably explains why there is a linear dose–response for the inhibitory effect of CPZ on TNF production *in vivo*, but the effect of endotoxic shock in terms of survival has a bell-shaped dose–response, for example, protection against LPS lethality is no longer observed at the higher doses of CPZ (Gadina *et al.*, 1991).

It should be mentioned that CPZ not only acts at the level of cytokine production but also at the level of their action. In fact, CPZ protects mice against the toxicity of recombinant IL-1 (Bertini *et al.*, 1989; Boraschi *et al.*, 1991) and inhibits the cytotoxicity of TNF (Libert *et al.*, 1991; Zinetti *et al.*, 1995).

Other phenothiazines share this inhibitory action (Bertini *et al.*, 1993). Interestingly, phenothiazines increase pituitary melanocyte-stimulating hormone (MSH) secretion and mimic its activity (Carter and Shuster, 1978). If we recall the anti-cytokine action of MSH, this may provide a mechanism for chlorpromazine's anti-cytokine action. In an opposite fashion, another widely used anti-psychotic agent, clozapine, induces TNF *in vitro* and *in vivo*, and this was proposed to explain fever that can occur upon administration of this drug (Hinze-Selch *et al.*, 1995; Pollmächer *et al.*, 1996). Benzodiazepines inhibit production of IL-1, IL-6, and TNF in mice, although this action seems restricted to peripheral and mixed but not central-type benzodiazepines, suggesting this may not necessarily be a CNS-mediated effect (Zavala *et al.*, 1990; Taupin *et al.*, 1993).

8.7 Neuroendocrine regulation of cytokine production

8.7.1 Corticosteroids and the hypothalamus–pituitary–adrenal axis

The hypothalamus–pituitary–adrenal axis (HPAA) is an integrated system constituted by the hypothalamus, the pituitary gland, and the adrenals, and its main function is to control of the levels of blood corticosteroids. The HPAA is usually represented as a cascade system, whereby activation of the hypothalamus (for instance by stress) causes release of hypothalamic peptide corticotropin-releasing hormone (CRH), which stimulates the release of adrenocorticotropic hormone (ACTH) by the pituitary. ACTH will be released into the blood and reach the adrenal glands to cause them to release corticosteroid (cortisol is the main corticosteroid in humans, while in mice corticosterone is the most important one). Corticosteroids, like all glucocorticoids, have a wide range of anti-inflammatory properties including inhibition of the synthesis and action of pro-inflammatory cytokines (Chapter 2). It has long been known that not only stress but also infections or injection of LPS increase blood corticosteroid levels by activating the HPAA, and this effect is inhibited in rats with complete hypothalamic deafferentiation (Ovadia *et al.*, 1989), demonstrating its central nature.

In the mid-eighties, Basedovsky and colleagues reported that IL-1 was a potent activator of the HPAA, acting at the hypothalamic level (Besedovsky *et al.*, 1986; Basedovsky and Del Rey, 1987; Berkenbosch *et al.*, 1987). This was early recognized as an immunoregulatory feedback linking IL-1 and glucocorticoids (Besedovsky *et al.*, 1986). HPAA is also

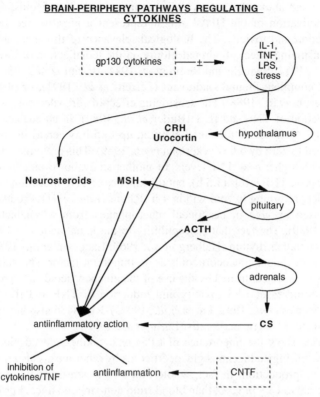

BRAIN-PERIPHERY PATHWAYS REGULATING CYTOKINES

Fig. 8.1 Cytokine regulation by the HPAA. The activation of the HPAA by IL-1 or TNF (potentiated by CNTF or IL-6) results in the cascade release of CRH, ACTH and corticosteroids (CS). Corticosteroids will inhibit cytokine synthesis and toxicity, while potentiating cytokine induction of liver acute-phase proteins (APP) and of pituitary MSH, which are also protective. ACTH may also directly inhibit TNF synthesis. The figure also outlines the possibility that CRH may also be a mediator of cytokine-induced fever and anorexia, and of the inhibitory feedback exerted by CS on the HPAA.

activated, although to a lesser extent, by injection of TNF (Benigni *et al.*, 1996). All gp130-user cytokines (IL-6, IL-11, LIF, cardiotrophin-1, oncostatin M, ciliary neurotrophic factor), while not significantly elevating corticosterone levels in mice, potentiate the elevation of corticosterone induced by IL-1 (Benigni *et al.*, 1995, 1996; Fantuzzi *et al.*, 1995a).

Studies with a monoclonal antibody to the type I IL-1 receptor have shown that IL-1 mediates the activation of HPAA observed during inflammation (Rivier *et al.*, 1989). Although in experimental models *in vitro*, IL-1 and IL-6 directly stimulated adrenocorticotropic hormone (ACTH) release from pituitary cells (Woloski *et al.*, 1985; Bernton *et al.*, 1987), the increase of blood GC *in vivo* seems mainly due to stimulation of hypothalamic cells to release corticotropin-releasing hormone (CRH) (Tsagarakis *et al.*, 1989). IL-1-induced elevation of GC levels is associated with increased CRH in the pituitary portal vessels and anti-CRH antibodies inhibited IL-1-induced GC, thus indicating that IL-1 exerts this effect through hypothalamic CRH (Sapolsky *et al.*, 1987; Bernardini *et al.*, 1990).

We have discussed above the anti-cytokine actions of glucocorticoids, and this suggests that the activation of the HPAA might represent a negative feedback to limit cytokine production and toxicity. The biological relevance of this mechanism is illustrated by the sensitizing effect of adrenalectomy on the lethal action of infections, LPS (Abernathy *et al.*, 1957; Swingle and Remington, 1944; Bertini *et al.*, 1988), turpentine (Krauss, 1962), complete Freund's adjuvant (Perretti *et al.*, 1991), or of recombinant TNF or IL-1 (Bertini *et al.*, 1988). The sensitizing effect of adrenalectomy was related to increased production of TNF and IL-1 (Butler *et al.*, 1989). In adrenalectomized mice injected with LPS, TNF levels remained elevated up to 5 h, whereas in sham-operated mice they returned to zero by 3 h (Zuckerman *et al.*, 1989). This prolonged induction was not associated with higher peak TNF levels. In another study, however, adrenalectomized mice had higher peak TNF levels (1.5 h), but the kinetics of TNF induction was similar to that of intact mice, returning to zero within 4 h (Parant *et al.*, 1991). Production of IL-1 was also increased *ex vivo* in peritoneal macrophages from adrenalectomized rats (Perretti *et al.*, 1989). The fact that susceptibility to the lethal action of LPS and TNF varies with the circadian rhythm (Halberg *et al.*, 1960; Langevin *et al.*, 1987) also supports a role for endogenous glucocorticoids as an important factor. The data on adrenalectomized animals were confirmed by the use of the glucocorticoids receptor antagonist RU38486, which increases LPS toxicity and induction of TNF and IL-6 (Lazar and Agarwal, 1986; Hawes *et al.*, 1992; Lazar *et al.*, 1992a). RU38486 also increased mortality in a mouse model of septic peritonitis (Lazar *et al.*, 1992b).

While these data show the importance of LPS- or cytokine-induced blood glucocorticoids levels, increasing endogenous glucocorticoids by other means also results in inhibition of cytokine production. In fact, whole blood from stressed mice produced less TNF, when exposed to LPS *in vitro*, than blood from non-stressed mice. Furthermore, the addition of a GC receptor antagonist restored normal TNF production in the stressed mice (Fantuzzi *et al.*, 1995). In addition, treating the mice with ACTH to increase serum corticosterone, reduced the TNF produced in response to an LPS injection (Fantuzzi *et al.*, 1995), and ACTH is still used as a therapeutic agent, although rarely, (Schimmer and Parker, 1996).

An impairment of the HPAA response correlates with higher susceptibility to TNF- and IL-1-mediated pathologies including experimental allergic encephalomyelitis (EAE) and arthritis. The role of endogenous GC in the susceptibility to EAE has been reviewed by Mason (Mason, 1991). EAE activates the HPAA as revealed by the increase in serum glucocorticoids. Adrenalectomized rats do not recover spontaneously from EAE, and adrenalectomy increases the mortality rate in this animal model (MacPhee *et al.*, 1989). Rat strains that are genetically resistant to the development of EAE have more marked HPAA activation to stressing stimuli, and adrenalectomy can render them normally susceptible to EAE. Lewis rats, which are genetically prone to streptococcal cell wall-induced arthritis, had markedly impaired ACTH and GC responses to streptococcal cell wall or IL-1 (Sternberg *et al.*, 1989). On the other hand, RU38486 induced susceptibility to streptococcal cell wall arthritis in normal rats. Thus, genetic susceptibility to arthritis might be related to a defective HPAA responsiveness to cytokines.

The activation of the HPAA by IL-1 can also have immunosuppressive effects. In fact, centrally injected IL-1 has an immunosuppressive effect, suppressing IL-1 production by splenic macrophages. This effect is inhibited not only by adrenalectomy, suggesting a role for the HPAA, but also by surgical interruption of the splenic nerve, suggesting a role of the sympathetic nervous system (Brown *et al.*, 1991). Centrally administered IL-1 also reduces NK cell activity, lymphocyte proliferation and IL-2 production (Sundar *et al.*, 1989, 1990). These immunosuppressive effects were prevented by anti-CRH antibodies and by pharmacological blockade of the sympathetic nervous system. Results were similar when the HIV envelope protein gp120 was injected intracerebroventricularly, leading to production of endogenous IL-1 in the brain (Sundar *et al.*, 1991).

8.7.2 Corticosteroid-independent effects of corticotropin-releasing hormone (CRH)

CRH is also a mediator, in a GC-independent fashion, of some of the effects of IL-1. Besides its role in ACTH release, CRH also acts as a neuropeptide within the CNS, mediating some responses to stress, including stress-induced anorexia (Brown *et al.*, 1986; Shibasaki *et al.*, 1988). Anti-CRH antibodies or CRH receptor antagonists attenuate IL-1 induced anorexia (Uehara *et al.*, 1989) and fever (Rothwell, 1989), suggesting that CRH is a central mediator for these effects. The finding that DEX inhibits IL-1-induced anorexia (Plata-Salaman, 1991) might also be explained through a down-regulation of CRH production. Regarding a direct effect of CRH on IL-1 production, reports contrast, indicating that CRH either inhibits or augmentats IL-1 production (Singh and Leu, 1990; Payne *et al.*, 1994). Various reports have described immunosuppressive or anti-inflammatory effects of exogenously administered CRH (Wei *et al.*, 1988; Labeur *et al.*, 1995; Correa *et al.*, 1997; Poliak *et al.*, 1997), and CRH transgenic mice have an immunosuppressive phenotype which is reversed by adrenalectomy (Boehme *et al.*, 1997). A recently described peptide homologous to CRH, urocortin (Vaughan *et al.*, 1995), was also shown to possess antiinflammatory activity (Turnbull *et al.*, 1996) and inhibit EAE (Poliak *et al.*, 1997).

However, the mechanism of anti-inflammatory action of CRH is unclear. Some reports suggest that CRH may have anti-inflammatory activities independently on endogenous corticosteroids (Kelley *et al.*, 1994; Poliak *et al.*, 1997). On the other hand, proinflammatory activities of CRH have been reported (Karalis *et al.*, 1991). Admininstration of urocortin or CRH inhibits LPS-induced TNF production (Agnello *et al.*, 1998). However, inhibition of corticosterone synthesis with cyanoketone did not prevent inhibition of TNF production by urocortin and this observation supports the hypothesis that antiinflammatory mechanisms of neuropeptides exist and work independently on the HPAA.

8.7.3 Melanocyte-stimulating hormone and other proopiomelanocortin peptides

Melanocyte-stimulating hormone (α-MSH) is a product of the pro-opiomelanocortin gene sharing the 1–13 amino acids with ACTH. This hormone has a wide spectrum of anti-cytokine actions and can be detected in the CNS, as well as in the circulation (reviewed in: Catania and Lipton, 1993; Lipton and Catania, 1997). When administered peripherally or intracerebroventricularly, MSH inhibits cytokine-induced fever (Murphy *et al.*, 1983) and, on a molar basis, is 25 000 times more potent than acetaminophen. MSH inhibits fever induced by LPS (Martin and Lipton, 1990), IL-1 (Murphy *et al.*, 1983; Daynes *et al.*, 1987), TNF, and IL-6 (Martin *et al.*, 1991). LPS injection also raises plasma MSH,

Table 8.4 Pathologies with elevated α-MSH levels

Endotoxemia in animal models (inhibition of MSH has worsening effect)
LPS-injected human volunteers (high MSH correlates with lower fever)
HIV infection (high MSH correlates with 6-month survival)
Rheumatoid arthritis (higher that in osteoarthritis)
Septic shock
Myocardial infarction and unstable angina

Table 8.5 Anti-inflammatory actions of α-MSH

Endotoxin fever
Endotoxic shock
Septic shock (cecal ligation and puncture)
ARDS in rats (intratracheal LPS)
Arthritis (rat adjuvant arthritis)
Skin inflammation (chemically induced in mice)
Hind paw inflammation

suggesting that this neuropeptide may provide an inhibitory feedback signal (Lipton *et al.*, 1991). Interestingly, this feedback mechanism is potentiated by DEX (Lipton *et al.*, 1991) and, in fact, anti-MSH antibodies worsen LPS fever (Clarke and Bost, 1989). Tables 8.4 and 8.5 list the various pathologies in which MSH is elevated and those where MSH administration has protective effects, respectively.

The mechanism of the anti-inflammatory action of MSH is complex and the data in the literature suggest both a direct and a centrally-mediated effect. The fact that MSH acts centrally is obvious in fever, but was also demonstrated in models of peripheral inflammation, such as that induced by picryl chloride in the mouse ear or in mice with hind paw inflammation. In these cases, it was reported that MSH was particularly effective when administered intracerebroventricularly (Catania and Lipton, 1993; Lipton and Catania, 1997). The anti-inflammatory effect of centrally-administered MSH was inhibited by β2 adrenergic receptor antagonists (see the inhibitory effect of beta-adrenergic agonists in Chapter 2).

Spinal cord transection inhibited the anti-inflammatory action of centrally administered MSH, but an anti-inflammatory action was still observed when the peptide was injected ip (Catania and Lipton, 1993; Lipton and Catania, 1997). Probably the strongest data supporting a direct, non-centrally-mediated, anti-inflammatory mechanism of MSH come from studies of the effect of MSH on cytokine production *in vitro*. MSH, like the other pro-opiomelanocortin peptide, ACTH, inhibits TNF production by LPS-stimulated human peripheral blood mononuclear cells (Lipton and Catania, 1997) and induces IL-10 production (Bhardwaj *et al.*, 1996). MSH also inhibits the induction of NO synthase *in vivo* (Lipton and Catania, 1997).

MSH is a 13-amino acid peptide but it is of particular importance for its pharmacological use that its anti-inflammatory activity can be reproduced by its C-terminal tripeptide (Lysine-Proline-Arginine) (Lipton and Catania, 1997). This could, thus, represent a candidate for both therapeutic use and drug design.

8.7.4 Miscellaneous hormones

The pituitary peptide growth hormone (GH) has been reported to inhibit the production of TNF and nuclear translocation of NF-kB in human monocytes or macrophages. This was observed both by adding recombinant human GH and by transfecting THP-1 cells with a GH-producing expression vector. This effect was specific for LPS-induced TNF, as PMA-induced TNF or NF-kB translocation were unaffected (Haeffner *et al.*, 1997).

8.7.5 Neurotransmitters and neurotransmitter receptor antagonists

The inhibitory effects of β-adrenoreceptor agonists on cytokine production have been discussed in Chapter 2. It should be noted, however, that α-adrenoceptor blockers inhibit TNF production *in vivo* (Bloksma *et al.*, 1982).On the other hand, serotonin was reported to induce production of TNF, IL-6, and TGF-beta (Pousset *et al.*, 1996), while antisero-toninergic agents inhibit TNF production (Bertini *et al.*, 1993).

References

Abernathy, R. S., Halberg, F., and Spink, W. W. (1957). Studies on mechanism of chloropromazine protection against Brucella endotoxin. *J. Lab. Clin. Med.*, **49**, 708–15.

Aderka, D., Le, J., and Vilcek, J. (1989). IL-6 inhibits lipopolysaccharide-induced tumor necrosis factor production in cultured human monocytes, U937 cells, and in mice. *J. Immunol.*, **143**, 3517–23.

Adorini, L., Gregori, S., Magram, J., and Trembleau, S. (1996). The role of IL-12 in the pathogenesis of Th1 cell-mediated autoimmune diseases. *Ann. NY Acad. Sci.*, **795**, 208–15.

Agnello, D., Bertini, R., Sacco, S., Meazza, C., Villa, P., and Ghezzi, P. (1998). Corticosteroid-independent inhibition of tumor necrosis factor production by the neuropeptide urocortin. *Am. J. Physiol.*, **38**, E757-E62.

Alheim, K. and Bartfai, T. (1998). The interleukin-1 system: receptors, ligands, and ICE in the brain and their involvement in the fever response. *Ann. NY Acad. Sci.*, **840**, 51–8.

Andersson, P. B., Perry, V. H., and Gordon, S. (1992). Intracerebral injection of proinflammatory cytokines or leukocyte chemotaxins induces minimal myelomonocytic cell recruitment to the parenchyma of the central nervous system. *J. Exp. Med.*, **176**, 255–9.

Baldessarini, R. J. (1985). Drugs and the treatment of psychiatric disorders. In *The pharmacological basis of therapeutics*, (7th edn), (ed. A. Goodman Gilman, L. S. Goodman, T. W. Rall, and F. Murad), pp. 387–445. Macmillan Publishing Co., New York.

Bandtlow, C. E., Meyer, M., Lindholm, D., Spranger, M., Heumann, R., and Thoenen, H. (1990). Regional and cellular codistribution of interleukin 1 beta and nerve growth factor mRNA in the adult rat brain: possible relationship to the regulation of nerve growth factor synthesis. *J. Cell. Biol.*, **111**, 1701–11.

Barone, F. C. and Feuerstein, G. Z. (1999). Inflammatory mediators and stoke: new opportunities for novel therapeutics. *J. Cereb. Blood Flow Metab.*, **19**, 819–34.

Basedovsky, H. and Del Rey, A. (1987). Neuroendocrine and metabolic responses induced by interleukin-1. *J. Neurosci. Res.*, **18**, 172–8.

Benigni, F., Fantuzzi, G., Sironi, M., Sacco, S., Pozzi, P., Dinarello, C. A. *et al.* (1995). Six different cytokines that share gp130 as a receptor subunit, induce serum amyloid A and potentiate the induction of interleukin-6 and the activation of the hypothalamus-pituitary-adrenal axis by interleukin-1. *Blood*, **87**, 1851–4.

Benigni, F., Faggioni, R., Sironi, M., Fantuzzi, G., Vandenabeele, P., Takahashi, N. *et al.* (1996). Tumor necrosis factor receptor p55 plays a major role in centrally-mediated increases of serum IL-6 and corticosterone after intracerebroventricular injection of TNF. *J. Immunol.*, **157**, 5563–8.

Benigni, F., Sacco, S., Pennica, D., and Ghezzi, P. (1996). Cardiotrophin-1 (CT-1) inhibits TNF production in the heart and serum of LPS-treated mice and *in vitro* in mouse blood cells. *Am. J. Pathol.*, **149**, 1847–50.

Berkenbosch, F., Van Oers, J., Del Rey, A., Tilders, F., and Basedovsky, H. (1987). Corticotropin-releasing factor-producing neurons in the rat activated by interleukin-1. *Science*, **238**, 524–6.

Berman, J. W., Guida, M. P., Warren, J., amat, J., and Brosnan, C. F. (1996). Localization of monocyte chemoattractant peptide-1 expression in the central nervous system in experimental autoimmune encephalomyelitis and trauma in the rat. *J. Immunol.*, **156**, 3017–23.

Bernardini, R., Calogero, A. E., Mauceri, G., and Chrousos, G. P. (1990). Rat hypothalamic corticotropin-releasing hormone secretion *in vitro* is stimulated by interleukin-1 in a eicosanoid-dependent manner. *Life Sci.*, **47**, 1601–7.

Bernasconi, S., Cinque, P., Peri, G., Sozzani, S., Crociati, A., Torri, W. *et al.* (1996). Selective elevation of monocyte chemotactic protein-1 in the cerebrospinal fluid of AIDS patients with cytomegalovirus encephalitis. *J. Infect. Dis.*, **174**, 1098–101.

Bernstein, I. L., Taylor, E. M., and Bentson, K. L. (1991). TNF-induced anorexia and learned food aversions are attenuated by area postrema lesions. *Am. J. Physiol.*, **260**, R906-R10.

Bernton, E. W., Beach, J. E., Holaday, J. W., Smallridge, R. C., and Fein, H. G. (1987). Release of multiple hormones by a direct action of interleukin-1 on pituitary cells. *Science*, **238**, 519–21.

Bertini, R., Bianchi, M., and Ghezzi, P. (1988). Adrenalectomy sensitizes mice to the lethal effects of interleukin 1 and tumor necrosis factor. *J. Exp. Med.*, **167**, 1708–12.

Bertini, R., Bianchi, M., and Ghezzi, P. (1989). Protective effect of chloropromazine against the lethality of interleukin 1 in adrenalectomized or actinomicin D-sensitized mice. *Biochem. Biophys. Res. Commun.*, **165**, 942–6.

Bertini, R., Garattini, S., Delgado, R., and Ghezzi, P. (1993). Pharmacological activities of chlorpromazine involved in the inhibition of tumor necrosis factor production *in vivo* mice. *Immunology*, **79**, 217–9.

Bertorelli, R., Adami, M., Di Santo, E., and Ghezzi, P. (1998). MK801 and dexamethasone decrease tumor necrosis factor (TNF) levels and reduce cerebral ischemia injury in rat brain. *Neuropharmacology*, **246**, 41–4.

Besedovsky, H., Del Rey, A., and Dinarello, C. A. (1986). Immunoregulatory feedback between interleukin-1 and glucocorticoid hormones. *Science*, **233**, 652–4.

Beutler, B. and van Huffel, C. (1994). Unraveling function in the TNF ligand and receptor families. *Science*, **264**, 667–8.

Bhardwaj, R. S., Schwarz, A., Becher, E., Mahnke, K., Aragane, Y., Schwarz, T. *et al.* (1996). Proopiomelanocortin-derived peptides induce IL-10 production in human monocytes. *J. Immunol.*, **156**, 2517–21.

Bloksma, N., Hofhuis, F., Benaissa-Trouw, B., and Willers, J. (1982). Endotoxin-induced release of tumour necrosis factor and interferon *in vivo* is inhibited by prior adrenoceptor blockade. *Cancer Immunol Immunother,* **14**, 41–5.

Bodnar, R. J., Pasternak, G. W., Mann, P. E., Paul, D., Warren, R., and Donner, D. B. (1989). Mediation of anorexia by human recombinant tumor necrosis factor through a peripheral action in the rat. *Cancer Res.*, **49**, 6280–4.

Boehme, S. A., Gaur, A., Crowe, P. D., Liu, X.-J., Tamraz, S., Wong, T. *et al.* (1997). Immunosuppressive phenotype of corticotropin-releasing factor transgenic mice is reversed by adrenalectomy. *Cell. Immunol.*, **176**, 103–12.

Boraschi, D., Villa, L., Ghiara, P., Tagliabue, A., Mengozzi, M., Solito, E. *et al.* (1991). Mechanism of acute toxicity of IL-1beta in mice. *Eur. Cytokine Netw.*, **2**, 61–7.

Breder, C. D., Dinarello, C. A., and Saper, C. B. (1988). Interleukin-1 immunoreactive innervation of the human hypothalamus. *Science*, **240**, 321–4.

Breder, C. D., Tsujimoto, M., Terano, Y., Scott, D. W., and Saper, C. B. (1993). Distribution and characterization of tumor necrosis factor-α-like immunoreactivity in the murine central nervous system. *J. Comp. Neurol.*, **337**, 543–67.

Breder, C. D., Hazuka, C., Ghayur, T., Klug, C., Huginin, M., Yasuda, K. *et al.* (1994). Regional induction of tumor necrosis factor α expression in the mouse brain after systemic lipopolysaccharide administration. *Proc. Natl. Acad. Sci.USA*, **91**, 11393–7.

Brenneman, D. E., McCune, S. K., and Gozes, I. (1993). Acquired immunodeficiency syndrome and the developing nervous system. *Internat. Rev. Neurobiol.*, **32**, 305–53.

Brosnan, C. F., Cannella, B., Battistini, L., and Raine, C. S. (1995). Cytokine localization in multiple sclerosis lesions: correlation with adhesion molecule expression and reactive nitrogen intermediates. *Neurology*, **45**, S16-S21.

Brown, M. R., Gray, T. S., and Fisher, L. A. (1986). Corticotropin-releasing factor receptor antagonist: effects on the autonomic nervous system and cardiovascular functions. *Regul. Pept.*, **16**, 321–9.

Brown, R., Li, Z., Vriend, C. Y., Nirula, R., Janz, L., Falk, J. *et al.* (1991). Suppression of splenic macrophage interleukin-1 secretion following intracerebroventricular injection of interleukin-1 β: evidence for pituitary-adrenal and sympathetic control. *Cell. Immunol.*, **132**, 84–93.

Bruce, A. J., Boling, W., Kindy, M. S., Peschon, J., Kraemer, P. J., Carpenter, M. K. *et al.* (1996). Altered neuronal and microglial responses to excitotoxic and ischemic brain injury in mice lacking TNF receptors. *Nature Medicine*, **2**, 788–94.

Brunetti, L., Preziosi, P., Ragazzoni, E., and Vacca, M. (1993). Involvement of nitric oxide in basal and interleukin-1 beta-induced CRH and ACTH release *in vitro*. *Life Sci.*, **53**, PL219-PL22.

Butler, L. D., Layman, N. K., Riedl, P. E., Cain, R. L., Shellhaas, J., Evans, G. F. *et al.* (1989). Neuroendocrine regulation of *in vivo* cytokine production and effects: I. *In vivo* regulatory networks involving the neuroendocrine system, interleukin-1 and tumor necrosis factor-α. *J. Neuroimmunol.*, **24**, 143–53.

Campbell, I. L., Eddleston, M., Kemper, P., Oldstone, M. B., and Hobbs, M. V. (1994). Activation of cerebral cytokine gene expression and its correlation with onset of reactive astrocyte and acute-phase response gene expression in scrapie. *J. Virol.*, **68**, 2383–7.

Carter, M. J. and Shuster, S. (1978). Melanocyte-stimulating hormone-mimetic action of the phenothiazines. *J. Pharm. Pharmac.*, **30**, 233–5.

Cash, E., Minty, A., Ferrara, P., Caput, D., Fradelizi, D., and Rott, O. (1994). Macrophage-inactivating IL-13 suppresses experimental autoimmune encephalomyelitis in rats. *J. Immunol.*, **153**, 4258–67.

Catania, A. and Lipton, J. M. (1993). Alpha-melanocyte stimulating hormone in the modulation of host reactions. *Endocrine Reviews*, **14**, 564–76.

Chai, Z., Gatti, S., Toniatti, C., Poli, V., and Bartfai, T. (1996). Interleukin (IL)-6 gene expression in the central nervous system is necessary for fever response to lipopolysaccharide or IL-1 beta: a study on IL-6-deficient mice. *J. Exp. Med.*, **183**, 311–6.

Chao, C. C. and Hu, S. (1994). Tumor necrosis factor-alpha potentiates glutamate neurotoxicity in human fetal brain cell cultures. *Dev. Neurosci.*, **16**, 172–9.

Chédid, L. (1954). Actions comparées de la prométhazine, de la chlorpromazine et de la cortisone chez la Souris recevant des doses mortelles d'une endotoxine bacterienne. *C. Rendu. Soc. Biol.*, **148**, 1039–43.

Clarke, B. L. and Bost, K. L. (1989). Differential expression of functional adrenocorticotropic hormone receptors by subpopulations of lymphocytes. *J. Immunol.*, **143**, 464–9.

Correa, S. G., Riera, C. M., Spiess, J., and Bianco, I. D. (1997). Modulation of the inflammatory response by corticotropin-releasing factor. *Eur. J. Pharmacol.*, **319**, 85–90.

Cousens, L. P., Orange, J. S., Su, E. C., and Biron, C. A. (1997). Interferon-α/β inhibition of interleukin 12 and interferon-g production *in vitro* and endogenously during viral infection. *Proc. Natl. Acad. Sci.USA*, **94**, 634–39.

Davatelis, G., Wolpe, S. D., Sherry, B., Dayer, J.-M., Chicheportiche, R., and Cerami, A. (1989). Macrophage inflammatory protein-1: a prostaglandin-independent endogenous pyrogen. *Science*, **243**, 1066–8.

Daynes, R. A., Robertson, B. A., Cho, B. H., Burnham, D. K., and Newton, R. (1987). α-melanocyte-stimulating hormone exhibits target cell selectivity in this capacity to affect interleukin-1-inducible responses *in vivo* and *in vitro*. *J. Immunol.*, **139**, 103–9.

DeRijk, R. H., Boelen, A., Tilders, F. J., and Berkenbosch, F. (1994). Induction of plasma interleukin-6 by circulating adrenaline in the rat. *Psychoneuroendocrinology*, **19**, 155–63.

Dinarello, C. A., Cannon, J. G., Wolff, S. M., Bernheim, H. A., Beutler, B., and Cerami, A. (1986). Tumor necrosis factor(cachectin) is an endogenous pyrogen and induces production of interleukin 1. *J. Exp. Med.*, **163**, 1433–1450.

Dinarello, C. A., Cannon, J. G., and Wolff, S. M. (1988). New concepts in the pathogenesis of fever. *Rev. Infect. Dis.*, **10**, 168–89.

Dinarello, C. A., Cannon, J. G., Mancilla, J., Bishai, I., Lees, J., and Coceani, F. (1991). Interleukin-6 as an endogenous pyrogen: induction of prostaglandin E_2 in brain but not in peripheral blood mononuclear cells. *Brain Res.*, **562**, 199–206.

Di Santo, E., Alonzi, T., Fattori, E., Poli, V., Ciliberto, G., Sironi, M. *et al.* (1996). Overexpression of IL-6 in the brain of transgenic mice increases central but not systemic proinflammatory cytokine production. *Brain Res.*, **740**, 239–44.

Di Santo, E., Alonzi, T., Poli, V., Fattori, E., Toniatti, C., Sironi, M. *et al.* (1997). Differential effects of IL-6 on systemic and central production of TNF. *Cytokine*, **9**, 300–6.

Donnelly, R. J., Friedhoff, A. J., Ber, B., Blume, A. J., and Vitek, M. P. (1990). Interleukin-1 stimulates the beta-amyloid precursor protein promoter. *Cell. Mol. Neurobiol.*, **10**, 485–95.

Duong, T. T., St Louis, J., Gilbert, J. J., Finkelman, F. D., and Strejan, G. H. (1992). Effect of anti-interferon-gamma and anti-interleukin-2 monoclonal antibody treatment on the development of actively and passively induced experimental allergic encephalomyelitis in the SJL/J mouse. *J. Neuroimmunol.*, **36**, 105–15.

Duong, T. T., Finkelman, F. D., Singh, B., and Strejan, G. H. (1994). Effect of anti-interferon-gamma monoclonal antibody treatment on the development of experimental allergic encephalomyelitis in resistant mouse strains. *J. Neuroimmunol.*, **53**, 101–7.

Emilie, D., Wijdens, J., Gisselbrecht, C., Jarrousse, B., Billaud, E., Blay, J.-V. *et al.* (1994). Administration of an anti-interleukin-6 monoclonal antibody to patients with acquired immunodeficiency syndrome and lymphoma: effect on lymphoma growth and on B clinical symptoms. *Blood*, **84**, 2472–9.

Engelmann, H., Holtmann, H., Brakenbusch, C., Avni, Y. S., Sarov, I., Nophar, Y. *et al.* (1990). Antibodies to a soluble form of a tumor necrosis factor (TNF) receptor have TNF-like activity. *J. Biol. Chem.*, **265**, 14497–504.

Fabry, Z., Fitzsimmons, K. M., Herlein, J. A., Moninger, T. O., Dobbs, M. B., and Hart, M. N. (1993). Production of the cytokines interleukin 1 and 6 by murine brain microvessel endothelium and smooth muscle pericytes. *J. Neuroimmunol.*, **47**, 23–34.

Fantuzzi, G., Benigni, F., Sironi, M., Conni, M., Carelli, M., Cantoni, L. *et al.* (1995a). Ciliary neurotrophic factor induces serum amyloid A, hypoglycemia and anorexia, and potentiates IL-1-induced corticosterone and IL-6 production in mice. *Cytokine*, **7**, 150–6.

Fantuzzi, G., Di Santo, E., Sacco, S., Benigni, F., and Ghezzi, P. (1995b). Role of the hypothalamus-pituitary-adrenal axis in the regulation of tumor necrosis factor production in mice: effect of stress and inhibition of endogenous glucocorticoids. *J. Immunol.*, **155**, 3552–5.

Fattori, E., Cappelletti, M., Costa, P., Sellitto, C., Cantoni, L., Carelli, M. *et al.* (1994). Defective inflammatory response in IL-6 deficient mice. *J. Exp. Med.*, **180**, 1243–50.

Fattori, E., Lazzaro, D., Musiani, P., Modesti, A., Alonzi, T., and Ciliberto, G. (1995). IL-6 expression in neurons of transgenic mice causes reactive astrocytosis and increase in ramified microglial cells but no neuronal damage. *Eur. J. Neurosci.*, **7**, 2441–9.

Gadina, M., Bertini, R., Mengozzi, M., Zandalasini, M., Mantovani, A., and Ghezzi, P. (1991). Protective effect of chlorpromazine on endotoxin toxicity and TNF production in glucocorticoid-sensitive and glucocorticoid-resistant models of endotoxic shock. *J. Exp. Med.*, **173**, 1305–10.

Gahring, L. C., Carlson, N. G., Kulmar, R. A., and Rogers, S. W. (1996). Neuronal expression of tumor necrosis factor alpha in the murine brain. *Neuroimmunomodulation.*, **3**, 289–303.

Gallo, P., Frei, K., Rordorf, C., Lazdins, J., Tavolato, B., and Fontana, A. (1989). Human immunodeficiency virus type 1 (HIV-1) infection of the central nervous system: an evaluation of cytokines in cerebrospinal fluid. *J. Neuroimmunol.*, **23**, 109–16.

Gately, M. K., Renzetti, L. M., Magram, J., Stern, A. S., Adorini, L., Gubler, U. *et al.* (1998). The interleukin-12/interleukin-12-receptor system: role in normal and pathologic immune responses. *Ann. Rev. Immunol.*, **16**, 495–521.

Gatti, S. and Bartfai, T. (1993). Induction of tumor necrosis factor-α mRNA in the brain after peripheral endotoxin treatment: comparison with interleukin-1 family and interleukin-6. *Brain Res.*, **624**, 291–4.

Gayle, M. A., Sims, J. E., Dower, S. K., and Slack, J. L. (1994). Monoclonal antibody 1994–01 (also known as Alva 42) reported to recognize type II IL-1 receptor is specific for HLA-DR alpha and beta chains. *Cytokine*, **6**, 83–6.

Gelin, J., Moldawer, L. L., Lönnroth, C., Sherry, B., Chizonnite, R., and Lundholm, K. (1991). Role of endogenous tumor necrosis factor α and interleukin 1 for experimental tumor growth and the development of cancer cachexia. *Cancer Res.*, **51**, 415–21.

Ghezzi, P., Garattini, S., Mennini, T., Bertini, R., Delgado Hernandez, R., Benigni, F. *et al.* (1996). Mechanism of inhibition of tumor necrosis factor production by chlorpromazine and its derivatives in mice. *Eur. J. Pharmacol.*, **317**, 369–76.

Gijbels, K., Van Damme, J., Proost, P., Put, W., Carton, H., and Billiau, A. (1990). Interleukin 6 production in the central nervous system during experimental autoimmune encephalomyelitis. *Eur. J. Immunol.*, **20**, 233–5.

Gijbels, K., Brocke, S., Abrams, J. S., and Steinman, L. (1995). Administration of neutralizing antibodies to interleukin-6 (IL-6) reduces experimental autoimmune encephalomyelitis and is associated with elevated levels of IL-6 bioactivity in central nervous system and circulation. *Mol..Med.*, **1**, 795–805.

Glabinski, A. R., Tani, M., Tuohy, V. K., Tuthill, R. J., and Ransohoff, R. M. (1995). Central nervous system chemokine mRNA accumulation follows initial leukocyte entry at the onset of acute murine experimental autoimmune encephalomyelitis. *Brain Behav. Immun.*, **9**, 315–30.

Glabinski, A. R., Balasingam, V., Tani, M., Kunkel, S. L., Strieter, R. M., Yong, V. W. *et al.* (1996). Chemokine monocyte chemoattractant protein-1 is expressed by astrocytes after mechanical injury to the brain. *J. Immunol.*, **156**, 4363–8.

Gloaguen, I., Costa, P., Demartis, A., Lazzaro, D., Di Marco, A., Graziani, R. *et al.* (1997). Ciliary neurotrophic factor corrects obesity and diabetes associated with leptin deficiency and resistance. *Proc. Natl. Acad. Sci.USA*, **94**, 6456–61.

Goldbach, J.-M., Roth, J., Störr, B., and Zeisberger, E. (1997). Influence of pentoxifylline on fevers induced by bacterial lipopolysaccharide and tumor necrosis factor-α in guinea pigs. *Eur. J. Pharmacol.*, **319**, 273–8.

Goldberg, R. M., Loprinzi, C. L., Mailliard, J. A., O'Fallo, J. R., Krook, J. E., Ghosh, C. *et al.* (1995). Pentoxifylline for treatment of cancer anorexia and cachexia? A randomized, double-blind, placebo-controlled trial. *J. Clin. Oncol.*, **13**, 2856–9.

Grau, G., Fajardo, L. F., Piguet, P.-F., Allet, B., Lambert, P.-H., and Vassalli, P. (1987). Tumor necrosis factor (cachectin) as an essential mediator in murine cerebral malaria. *Science*, **237**, 210–13.

Griffin, W. S., Stanley, L. C., Ling, C., White, L., MacLeod, V., Perrot, L. J. *et al.* (1989). Brain interleukin 1 and S-100 immunoreactivity are elevated in Down's syndrome and Alzheimer's disease. *Proc. Natl. Acad. Sci.USA*, **86**, 7611–5.

Grimaldi, L. M. E., Martino, G. V., Franciotta, D. M., Brustia, R., Castagna, A., Pristerà, R. *et al.* (1991). Elevated alpha-tumor necrosis factor levels in spinal fluid from HIV-1-infected patients with central nervous system involvement. *Ann. Neurol.*, **29**, 21–5.

Hack, V., Gross, A., Kinscherf, R., Bockstette, M., Fiers, W., Berke, G. *et al.* (1996). Abnormal glutathione and sulfate levels after interleukin 6 treatment and in tumor-induced cachexia. *FASEB J.*, **10**, 1219–26.

Haeffner, A., Thieblemont, N., Déas, O., Marelli, O., Charpentiar, B., Senik, A. *et al.* (1997). Inhibitory effect of growth hormone on TNF-α secretion and nuclear factor-kB translocation in lipopolysaccharide-stimulated human monocytes. *J. Immunol.*, **158**, 1310–4.

Halberg, F., Johnson, E. A., Brown, B. W., and Bittner, J. J. (1960). Susceptibility rhythm to *E. coli* endotoxin and bioassay. *Proc. Soc. Exp. Biol.*, **103**, 142–7.

Hauser, S. L., Doolittle, T. H., Lincoln, R., Brown, R. H., and Dinarello, C. A. (1990). Cytokine accumulation in CSF of multiple sclerosis patients: frequent detection of interleukin-1 and tumor necrosis factor but not interleukin-6. *Neurology*, **40**, 1735–9.

Hawes, A. S., Rock, C. S., Keogh, C. V., Lowry, S. F., and Calvano, S. E. (1992). *In vivo* effects of the antiglucocorticoid RU 486 on glucocorticoid and cytokine response to *Escherichia coli* endotoxin. *Infect. Immun.*, **60**, 2641–7.

Hellerstein, M. K., Meydani, S. N., Meydani, M., and Dinarello, C. A. (1989). Interleukin-1-induced anorexia in rat. *J. Clin. Invest.*, **84**, 228–35.

Hinze-Selch, D., Mullington, J., and Pollmächer, T. (1995). Sleep during clozapine-induced fever in a schizophrenic patient. *Biological Psychiatry*, **38**, 690–3.

Hofman, F. M., Hinton, D. R., Johnson, K., and Merril, J. E. (1989). Identification of lymphotoxin and tumor necrosis factor identified in multiple sclerosis brain *J. Exp. Med.*, **170**, 607–12.

Horuk, R., Martin, A. W., Wang, Z., Schweitzer, L., Gerassimides, A., Guo, H. *et al.* (1997). Expression of chemokine receptors by subsets of neurons in the central nervous system. *J. Immunol.*, **158**, 2882–90.

Houssiau, F. A., Bukasa, K., Sindic, C. J. M., Van Damme, J., and Van Snick, J. (1988). Elevated levels of the 26K human hybridoma growth factor (interleukin 6) in cerebrospinal fluid of patients with acute infection of the central nervous system. *Clin. Exp. Immunol.*, **71**, 320–3.

Huitinga, I., Van Rooijen, N., de Groot, C. J. A., Uitdehaag, B. M. J., and Dijkstra, C. D. (1990). Suppression of experimental allergic encephalomyelitis in Lewis rats after elimination of macrophages. *J. Exp. Med.*, **172**, 1025–33.

Issazadeh, S., Mustafa, M., Ljingdal, A., Hojeberg, B., Dagerlind, A., Elde, R. *et al.* (1995). Interferon g, interleukin 4 and transforming growth factor β in experimental autoimmune encephalomyelitis in Lewis rats: dynamics of cellular mRNA expression in the central nervous system and lymphoid cells. *J. Neurosci. Res.*, **40**, 579–90.

Jeding, I., Evans, P. J., Akanmu, D., Dexter, D., Spencer, J. D., Aruoma, O. I. *et al.* (1995). Characterization of the potential antioxidant and pro-oxidant actions of some neuroleptic drugs. *Biochem. Pharmacol.*, **49**, 359–65.

Kapas, L., Hong, L., Cady, A. B., Opp, M. R., Postlethwaite, A. E., Seyer, J. M. *et al.* (1992). Somnogenic, pyrogenic, and anorectic activities of tumor necrosis factor-alpha fragments. *Am. J. Physiol.*, **263**, R708-R15.

Kapas, L., Shibata, M., Kimura, M., and Krueger, J. M. (1994). Inhibition of nitric oxide synthesis suppresses sleep in rabbits. *Am. J. Physiol.*, **266**, R151-R7.

Karalis, K., Sano, H., Redwine, J., Listwak, S., Wilder, R. L., and Chrousos, G. P. (1991). Autocrine or paracrine inflammatory actions of corticotropin-releasing hormone *in vivo*. *Science*, **254**, 421–3.

Karanth, S., Lyson, K., and McCann, S. M. (1993). Role of nitric oxide in interleukin 2-induced corticotropin-releasing factor release from incubated hypothalami. *Proc. Natl. Acad. Sci.USA*, **90**, 3383–87.

Karpus, W. J., Lukacs, N. W., McRae, B. L., Strieter, R. M., Kunkel, S. L., and Miller, S. D. (1995). An important role for the chemokine macrophage inflammatory protein-1 alpha in the pathogenesis of the T cell-mediated autoimmune disease, experimental autoimmune encephalomyelitis. *J. Immunol.*, **155**, 5003–10.

Kassiotis, G., Pasparakis, M., Kollias, G. and Probert, L. (1999). TNF accelerates the onset but does not alter the incidence and severity of myelin basic protein-induced experimental autoimmune encephalomyelitis. *Eur. J. Immunol.* **29**, 774–80.

Kelley, D. M., Lichtenstein, A., Wang, J., Taylor, A. N., and Dubinett, S. M. (1994). Corticotropin-releasing factor reduces lipopolysaccharide-induced pulmonary vascular leak. *Immunopharmacol. Immunotoxicol.*, **16**, 139–48.

Krauss, S. (1962). Response of serum haptoglobin to inflammation in adrenalectomized rats. *Proc. Soc. Exp. Biol. Med.*, **112**, 552–4.

Kuriyama, K., Hori, T., Mori, T., and Nakashima, T. (1990). Actions of interferon alpha and inter-leukin- 1 beta on the glucose-responsive neurons in the ventromedial hypothalamus. *Brain Res. Bull.*, **24**, 803–10.

Labeur, M. S., Artz, E., Wiegers, G. J., Holsboer, F., and Reul, J. M. H. M. (1995). Long-term intracerebroventricular corticotropin-releasing hormone administration induces distinct changes in rat splenocyte activation and cytokine expression. *Endocrinology*, **136**, 2678–88.

Langevin, T., Young, J., Walker, K., Roemeling, R., Nygaard, S., and Hrunhesky, W. J. M. (1987). The toxicity of tumor necrosis factor (TNF) is reproducibly different at specific times of the day. *Proc. Am. Ass. Cancer*, **28**, 398–0.

Lazar, G. and Agarwal, M. K. (1986). The influence of a novel glucocorticoid antagonist on endo-toxin lethality in mice strains. *Biochem. Med. Metab. Biol*, **36**, 70–4.

Lazar, G. J., Duda, E., and Lazar, G. (1992a). Effect of RU 38486 on TNF production and toxicity. *FEBS Lett.*, **308**, 137–40.

Lazar, G. J., Lazar, G., and Agarwal, M. K. (1992b). Modification of septic shock in mice by the antiglucocorticoid RU 38486. *Circ. Shock*, **36**, 180–4.

Leist, T. P., Frei, K., Kam-Hansen, S., Zinkernagel, R. M., and Fontana, A. (1988). Tumor necrosis factor alpha in cerebrospinal fluid during bacterial, but not viral, meningitis *J. Exp. Med.*, **167**, 1743–8.

LeMay, L. G., Vander, A. J., and Kluger, M. J. (1990). The effect of psychological stress on plasma interleukin-6 activity in rats. *Physiol. Behav.*, **47**, 957–61.

Leonard, J. P., Waldburger, K. E., and Goldman, S. J. (1995). Prevention of experimental autoim-mune encephalomyelitis by antibodies against interleukin 12. *J. Exp. Med.*, **181**, 381–6.

Leppert, D., Waubant, E., Bürk, M. R., Oksenberg, J. R., and Hauser, S. L. (1996). Interferon beta-1b inhibits gelatinase secretion and *in vitro* migration of human T cells: a possible mechanism for treatment efficacy in multiple sclerosis. *Ann. Neurol.*, **40**, 846–52.

Libert, C., Van Bladel, S., Brouckaert, P., and Fiers, W. (1991). The influence of modulating sub-stances on tumor necrosis factor and intereukin-6 levels after injection of murine tumor necrosis factor or lipopolysaccharide in mice. *J. Immunother.*, **10**, 227–35.

Licinio, J. and Wong, M. L. (1992). Neutrophil-activating peptide-1/interleukin-8 mRNA is local-ized in rat hypothalamus and hippocampus. *Neuroreport.*, **3**, 753–6.

Lipton, J. M. and Catania, A. (1997). Anti-inflammatory actions of the neuroimmunomodulator α-MSH. *Immunol. Today*, **18**, 140–5.

Lipton, J. M., Macaluso, A., Hitz, M. E., and Catania, A. (1991). Central administration of the peptide alpha-MSH inhibits inflammation in the skin. *Peptides*, **12**, 795–8.

Liu, T., Clark, R. K., McDonnel, P. C., Young, P. R., White, R. F., Barone, F. C. *et al.* (1994). Tumor necrosis factor-α expression in ischemic neurons. *Stroke*, **25**, 1481–8.

Long, N. C., Otterness, I., Kunkel, S. L., Vander, A. J., and Kluger, M. J. (1990). Roles of interleukin 1β and tumor necrosis factor in lipopolysaccharide fever in rats. *Am. J. Physiol.*, **259**, R724–R8.

Long, N. C., Vander, A. J., Kunkel, S. L., and Kluger, M. J. (1990). Antiserum against tumor necro-sis factor increases stress hyperthermia in rats. *Am. J. Physiol.*, **258**, R591–R5.

Lublin, F. D., Knobler, R. L., Kalman, B., Goldhaber, M., Marini, J., Perrault, M. *et al.* (1993). Monoclonal anti-gamma interferon antibodies enhance experimental allergic encephalomyelitis. *Autoimmunity Journal*, **16**, 267–74.

Luheshi, G., Hopkins, S. J., Lefeuvre, R. A., Dascombe, M. J., Ghiara, P., and Rothwell, N. J. (1993). Importance of brain IL-1 type II receptors in fever and thermogenesis in the rat. *Am. J. Physiol.*, **265**, E585-E91.

Lyson, K. and McCann, S. M. (1992). Involvement of arachidonic acid cascade pathways in inter-leukin-6-stimulated corticotropin-releasing factor release *in vitro*. *Neuroendocrinology*, **55**, 708–13.

MacPhee, I. A. M., Antoni, F. A., and Mason, D. W. (1989). Spontaneous recovery of rats from experimental allergic encephalomyelitis is dependent on regulation of the immune system by endogenous adrenal corticosteroids *J. Exp. Med.*, **169**, 431–45.

Martin, L. W. and Lipton, J. M. (1990). Acute phase response to endotoxin: rise in plasma α-MSH and effects of α-MSH injection. *Am. J. Physiol.*, **259**, R768-R2.

Martin, L. W., Catania, A., Hiltz, M. E., and Lipton, J. M. (1991). Neuropeptide α-MSH antago-nizes IL-6- and TNF-induced fever. *Peptides*, **12**, 297–304.

Mason, D. (1991). Genetic variation in the stress response: susceptibility to experimental allergic encephalomyelitis and implications for human inflammatory disease. *Immunol. Today*, **12**, 57–60.

Masotto, C., Caspani, G., De Simoni, M. G., Mengozzi, M., Scatturin, M., Sironi, M. *et al.* (1992). Evidence for a different sensitivity to various central effects of interleukin-1β in mice. *Brain Res. Bull.*, **28**, 161–5.

Meda, L., Cassatella, M. A., Szendrei, G. I., Otvos Jr, L., Baron, P., Villalba, M. *et al.* (1995). Activation of microglial cells by β-amyloid protein and interferon-g. *Nature*, **374**, 647–50.

Meistrell III, M. E., Cockroft, K. M., Botchinka, G. I., Di Santo, E., Bloom, O., Murthy, J. *et al.* (1997). TNF is a brain damaging cytokine in stroke. *Shock*, **8**, 341–8.

Mendel, I., Katz, A., Kozak, N., Ben-Nun, A., and Revel, M. (1998). Interleukin-6 functions in autoimmune encephalomyelitis: a study in gene-targeted mice. *Eur. J. Immunol.*, **28**, 1727–37.

Mengozzi, M., Fantuzzi, G., Faggioni, R., Marchant, A., Goldman, M., Orencole, S. *et al.* (1994). Chlorpromazine specifically inhibits peripheral and brain TNF production, and up-regulates interleukin 10 production in mice. *Immunology*, **82**, 207–10.

Minami, M., Kuraishi, Y., and Satoh, M. (1991). Effects of kainic acid on messenger RNA levels of IL-1 beta, IL-6, TNF alpha and LIF in the rat brain. *Biochem. Biophys. Res. Commun.*, **176**, 593–8.

Moiola, L., Galbiati, F., Martino, G., Amadio, S., Brambilla, E., Comi, G. *et al.* (1998). IL-12 is involved in the induction of experimental autoimmune myasthenia gravis, an antibody-medi-ated disease. *Eur. J. Immunol.*, **28**, 2487–97.

Murphy, M. T., Richards, D. B., and Lipton, J. M. (1983). Antipyretic potency of centrally adminis-tered alpha-melanocyte stimulating hormone. *Science*, **221**, 192–3.

Mustafa, M. M., Mrstola, J., Ramilo, O., Saez-Llorens, X., Risser, R. C., and McCracken, G. H. J. (1989). Increased endotoxin and interleukin-1 beta concentrations in cerebrospinal fluid of infants with coliform meningitis and ventriculitis associated with intraventricular gentamicin therapy. *J. Infect. Dis.*, **160**, 891–5.

Mustafa, M. M., Ramilo, O., Olsen, K. D., Franklin, P. S., Hansen, E. J., Beutler, B. *et al.* (1989). Tumor necrosis factor in mediating experimental Haemophilus influenzae type B meningitis. *J. Clin. Invest.*, **84**, 1253–9.

Mustafa, M. M., Ramilo, O., Saez-Llorens, X., Olsen, K. D., Magness, R. R., and McCracken, G. H. J. (1990). Cerebrospinal fluid prostaglandins, interleukin-1 beta and tumor necrosis factor in bacterial meningitis. Clinical and laboratory correlation in placebo-treated and dexametha-sone-treated patients. *Am. J. Dis. Child.*, **144**, 883–7.

Nagai, M., Saigusa, T., Shimada, Y., Inagawa, H., Oshima, H., and Iriki, M. (1988). Antibody to tumor necrosis factor (TNF) reduces endotoxin fever. *Experientia*, **44**, 606–7.

Nataf, S., Louboutin, J. P., Chabannes, D., Feve, J. R., and Muller, J. Y. (1993). Pentoxifylline inhibits experimental allergic encephalomyelitis. *Acta Neurol. Scand.*, **88**, 97–9.

Odio, C. M., Faingezicht, I., Paris, M., Nassar, M., Baltodano, A., Rogers, J. *et al.* (1991). The beneficial effects of early dexamethasone administration in infacts and children with bacterial meningitis. *New Engl. J. Med.*, **324**, 1525–31.

Okuda, Y., Sakoda, S., Fujimura, H., and Yanagihara, T. (1996). Pentoxifylline delays the onset of experimental allergic encephalomyelitis in mice by modulating cytokine production in peripheral blood mononuclear cells. *Immunopharmacology*, **35**, 141–8.

Okuda, Y., Sakoda, S., Bernard, C. C., Fujimura, H., Saeki, Y., Kishimoto, T. *et al.* (1998). IL-6-deficient mice are resistant to the induction of experimental autoimmune encephalomyelitis provoked by myelin oligodendrocyte glycoprotein. *Int. Immunol.*, **10**, 703–8.

Oldenburg, H. S. A., Rogy, M. A., Lazarus, D. D., Van Zee, K. J., Keeler, B. B., Chizzonite, R. A. *et al.* (1993). Cachexia and the acute-phase protein response in inflammation are regulated by interleukin-6. *Eur. J. Immunol.*, **23**, 1889–94.

Oliff, A., Defeo-Jones, D., Boyer, M., Martinez, D., Kiefer, D., Vuocolo, G. *et al.* (1987). Tumors secreting human TNF/cachectin induce cachexia in mice. *Cell*, **50**, 555–63.

Olsson, T. (1995). Cytokine-producing cells in experimental autoimmune encephalomyelitis and multiple sclerosis. *Neurology*, **45** (supplement 6), S11–S5.

Opp, M. R. and Krueger, J. M. (1991). Interleukin 1-receptor antagonist blocks interleukin 1-induced sleep and fever. *Am. J. Physiol.*, **260**, R453–R7.

Opp, M., Obal, J., Cady, A. B., Johannsen, L., and Krueger, J. M. (1989). Interleukin-6 is pyrogenic but not somnogenic. *Physiol. Behav.*, **45**, 1069–72.

Ovadia, H., Abramsky, O., Barak, V., Conforti, N., Saphier, D., and Weidenfeld, J. (1989). Effect of interleukin-1 on adrenocortical activity in intact and hypothalamic deafferentated male rats. *Exp. Brain Res.*, **76**, 246–9.

Panitch, H. S., Hirsch, R. L., Schindler, J., and Johnson, K. P. (1987). Treatment of multiple sclerosis with gamma interferon: exacerbations associated with activation of the immune system. *Neurology*, **37**, 1097.

Parant, M., Le Contel, C., Parant, F., and Chedid, L. (1991). Influence of endogenous glucocorticoid on endotoxin-induced production of circulating TNF-alpha. *Lymphokine Cytokine Res.*, **10**, 265–71.

Payne, L. C., Weigent, D. A., and Blalock, J. E. (1994). Induction of pituitary sensitivity to interleukin-1: a new function for corticotropin-releasing hormone. *Biochem. Biophys. Res. Commun.*, **198**, 480–4.

Perretti, M., Becherucci, C., Scapigliati, G., and Parente, L. (1989). The effect of adrenalectomy on interleukin-1 release *in vitro* and *in vivo*. *Br. J. Pharmacol.*, **98**, 1137–42.

Perretti, M., Mugridge, K. G., Becherucci, C., and Parente, L. (1991). Evidence that interleukin-1 and lipoxygenase metabolites mediate the lethal effect of complete Freund's adjuvant in adrenalectomized rats. *Lymphokine Cytokine Res.*, **10**, 239–43.

Plata-Salaman, C. R. (1991). Dexamethasone inhibits food intake suppression induced by low doses of interleukin-1 β administered intracerebroventricularly. *Brain Res. Bull.*, **27**, 737–8.

Plata-Salaman, C. R., Oomura, Y., and Kai, Y. (1988). Tumor necrosis factor and interleukin-1β: suppression of food intake by direct action in the central nervous system. *Brain Res.*, **448**, 106–14.

Poliak, S., Mor, F., Conlon, P., Wong, T., Ling, N., Rivier, J. *et al.* (1997). The neuropeptides corticotropin-releasing factor and urocortin suppress encephalomyelitis via effects on both the hypothalamic-pituitary-adrenal axis and the immune system. *J. Immunol.*, **158**, 5751–6.

Pollmächer, T., Hinze-Selch, D., and Mullington, J. (1996). Effects of clozapine on plasma cytokine and soluble cytokine rreceptor levels. *J. Clin. Psychopharmacol.*, **16**, 403–9.

Pousset, F., Fournier, J., Legoux, P., Keane, P., Shire, D., and Soubrie, P. (1996). Effect of serotonin on cytokine mRNA expression in rat hippocampal astrocytes. *Mol. Brain Res.*, **38**, 54–62.

Racke, M. K., Burnett, D., Pak, S.-L., Albert, P. S., Cannella, P., Raine, C. S. *et al.* (1995). Retinoid treatment of experimental allergic encephalomyelitis. IL-4 production correlates with improved disease course. *J. Immunol.*, **154**, 450–8.

Raine, C. S. (1994). The immunology of the multiple sclerosis lesion. *Ann. Neurol.*, **36**, S61-S72.

Relton, J. K. and Rothwell, N. J. (1992). Interleukin-1 receptor antagonist inhibits ischemic and excitotoxic neuronal damage in the rat. *Brain Res.Bull.*, **29**, 243–6.

Renno, T., Krakowski, M., Piccirillo, C., Lin, J., and Owens, T. (1995). TNF-α expression by resident microglia and infiltrating leukocytes in the central nervous system of mice with experimental allergic encephalomyelitis. *J. Immunol.*, **154**, 944–53.

Riccardi-Castagnoli, P., Pirami, L., Righi, M., Sacerdote, P., Locatelli, V., Bianchi, M. *et al.* (1990). Cellular sources and effects of tumor necrosis factor-alpha on pituitary cells and in the central nervous system. *Ann. NY Acad. Sci.*, **594**, 156–68.

Rieckmann, P., Albrecht, M., Kitze, B., Webver, T., Tumani, H., Brooks, A. *et al.* (1995). Tumor necrosis factor-α messenger RNA expression in patients with relapsing-remitting multiple sclerosis is associated with disease activity. *Ann. Neurol.*, **37**, 82–8.

Rivier, C., Chizzonite, R., and Vale, W. (1989). In the mouse, the activation of the hypothalamic-pituitary-adrenal axis by a lipopolysaccharide (endotoxin) is mediated through interleukin-1. *Endocrinology*, **125**, 2800–5.

Rodriguez, M., Pavelko, K. D., McKinney, C. W., and Leibowitz, J. L. (1994). Recombinant human IL-6 suppresses demyelination in a viral model of multiple sclerosis. *J. Immunol.*, **153**, 3811–20.

Rothwell, N. J. (1989). CRF is involved in the pyrogenic and thermogenic effects of interleukin 1 beta in the rat. *Am. J. Physiol.*, **256**, E111–E5.

Rothwell, N. J., Busbridge, N. J., Lefeuvre, R. A., Hardwick, A. J., Gauldie, J., and Hopkins, S. J. (1991). Interleukin 6 is a centrally acting endogenous pyrogen in the rat. *Can. J. Physiol. Pharmacol.*, **69**, 1465–9.

Rothwell, N., Allan, S., and Toulmond, S. (1997). The role of interleukin 1 in acute neurodegeneration and stroke: pathophysiological and therapeutic implications. *J. Clin. Invest.*, **100**, 2648–52.

Rott, O., Cash, E., and Fleischer, B. (1993). Phosphodiesterase inhibitor pentoxifylline, a selective suppressor of T helper type 1, but not type 2, associated lymphokine production, prevents induction of experimental autoimmune encephalomyelitis in Lewis rats. *Eur. J. Immunol.*, **23**, 1745–51.

Rott, O., Fleischer, B., and Cash, E. (1994). Interleukin-10 prevents experimental allergic encephalomyelitis in rats. *Eur. J. Immunol.*, **24**, 1434–40.

Ruddle, N. H., Bergman, C. M., McGrath, K. M., Lingenheld, E. G., Grunnet, M. L., and Padula, S. J. (1990). An antibody to lymphotoxin and tumor necrosis factor prevents transfer of experimental allergic encephalomyelitis. *J. Exp. Med.*, **172**, 1193–200.

Rudick, R. A., Ransohoff, R. M., Peppler, R., Medendorp, S. V., Lehmann, P., and Alam, J. (1996). Interferon beta induces interleukin-10 expression: relevance to multiple sclerosis. *Ann. Neurol.*, **40**, 618–27.

Rusconi, F., Parizzi, F., Garlaschi, L., Assael, B. M., Sironi, M., Ghezzi, P. *et al.* (1991). Interleukin 6 activity in infants and children with bacterial meningitis. *Pediatr. Infect. Dis. J.*, **10**, 117–21.

Ruuls, S. R., de Labie, M. C. D. C., Weber, K. S., Botman, C. A. D., Groenestein, R. J., Dijkstra, C. D. *et al.* (1996). The lenght of treatment determines whether IFN-β prevents or aggravates experimental autoimmune encephalomyelitis in Lewis rats. *J. Immunol.*, **157**, 5721–31.

Saez-Llorens, X., Ramilo, O., Mustafa, M. M., Mertsola, J., de Alba, C., Hansen, E. *et al.* (1990). Pentoxifylline modulates meningeal inflammation in experimental bacterial meningitis. *Animicrob. Agents Chemother.*, **34**, 837–43.

Samoilova, E. B., Horton, J. L., Hilliard, B., Liu, T. S., and Chen, Y. (1998). IL-6-deficient mice are resistant to experimental autoimmune encephalomyelitis: roles of IL-6 in the activation and differentiation of autoreactive T cells. *J. Immunol.*, **161**, 6480–6.

Sapolsky, R., Rivier, C., Yamamoto, G., Plotsky, P., and Vale, W. (1987). Interleukin-1 stimulates the secretion of hypothalamic corticotropin-releasing factor. *Science*, **238**, 522–4.

Saukkonen, K., Sande, S., Cioffe, C., Wolpe, S., Sherry, B., Cerami, A. *et al.* (1990). The role of cytokines in the generation of inflammation and tissue damage in experimental Gram-positive meningitis *J. Exp. Med.*, **171**, 439–48.

Schimmer, B. P. and Parker, K. L. (1996). Adrenocorticotropic hormone; adrenocortical steroids and their synthetic analogs; inhibitors of the synthesis and action of adrenocortical hormones. In *Goodman & Gilman's the pharmacological basis of therapeutics*, (9th edn), (ed.. J. G. Hardman, L. E. Limbird, P. B. Molinoff, R. W. Ruddon, and A. Goodman Gilman), pp. 1459–85. McGraw-Hill, New York.

Schobitz, B., Holsboer, F., Kikkert, R., Sutanto, W., and De Kloet, E. R. (1992). Peripheral and central regulation of IL-6 gene expression in endotoxin-treated rats. *Endocr. Regul.*, **26**, 103–9.

Schuman, E. M. and Madison, D. V. (1994). Nitric oxide and synaptic function. *Annu. Rev. Neurosci.*, **17**, 153–83.

Sébire, G., Emilie, D., Wallon, C., Hery, C., Devergne, O., Delfraissy, J. F. *et al.* (1993). *In vitro* production of IL-6, IL-1 beta, and tumor necrosis factor-alpha by human embryonic microglial and neural cells. *J. Immunol.*, **150**, 1517–23.

Selmaj, K. W. and Raine, C. S. (1995). Experimental autoimmune encephalomyelitis: immunotherapy with anti-tumor necrosis factor antibodies and soluble tumor necrosis factor receptors. *Neurology*, **45**, S44-S9.

Shapiro, L., Zhang, X.-X., Rupp, R. P., Wolff, S. M., and Dinarello, C. A. (1993). Ciliary neurotrophic factor is an endogenous pyrogen. *Proc. Natl. Acad. Sci.USA*, **90**, 8614–8.

Sharief, M. K. and Hentges, R. (1991). Association between tumor necrosis factor-α production and disease progression in patients with multiple sclerosis. *New Engl. J. Med.*, **325**, 467–72.

Sherry, B. A., Gelin, J., Fong, Y., Marano, M., Wei, H., Cerami, A. *et al.* (1989). Anticachectin/tumor necrosis factor-a antibodies attenuate development of cachexia in tumor models. *FASEB J.*, **3**, 1956–62.

Shibasaki, T., Yamauchi, N., Kato, Y., Masuda, A., Imaki, T., Hotta, M. *et al.* (1988). Involvement of corticotropin-releasing factor in restraint stress-induced anorexia and reversion of the anorexia by somatostatin in the rat. *Life Sci.*, **43**, 1103–10.

Singh, W. K. and Leu, S.-J. C. (1990). Enhancing effect of corticotropin-releasing neurohormone on the production of interleukin-1 and interleukin-2. *Neurosci. Lett.*, **120**, 151–4.

Sinz, E. H., Kochanek, P. M., Dixon, C. E., Clark, R. S., Carcillo, J. A., Schiding, J. K. *et al.* (1999). Inducible nitric oxide synthase is an endogenous neuroprotectant after traumatic brain injury in rats and mice. *J. Clin. Invest.*, **104**, 647–56.

Sirko, S. P., Bishai, I., and Coceani, F. (1989). Prostaglandin formation in the hypothalamus *in vivo*: effect of pyrogens. *Am. J. Physiol.*, **256**, R616-R24.

Slater, T. F. (1968). The inhibitory effects '*in vitro*' of phenothiazines and other drugs on lipid peroxidation systems in rat liver microsomes and their relationships to liver necrosis produced by carbon tetrachloride. *Biochem. J.*, **106**, 155–60.

Smith, B. K. and Kluger, M. J. (1992). Human IL-1 receptor antagonist partially suppresses LPS fever but not plasma levels of IL-6 in Fischer rats. *Am. J. Physiol.*, **263**, R653-R5.

Sommer, N., Löschmann, P.-A., Northoff, G. H., Weller, M., Steinbrecher, A., Steinbach, J. P. *et al.* (1995). The antidepressant rolipram suppresses cytokine production and prevents autoimmune encephalomyelitis. *Nature Medicine*, **1**, 244–8.

Steinman, L. (1997). Some misconceptions about understanding autoimmunity through experiments with knockouts. *J. Exp. Med.*, **185**, 2039–41.

Sternberg, E. M., Hill, J. M., Chrousos, G. P., Kamilaris, T., Listwak, S. J., Gold, P. W. *et al.* (1989). Inflammatory mediator-induced hypothalamic-pituitary-adrenal axis activation is defective in streptococcal cell wall arthritis-susceptible Lewis rats. *Proc. Natl. Acad. Sci. USA*, **86**, 2374–8.

Stovroff, M. C., Fraker, D. L., Svedenborg, J. A., and Norton, J. A. (1988). Cachectin/tumor necrosis factor: a possible mediator of cancer anorexia in the rat. *Cancer Res.*, **48**, 4567–72.

Sundar, S. K., Becker, K. J., Cierpial, M. A., Carpenter, M. D., Rankin, L. A., Fleener, S. L. *et al.* (1989). Intracerebroventricular infusion of interleukin 1 rapidly decreases peripheral cellular immune responses. *Proc. Natl. Acad. Sci. USA*, **86**, 6398–402.

Sundar, S. K., Cierpial, M. A., Kilts, C., Ritchie, J. C., and Weiss, J. M. (1990). Brain IL-1-induced immunosuppression occurs through activation of both pituitary-adrenal axis and sympathetic nervous system by corticotropin-releasing factor. *J. Neurosci.*, **10**, 3701–6.

Sundar, S. K., Cierpial, M. A., Kamaraju, L. S., Long, S., Hsieh, S., Lorenz, C. *et al.* (1991). Human immunodeficiency virus glycoprotein (gp120) infused into rat brain induces interleukin 1 to elevate pituitary-adrenal activity and decrease peripheral cellular immune responses. *Proc. Natl. Acad. Sci. USA*, **88**, 11246–50.

Swingle, W. W. and Remington, J. W. (1944). Role of adrenal cortex in physiological processes. *Physiol. Rev.*, **24**, 89–127.

Tada, M., Suzuki, K., Yamakawa, Y., Sawamura, Y., Abe, H., van Meir, E. *et al.* (1993). Human glioblastoma cells produce 77 amino acid interleukin-8 (IL-8(77)). *J. Neurooncol.*, **16**, 25–34.

Tani, M., Fuentes, M. E., Peterson, J. W., Trapp, B. D., Durham, S. K., Loy, J. K. *et al.* (1996). Neutrophil infiltration, glial reaction, and neurological disease in transgenic mice expressing the chemokine N51/KC in oligodendrocytes. *J. Clin. Invest.*, **98**, 529–39.

Tarazona, R., Gonzàles-Garcia, A., Zamzami, N., Marchetti, P., Frechin, N., Gonzalo, J. A. *et al.* (1995). Chlorpromazine amplifies macrophage dependent IL-10 production *in vivo*. *J. Immunol.*, **154**, 861–70.

Taupin, V., Gogusev, J., Descamps Latscha, B., and Zavala, F. (1993). Modulation of tumor necrosis factor-alpha, interleukin-1 beta, interleukin-6, interleukin-8, and granulocyte/macrophage colony-stimulating factor expression in human monocytes by an endogenous anxiogenic benzodiazepine ligand, triakontatetraneuropeptide: evidence for a role of prostaglandins. *Mol. Pharmacol.*, **43**, 64–9.

Tazi, A., Dantzer, R., Crestani, F., and Le Moal, M. (1988). Interleukin-1 induces conditioned taste aversion in rats: a possible explanation for its pituitary-adrenal stimulating activity. *Brain Res.*, **473**, 369–71.

The IFN-β Multiple Sclerosis Study Group and the University of British Columbia MS/MRI Analysis Group. (1995). Interferon beta-1b in the treatment of multiple sclerosis: final outcome of the randomized controlled trial. *Neurology*, **45**, 1277–85.

Tracey, K. J. and Cerami, A. (1992). Tumor necrosis factor and regulation of metabolism in infection: role of systemic versus tissue levels. *Proc. Soc. Exp. Biol. Med.*, **200**, 233–9.

Tracey, K. J., Morgello, S., Koplin, B., Fahey, T. J. I., Fox, J., Aledo, A. *et al.* (1990). Metabolic effects of cachectin/tumor necrosis factor are modified by site of production: cachectin/tumor necrosis factor-secreting tumor in skeletal muscle induces chronic cachexia, while implantation in brain induces predominately acute anorexia. *J. Clin. Invest.*, **86**, 2014–24.

Tsagarakis, S., Gillies, G., Rees, L. H., Besser, M., and Grossman, A. (1989). Interleukin-1 directly stimulates the release of corticotropin releasing factor from rat hypotalamus. *Neuroendocrinology*, **49**, 98–101.

Turnbull, A. V., Vale, W., and Rivier, C. (1996). Urocortin, a corticotropin-releasing factor-related mammalian peptide, inhibits edema due to thermal injury in rats. *Eur. J. Pharmacol.*, **303**, 213–6.

Uehara, A., Sekiya, C., Takasugi, Y., Namiki, M., and Arimura, A. (1989). Anorexia induced by interleukin 1: involvement of corticotropin-releasing factor. *Am. J. Physiol.*, **257**, R613-R7.

Vadas, P., Stefansky, E., and Pruzanski, W. (1986). Potential therapeutic efficacy of inhibitors of phospholipase A2 in septic shock. *Agents Actions*, **19**, 194–202.

Van Dam, A. M., Malinowsky, D., Lenczowski, M. J., Bartfai, T., and Tilders, F. J. (1998). Interleukin 1 (IL-1) type I receptors mediate activation of rat hypothalamus-pituitary-adrenal axis and interleukin 6 production as shown by receptor type selective deletion mutants of IL-1beta. *Cytokine*, **10**, 413–7.

Vandenabeele, P. and Fiers, W. (1991). Is amyloidogenesis during Alzheimer's disease due to an IL-1/IL-6-mediated 'acute phase response' in the brain? *Immunol. Today*, **12**, 217–9.

Van Gool, J., Van Vugt, H., helle, M., and Aarden, L. A. (1990). The regulation among stress, adrenalin, interleukin 6 and acute phase protein in the rat. *Clin. Immunol. Immunopathol.*, **57**, 200–10.

Vaughan, J., Donaldson, C., Bittencourt, J., Perrin, M. H., Lewis, K., Sutton, S. *et al.* (1995). Urocortin, a mammalian neuropeptide related to fish urotensin I and to corticotropin-releasing factor. *Nature*, **378**, 287–92.

Voorthuis, J. A. C., Uitdehaag, B. M. J., de Groot, C. J. A., Goede, P. H., Van der Meide, P. H., and Dijikstra, C. D. (1990). Suppression of experimental allergic encephalomyelitis by intraventricular administration of interferon-gamma in Lewis rats. *Clin. Exp. Immunol.*, **81**, 183–8.

Wei, E. T., Serda, S., and Tian, J. Q. (1988). Protective actions of corticotropin-releasing factor on thermal injury to rat pawsking. *J. Pharmacol. Exp. Ther.*, **247**, 1082–5.

Wolfe, L. S. and Coceani, F. (1979). The role of prostaglandins in the central nervous system. *Ann. Rev. Physiol.*, **41**, 669–84.

Woloski, B. M. R. N. J., Smith, E. M., Meyer, W. J. I., Fuller, G. M., and Blalock, J. E. (1985). Corticotropin-releasing activity of monokines. *Science*, **230**, 1035–7.

Wood, J. A., Wood, P. L., Ryan, R., Graff-Radford, N. R., Pilapil, C., Robitaille, Y. *et al.* (1993). Cytokines induced in Alzheimer's temporal cortex: no changes in mature IL-1 β or IL-1RA but increases in the associated acute phase proteins IL-6, alpha 2-macroglobulin and C-reactive protein. *Brain Res.*, **629**(2), 245–52.

Woodroofe, M. N. (1995). Cytokine production in the central nervous system. *Neurology*, **45**, 6–10.

Zampronio, A. R., Souza, G. E. P., Silva, C. A. A., Cunha, F. Q., and Ferreira, S. H. (1994). Interleukin-8 induces fever by a prostaglandin-independent mechanism. *Am. J. Physiol.*, **266**, R1670-R4.

Zavala, F., Taupin, V., and Descamps-Latscha, B. (1990). *In vivo* treatment with benzodiazepines inhibits murine phagocyte oxidative metabolism and production of interleukin 1, tumor necrosis factor and interleukin 6. *J. Pharmacol. Exp. Ther.*, **255**, 442–50.

Zetterstrom, M., Lundkvist, J., Malinowsky, D., Eriksson, G., and Bartfai, T. (1998). Interleukin-1-mediated febrile responses in mice and interleukin-1 beta activation of NFkappaB in mouse primary astrocytes, involves the interleukin-1 receptor accessory protein. *Eur. Cytokine Netw.*, **9**, 131–8.

Zhou, D., Kusnecov, A. W., Shurin, M. R., De Paoli, M., and Rabin, B. S. (1993). Exposure to physical and psychological stressors elevates plasma interleukin 6: relationship to the activation of hypothalamic-pituitary-adrenal axis. *Endocrinology*, **133**, 2523–30.

Zilberstein, A., Ruggieri, R. M., Korn, J. H., and Revel, M. (1986). Structure and expression of cDNA and genes for human interferon-β2, a distinct species inducible by growth-stimulatory cytokines. *EMBO J.*, **5**, 2529–37.

Zinetti, M., Galli, G., Demitri, M. T., Fantuzzi, G., Minto, M., Ghezzi, P. *et al.* (1995). Chlorpromazine inhibits tumor necrosis factor synthesis and cytotoxicity *in vitro*. *Immunology.*, **86**, 416–21.

Zuckerman, S. H., Shellhaas, J., and Butler, L. D. (1989). Differential regulation of lipopolysaccharide-induced interleukin 1 and tumor necrosis factor synthesis: effects of endogenous and exogenous glucocorticoids and the role of the pituitary-adrenal axis. *Eur. J. Immunol.*, **19**, 301–5.

9 *Cardiovascular system*

Blood vessels have long been considered blood containers, whose main property was to contract and to regulate pressure. This 'passive' view particularly emphasized the negative properties of vessels and of endothelial cells (EC), the most important being that they are a non-thrombogenic substrate for blood. As such, vascular cells were considered to participate in tissue reactions mainly as targets for injurious agents. The possibility of isolating and culturing vascular cells, particularly EC, from various tissues opened the way to studying their complex reactions to a variety of activating stimuli. Vascular cells have thus emerged as active participants in many physiological and pathological processes.

It is now evident that hemostasis, inflammatory reactions, and immunity involve close interactions between immunocompetent cells and vascular endothelium. The ontogeny and function of white blood cells require an intimate relationship with vascular EC. Cytokines mediate these complex interactions between leukocytes and vascular elements (Mantovani and Dejana, 1989; Mantovani *et al.*, 1992, 1997).

EC are strategically located at the interface between blood and tissues. Besides responding rapidly—in seconds to minutes—to agonists such as histamine and thrombin, vascular cells, when exposed to cytokines, undergo profound functional alterations that involve gene expression and protein synthesis, require hours to develop, and are relatively long-lasting. This functional reprogramming of EC has been referred to as 'activation', in analogy with the terminology long used for the monocyte–macrophage lineage.

Vascular cells are both a target for, and a source of, cytokines and these soluble polypeptide mediators serve as communication signals with leukocytes—the primary producers of these molecules—as well as with diverse tissues and organs. Here we will concisely review the response elicited by cytokines in vascular cells and analyze how vessel-wall elements participate in cytokine cascades by producing copious amounts of some of these polypeptide mediators. The role of cytokines in selected pathologies, which affect vascular elements and the possibility of cytokine targeted therapies, will then be discussed.

9.1 Vascular cell responses to cytokines

The spectrum of responses elicited by different cytokines in vascular cells, particularly EC, is vast and varied. Different cytokines activate distinct, largely non-overlapping, sets of functions that can be grouped into programs of activation/differentiation (Fig. 9.1). These programs are activated by cytokine receptors on EC (Fig. 9.2).

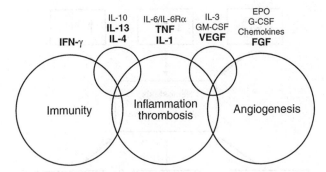

Fig. 9.1 Distinct but overlapping sets of functions activated by cytokines in endothelial cells (EC). VEGF, vascular endothelium growth factor; FGF, fibroblast growth factor; EPO, erythropoietin;chemokines have both + and – effects on EC. Bold and plain indicate the relative strength of activation. Reproduced with minor modifications from Mantovani *et al.*, (1997) *Immunology Today* **18**, 231–9.

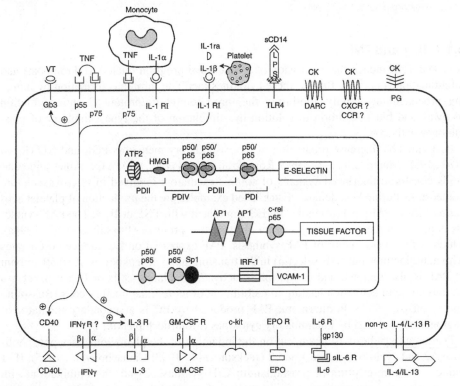

Fig. 9.2 Cytokine receptors expressed on in endothelial cells (EC). Question marks indicate controversy (CCR or CXCR chemokine receptor) or lack of identification of the receptor or type of receptor (CC, CXC, or LPS receptor) or lack of specific studies in EC (IFNγ receptor). The location of the receptor does not imply a different distribution on the luminal and abluminal surfaces of EC. A schematic representation of the promoters of three genes expressed in EC is shown in the nucleus. Abbreviations: CK, chemokine; DARC, Duffy antigen receptor for chemokines; Gb3, globotriaosylceramide; L, ligand; LPS, lipopolysaccharide; non γc, non-common γ chain; PD, positive regulatory domain; PG, proteoglycans; R, receptor; VT, verotoxin Reproduced with minor modifications from Mantovani *et al.*, (1997) *Immunology Today* **18**, 231–9.

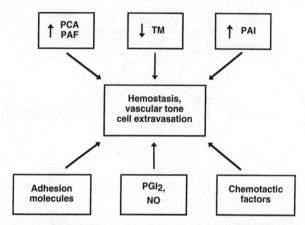

Fig. 9.3 A schematic view of prothrombotic, pro-inflammatory functions activated by IL-1 and TNF. Abbreviations: PCA, procoagulant activity; TM, thrombomodulin; PAF, platelet-activating factor; PAI, plasminogen activator inhibitor.

9.1.1 IL-1 and TNF

IL-1 and TNF induce the expression of a functional program related to thrombosis and inflammation (Fig. 9.3). Briefly, these cytokines facilitate thrombus formation by inducing procoagulant activity, inhibiting the thrombomodulin/protein C anticoagulation pathway and blocking fibrin dissolution by stimulation of the type I inhibitor of plasminogen activator.

IL-1 and TNF increase production of the vasodilatory mediators PGI_2 and NO (Rossi *et al.*, 1985; Mantovani *et al.*, 1992; Rosenkranz Weiss *et al.*, 1994). Cytokines and autacoids constitute interlaced systems of soluble mediators involved in microvasculature homeostasis during host defense. Established examples are the production of platelet activating factor (PAF) or prostanoids by EC stimulated with TNF or IL-1. The PAF synthesis depends on the neo-synthesis of an elastase-like protease (Bussolino *et al.*, 1994a), which is the final effector of PAF synthesis. PAF expressed on EC surface co-operates with adhesion molecules (E-selectin) in the transmigration of leukocytes. A small amount of PAF is also secreted and can prime or activate circulating cells or EC: it triggers a vicious circle of activation leading to recruitment of more inflammatory cells (Bussolino and Camussi, 1995). Furthermore, PAF produced by EC is a secondary mediator of angiogenesis induced by inflammatory cytokines (Montrucchio *et al.*, 1994).

Prostanoid synthesis is dependent on the induction of the pivotal enzymes phospholipase A2 and cyclo-oxygenase 1 and 2 (Jackson *et al.*, 1993; Camacho *et al.*, 1995). IL-1 induces the transcription of prostaglandin G/H synthase 2 and, in combination with aspirin, increases the synthesis of a new class of lipoxins during EC–leukocyte interactions, with an inhibitory effect on neutrophil adhesion (Claria and Serhan, 1995).

NO is a representative of a class of autacoids serving a variety of functions in several tissues, including the vasculature, and acting through an independent receptor mechanism (Nathan and Xie, 1994). NO synthase (NOS) type II (inducible, Ca^{++}-independent isoform) and type III (constitutive, EC-isoform) are present in EC, and catalyze the conversion of arginine into citrulline and NO. The latter continuously produces 'quanta' of

NO, which participates particularly in the regulation of vascular tone (Nathan and Xie, 1994).

In humans, experiments on EC from large vessels indicate that inflammatory cytokines increase the activity of NOS III and the synthesis of NO (Werner Felmayer *et al.*, 1993; Rosenkranz Weiss *et al.*, 1994). The effect of inflammatory cytokines on metabolic pathways leading to NO formation involves a loss of stability of NOSIII mRNA (Rosenkranz Weiss *et al.*, 1994), an increase of GTP cyclohydrolase I, the rate-limiting enzyme of tetrahydrobiopterin synthesis, and of tetrahydrobiopterin, a cofactor for the full activity of NOS III (Werner Felmayer *et al.*, 1993; Rosenkranz Weiss *et al.*, 1994). However, the increase of tetrahydrobiopterin is compensated by a decrease in stability of NOS III mRNA (Yoshizumi *et al.*, 1993), necessary to counteract the toxic effect of NO and its metabolite peroxynitrite on EC themselves.

Several laboratories have demonstrated that the enhancement of NO production in murine, rat, porcine, and bovine EC, in response to cytokine challenge, is mediated by transcription of the NOS II gene (Radomski *et al.*, 1990; Lamas *et al.*, 1992; Suschek *et al.*, 1993; Balligand *et al.*, 1995). This gene's promoter contains cis-acting DNA elements that are targets for the cytokine-activated transcription factors NF-kB/Rel and IRF (Kamijo *et al.*, 1994; Martin *et al.*, 1994). Recent data point to a role of Sp1 and GATA factors in endothelial basal transcription of the NOS III gene (Zhang *et al.*, 1995). Unequivocal information on the role of this NOS isoform in human EC is lacking at present, since experiments have only been done on EC from large vessels. However, NOS II is presumably operative in human microvasculature, after induction by inflammatory cytokines, because it has been detected in EC lining the vessels in synovia of patients with rheumatoid arthritis (Sakurai *et al.*, 1995) and in brain tumours (Cobbs *et al.*, 1995).

The ability of different cytokines alone, or in combination, to induce NO production is disputed. In human EC, at least three cytokines (IL-1, TNF, and IFNγ) are required to enhance NO synthesis (Rosenkranz Weiss *et al.*, 1994). In other species, only one cytokine is needed to elicit NO synthesis (Lamas *et al.*, 1992; Balligand *et al.*, 1995). Thus in humans a complex and refined mechanism for NO synthesis in EC may have developed during evolution.

The complexity of this phenomenon is highlighted by the opposite effects of one cytokine in different animal species or on different NOS isoforms. For instance IFN-γ is required for NO synthesis in human EC (Rosenkranz Weiss *et al.*, 1994), but is an inhibitor in bovine EC stimulated with TNF (Lamas *et al.*, 1992). Furthermore, TGFß inhibits NOS II (Murata *et al.*, 1995), but up-regulates NOS III (Inoue *et al.*, 1995).

NO produced by EC acts in an autocrine and paracrine manner. For example, alteration of NO levels in EC has EC themselves as a primary target and modifies their biological properties. The inhibition of basal production of NO by competitive analogues of arginine increases leukocyte adhesion to the EC surface, by a mechanism partly dependent on the up-regulation of VCAM-1, and on PAF synthesis (Niu *et al.*, 1994; De Caterina *et al.*, 1995). Furthermore, treatment of EC with NO donors reduces the expression of VCAM-1 induced by IL-1, IL-4, TNF, or LPS (De Caterina *et al.*, 1995). NO also reduces the expression of other adhesion molecules (ICAM-1 and E-selectin) and secretable cytokines (IL-6, MCP-1, IL-8, and M-CSF) (De Caterina *et al.*, 1995; Peng *et al.*, 1995b; Zeiher *et al.*, 1995; Villarete and Remick, 1995). These effects do not appear to involve stimulation of guanylate cyclase, NO's classical intracellular target, but are mediated by inhibition of NF-kB through the induction and stabilization of NF-kB inhibitor (De Caterina *et al.*, 1995; Peng *et al.*, 1995a). The finding that inhibition of endogenous, cytokine-independent NO production by arginine analogues could activate NF-kB suggests that constitutively produced NO may play an important physiological role, tonically inhibiting the expression of NF-kB-dependent pro-inflammatory genes (Niu *et al.*, 1994; De Caterina *et al.*, 1995; Peng *et al.*, 1995a). Moreover, NO produced by cytokine stimulation attenuates the inflammatory effects of these molecules.

However, NO is not only an intracellular regulator of EC function, but is instrumental in EC response. For example, NO-dependent killing of *Schistosoma mansoni* has been described in murine EC stimulated with IFN-γ, IL-1 or TNF (Oswald *et al.*, 1994). NO participates in the long-term morphogenetic program of the vasculature, in delayed hypersensitivity responses, chronic inflammation and atherogenesis. It enhances the motility of EC, inhibits the proliferation of vascular smooth cells, is angiogenic *in vivo* and reduces neointima formation (Ziche *et al.*, 1994; Fukuo *et al.*, 1995; von der Leyen *et al.*, 1995). In septic shock, NO produced by EC co-operates in the pathogenesis of the depression of myocardial contractile function (Sato *et al.*, 1995; Schulz *et al.*, 1995).

Inflammatory cytokines promote leukocyte extravasation by altering the rheology of microcirculation, by inducing adhesion molecules (E-selectin, vascular cell adhesion molecule-1, VCAM-1, and intercellular adhesion molecule-1, ICAM-1) and chemotactic cytokines. The regulated expression of adhesion molecules in the multistep process of recruitment has been the topic of recent extensive reviews and chemokine production is discussed below. TNF and IFNγ cause redistribution of CD31 on the EC surface (Romer *et al.*, 1995) and this may be important, given this molecule's role in transmigration. IL-1 and TNF cause production of platelet activating factor (PAF) in EC (Mantovani *et al.*, 1992). A serine protease is involved in PAF synthesis in activated EC (Heller *et al.*, 1992; Bussolino *et al.*, 1994a). PAF can act on leukocytes as well as on EC themselves (Bussolino *et al.*, 1994c). PAF is not important for leukocyte adhesion, but primes leukocytes and facilitates transmigration (Hill *et al.*, 1994).

The membrane attack complex of complement (C) boosts TNF-induced expression of adhesion molecules (Kilgore *et al.*, 1995) and induces tissue factor by inducing IL-1α (Saadi *et al.*, 1995). In turn, IL-1 increases the production of C3 and factor B by EC (Coulpier *et al.*, 1995). Inactive MAC also activates expression of adhesion molecules and chemokines in EC (Tedesco *et al.*, 1997). The first long pentraxin PTX3, also known as TSG14, is one of the many genes identified in cytokine-activated EC (Breviario *et al.*, 1992; Introna *et al.*, 1996). This secreted molecule consists of a C-terminal domain, encoded by the 3rd exon, with sequence and structural similarity to classical pentraxins (e.g. CRP), coupled with an unrelated N-terminal portion. PTX3 is produced *in vitro* by various cell types, particularly EC and mononuclear phagocytes. After LPS administration to mice, PTX3 is expressed predominantly by heart and skeletal muscle EC (Introna *et al.*, 1996). Recent results suggest that PTX3 binds C1q and thus may be a mechanism of regulation of innate immunity (Bottazzi *et al.*, 1997).

9.1.2 IL-6

Various stimuli induce production not of IL-11 but of copious amounts of IL-6 and leukemia inhibitory factor (LIF) (Sironi *et al.*, 1989; Grosset *et al.*, 1995) in EC (Mantovani *et al.*, 1992). IL-6 production is elicited by IL-1, TNF, IL-4, IL-13, oncostatin M, IL-17 (Fossiez *et al.*, 1996), infectious agents and their products, and hypoxia (Yan *et al.*, 1995; for review see: Mantovani *et al.*, 1997). NFIL-6 is involved in the latter response (Yan *et al.*, 1995).

Original studies on IL-6 production by human umbelical vein EC (HUVEC) concluded that this cytokine did not affect several EC functions (Sironi *et al.*, 1989), and this has been repeatedly confirmed, despite indications that this molecule is involved in angiogenesis and tumor vessel formation. Observations in IL-6-deficient knock-out mice prompted a re-examination of the interaction of IL-6 with EC. HUVEC express the signal transducing the gp130 chain but not the IL-6R chain (Fig. 9.2). Soluble IL-6R and IL-6 alone did not affect EC function, but the two together induced chemokine production in EC, with no other measurable response. IL-6/IL-6R complexes activated STAT3 in EC (Modur *et al.*, 1997; Romano *et al.*, 1997). Thus, recent *in vitro* and *in vivo* data suggest that IL-6 plays an unsuspected role as a pathway of amplification of leukocyte recruitment and that, in concert with its soluble receptor, it activates a unique functional program in EC. This finding may underlie attenuation of inflammatory diseases (rheumatoid arthritis, allergic encephalomyelitis) observed in IL-6 gene targeted mice and the activity of anti-IL-6 antibodies observed in humans (see Chapter 7).

9.1.3 Bacterial products and toxins

Bacterial lipopolysaccharides (LPS) elicits a spectrum of EC responses similar to that of IL-1 and TNF (Mantovani *et al.*, 1992). EC, which are CD14⁻, interact with soluble CD14 and LPS-binding protein, both present in plasma (Haziot *et al.*, 1993; Pugin *et al.*, 1993a; Read *et al.*, 1993; von Asmuth *et al.*, 1993; Goldblum *et al.*, 1994). While EC can be directly activated by LPS, the indirect pathway involving mononuclear phagocyte activation and production of inflammatory cytokines is more effective in LPS stimulation of EC (Pugin *et al.*, 1993b). EC express Toll-like receptor 4 (TLR-4), but not TLR-2, which activates the MyD88/IL-1 receptor activated kinase (IRAK) pathway (Zhang *et al.*, 1999).

The *Lexosceles* venom toxin causes selective expression of IL-8, granulocyte-macrophage colony stimulating factor (GM-CSF) and E-selectin but not of IL-6 or ICAM-1 (Patel *et al.*, 1994). *Staphylococcus aureus*, a gram-positive bacterium, interacts with EC and after internalization induces IL-1 and IL-6 production (Yao *et al.*, 1995).

Infection with *E. coli* producing verocytotoxin (also known as Shiga toxin) is causally related to the subsequent development of hemolytic uremic syndrome (Remuzzi and Ruggenenti, 1995). Verocytotoxin directly activates EC in a prothrombotic proinflammatory sense, acting synergistically with IL-1 and TNF (van de Kar *et al.*, 1992, 1995). These cytokines boost the expression of receptors for verocytotoxin by enhancing galactosyltransferase and increasing globotriaosylceramide (Gb3) (van de Kar *et al.*, 1995), thus providing a molecular basis for synergism (van de Kar *et al.*, 1992). *Cowdria rumirantum* infects EC and elicits IL-1, IL-8, and IL-6 (Bourdoulous *et al.*, 1995). EBV infects EC and EBV cell lines induce IL-6 production (Jones *et al.*, 1995). *Rickettsia conorii*, the agent of Mediterranean spotted fever, induces IL-6 and IL-8 production through IL-1 (Kaplanski *et al.*, 1995). Various viruses, including CMV for instance, alter cytokine production (Almeida *et al.*, 1994).

9.1.4 Hematopoietic growth factors

The hematopoietic growth factors GM-CSF, G-CSF, IL-3, and erythropoietin affect EC (Bussolino *et al.*, 1994b). These factors are relatively weak agonists, which affect migration and proliferation, and amplify EC responsiveness to other signals (Bussolino *et al.*,

1994b); in the same studies M-CSF, IL-5, and IL-6 were inactive. However, in two studies, M-CSF induced expression of monocyte chemotactic protein-1 (MCP-1) in EC (Shyy *et al.*, 1993) (see above). We did not detect c-fms mRNA, encoding the M-CSF receptor, in HUVEC (unpublished data). Analysis of receptor expression showed that EC express c-kit and the ß chain common to the GM-CSF, IL-3, and IL-5 receptors. They also have detectable mRNA for αIL-3 and αGM, but not for αIL-5. It was suggested that the ability of various hemopoietic cytokines to affect EC is a 'memoire' from common ancestors, reflecting the common ontogenetic origin of hematopoietic and endothelial elements in blood islands (Bussolino *et al.*, 1994b). EC express the IL-3Rα chain, and TNF and IFNγ augment its expression (Korpelainen *et al.*, 1995). IL-3 and TNF act synergistically in terms of induction of IL-8 and adhesion molecules and the same occurs with IFNγ in terms of class II MHC.

9.1.5 Interferons and IL-12

IFNγ was the first molecularly identified cytokine shown to affect EC (Pober and Cotran, 1990). IFNγ induces EC expression of MHC class II antigens and the invariant chain, and increases class I. It also amplifies responses to TNF, slowly stimulates ICAM-1 expression, and boosts LPS-induced production of IL-1. EC express CD40 and IFNγ, as well as IFNß, IL-1 and TNF augment its expression (Hollenbaugh *et al.*, 1995; Karmann *et al.*, 1995; Yellin *et al.*, 1995). Engagement of CD40 amplifies the induction of adhesion molecules (Karmann *et al.*, 1995). Thus, ping-pong stimulation may occur when cells expressing CD40L (leukocytes and platelets) interact with EC.

IL-12 is a heterodimer active on T cells and NK cells, with activity against a variety of murine tumors. This cytokine has potent anti-angiogenic activity *in vivo* (Voest *et al.*, 1995). In a mouse opportunistic vascular tumor, IL-12 is the most effective single agent studied to date (Vecchi *et al.*, unpublished data). Circumstantial evidence suggests that IL-12 does not act *per se* on EC, but rather by inducing IFNγ (Voest *et al.*, 1995). IFNs have long been known to have anti-angiogenic activity and IFNα is used in the treatment of human hemangiomas (Ezekowitz *et al.*, 1992). IFNγ may act on EC through induction of the C-X-C chemokine IP-10 (see below). Thus, IL-12 may set in motion a cytokine cascade involving IFNγ and IP10, which eventually results in inhibition of angiogenesis.

9.1.6 IL-4 and IL-13

IL-4 has growth factor activity and induces uPA in micro but not macrovascular EC (Mantovani *et al.*, 1992; Wojta *et al.*, 1993). IL-4 and IL-13, but not IL-10, inhibited the induction of RANTES expression in EC stimulated by IFNγ and TNF (Marfaingkoka *et al.*, 1995). IL-4 selectively induces VCAM-1 and inhibits ICAM-1 and E-selectin expression. IL-4 is a weak inducer of IL-6 and MCP-1 in EC and amplifies production of these mediators in concert with other stimuli (Mantovani *et al.*, 1992). IL-13 has similar activities on EC (Sironi *et al.*, 1994). Sharing receptor components may underlie the similarity of action of IL-4 and IL-13 in EC (see Chapter 6). These cytokines have divergent effects on monocytes (where they inhibit), and EC (where they amplify the production of certain cytokines). Stimulation of certain EC functions may be important in the induction and local expression of Th2 type responses, by, for instance, inducing recruitment of eosinophils and basophils and favoring the transition to the late phase reaction.

9.1.7 IL-10

Information on the interaction of IL-10 with vascular endothelium is scanty and fragmentary. This cytokine was a weak stimulus for expression of chemokines, and IL-6 in mouse Polyoma middle T (PmT) immortalized EC lines and amplified the action of IL-1 and TNF (Sironi *et al.*, 1993). This effect was associated with prolongation of the mRNA half life. Stimulation of HUVEC was variable and not reproducible. Under the same conditions, IL-10 inhibited pro-inflammatory cytokine production in human and murine mononuclear phagocytes. This dissociation of effects (inhibition versus co-stimulation) is reminiscent of the activity of IL-4 and IL-13 (see above). IL-10 was reported to inhibit antigen presentation by human dermal microvascular EC (Vora *et al.*, 1994) and induction of tetrahydrobiopterin in HUVEC (Schoedon *et al.*, 1993). The effects of IL-10 on IL-8 production have been the subject of conflicting reports (Debeaux *et al.*, 1995; Chen and Manning, 1996). IL-10 inhibited the ability of LPS to amplify apoptosis of EC by irradiation (Eissner *et al.*, 1995). In one study (Krakauer, 1995), IL-10 inhibited induction of adhesion molecules by IL-1α.

9.1.8 Chemokines

By and large, the spectrum of action of chemokines is restricted to leukocytes, but recent evidence suggests that some members of this superfamily of inflammatory mediators affect EC function. IL-8, groα and other CXC chemokines were reported to induce EC migration and proliferation *in vitro* and to be angiogenic *in vivo* (Wen *et al.*, 1989; Koch *et al.*, 1992; Strieter *et al.*, 1992). The expression of high-affinity receptors and responsiveness to IL-8 of EC has been investigated, but with conflicting resuts (Petzelbauer *et al.*, 1995; Schonbeck *et al.*, 1995). Platelet factor 4, a CXC chemokine contained in the α granules of platelets, inhibits growth factor-induced proliferation of EC and angiogenesis (Maione *et al.*, 1990). Interferon γ-inducible protein 10 (IP 10) also had angiostatic properties *in vivo*, though results are conflicting as regards its capacity to inhibit bFGF-induced proliferation of HUVEC *in vitro* (Angiolillo *et al.*, 1995; Luster *et al.*, 1995). IP-10 induced through IFNγ may be the ultimate mediator of the anti-angiogenic activity of IL-12 (Voest *et al.*, 1995). A 3-amino acid motif (Glu–Leu–Arg) (ELR) is highly conserved in all members of the CXC family, which activate neutrophils. Recent results, including the action of ELR$^+$ versus ELR$^-$ molecules and the activity of IL-8 muteins, suggest that the presence or absence of an ELR motif dictates whether CXC chemokines induce or inhibit angiogenesis (Strieter *et al.*, 1995). However, the observation that groß inhibits angiogenesis is not consistent with this (Cao *et al.*, 1995). Three types of chemokine binding sites have been identified (Mantovani *et al.*, 1996) (Fig. 9.2). Chemokines activate leukocytes through seven-transmembrane domain, G-protein coupled receptors. A promiscuous chemokine receptor identical to the Duffy blood group antigen has been identified on erythrocytes, where it may act as a sink for chemokines leaking from inflamed tissues. This promiscuous receptor is expressed by EC at postcapillary venules *in vivo*, but not by endothelial cells *in vitro* (Peiper *et al.*, 1995; Mantovani *et al.*, 1996). The receptor structure is that of a seven-transmembrane-type molecule, but there is no clear evidence of signalling activity. Finally, chemokines bind heparin and heparin-like proteoglycans, and on EC these molecules present at least certain chemokines to leukocytes in the multistep process of recruitment. The molecular basis of the pro- and anti-angiogenic has not been clearly established. The expression of classic chemokine serpentine receptors in EC is controversial (Wen *et al.*, 1989; Maione *et al.*, 1990; Rot, 1992; Heinrich *et al.*, 1993; Angiolillo *et al.*, 1995; Luster *et al.*, 1995; Petzelbauer *et al.*, 1995) but there is evidence that EC express CXCR2 and CXCR4. Genetic inactivation of CXCR4 and of its ligand SDF1 resulted in defective formation of the vascular tree of the gastrointestinal tract (Tachibana *et al.*, 1998).

9.2 The cytokine repertoire of vascular cells

Vascular cells, particularly EC, are important producers of various polypeptide mediators that regulate the hematopoietic system, the differentiation of T and B cells, and the extravasation of leukocytes at inflammatory sites. Here we briefly summarize information on the production by EC of cytokines that affect leukocytes. TGFß, a product and a regulator of EC (Sporn *et al.*, 1987; Mantovani and Dejana, 1989; Gamble and Vadas, 1991), is not considered here (see Chapter 6).

9.2.1 IL-1 and IL-6

IL-1, a cytokine that profoundly affects vascular cells (see above), is also a product of vessel wall elements (Mantovani and Dejana, 1989; Pober and Cotran, 1990; Libby and Hansson, 1991). Inducers of IL-1 production by vascular cells include LPS, TNF and IL-1 itself. *In vitro* passage of EC results in spontaneous expression of the IL-1α message and refractoriness to activation by exogenous IL-1. IL-1 gene expression and protein were also detected *in vivo* after inoculation of LPS and feeding an atherogenic diet (Clinton *et al.*, 1991; Moyer *et al.*, 1991). Endothelial cells produce IL-1, but efforts to demonstrate expression of the IL-1 receptor antagonist (IL-1ra) in umbilical vein cells gave negative results (Bertini *et al.*, 1992). IL-1ra blocks the action of IL-1 on EC, and these cells may be a major target for the therapeutic activity of this molecule *in vivo*.

On exposure to inflammatory signals and superinduction by protein synthesis inhibitors, vascular SMC, but not EC, can express TNF mRNA and protein (Warner and Libby, 1989). SMC and EC produce high levels of IL-6 (Sironi *et al.*, 1989). Variable levels of spontaneous IL-6 production can usually be detected and are markedly increased by exposure to IL-1, TNF, and LPS. IL-1 acts on T cells at least partly by inducing IL-6. There is evidence that IL-6, acting in concert with soluble IL-6 receptor, is an important, amplifying agent of chemokine production *in vivo* (Romano *et al.*, 1997). Production of IL-6 is amplified by co-stimulation with IL-4 or IL-13 (Howell *et al.*, 1991; Rollins and Pober, 1991; Colotta *et al.*, 1992). IL-6 is also induced by IL-17 (Fossiez *et al.*, 1996). Hypoxia induces IL-6 production in EC and NFIL-6 plays a central role in this (Yan *et al.*, 1995). IL-6 is a pleiotropic cytokine that affects T and B lymphocytes and the production of acute-phase proteins by liver. The production of IL-6 by EC integrates these cells in immunological circuits and in the regulation of the acute-phase response. IL-1 also induces the production of leukemia inhibitory factor (LIF) (Grosset *et al.*, 1995), but not of IL-11 (Suen *et al.*, 1994).

9.2.2 Colony stimulating factors (CSF)

EC are an important source of CSF. Hematopoietic growth factors produced by EC include stem cell factor (Meininger *et al.*, 1995), G-CSF, GM-CSF, and M-CSF. CSF production is induced or boosted by a variety of stimuli including LPS, IL-1 and TNF (Mantovani and Dejana, 1989; Pober and Cotran, 1990; Libby and Hansson, 1991) and minimally modified low-density lipoproteins (MM-LDL) (Rajavashisth *et al.*, 1990). By producing CSF as well as IL-1 and IL-6, which have CSF activity, EC participate in the regulation of hematopoiesis. Because EC respond to certain CSF molecules (G-CSF, GM-CSF, and erythropoietin), autocrine and paracrine circuits involving EC and CSF could be important in the generation and maintenance of an appropriate bone marrow mileu.

9.2.3 Chemokines

EC produce various chemokines in response to signals representative of inflammatory reactions, immunity and thrombosis (Mantovani *et al.*, 1992). Inflammatory cytokines (IL-1 and TNF) and bacterial LPS induce expression and release of IL-8 and groα (Gimbrone *et al.*, 1989; Schroder and Christophers, 1989; Strieter *et al.*, 1989; Wen *et al.*, 1989; Dixit *et al.*, 1990; Rollins *et al.*, 1990; Sica *et al.*, 1990a, 1990b). Monocyte-associated IL-1α induces IL-8 expression in EC through via a juxtacrine mechanism (Kaplanski *et al.*, 1994). Induction of IL-8 expression is associated with and depends on gene transcription (Sica *et al.*, 1990a). IL-4 and IL-13 are weak inducers of IL-8 expression and amplify induction by inflammatory cytokines (Howell *et al.*, 1991; Rollins and Pober, 1991; Colotta *et al.*, 1992; Korpelainen *et al.*, 1993; Sironi *et al.*, 1994). Histamine induces IL-8 production in EC (Jeannin *et al.*, 1994). Hypoxia has been shown to induce IL-8 and MCP-1 expression in EC, a finding potentially relevant for pathological conditions in which leukocyte activation and recruitment may amplify tissue damage (Kaplanski *et al.*, 1993; Karakurum *et al.*, 1994). Platelets contain IL-1 and induce IL-8 gene expression when they interact with vascular EC (Kaplanski *et al.*, 1993). Fibrin induces IL-8 in EC (Qi and Kreutzer, 1995). Recent results suggest that activated EC store IL-8 in their Weibel-Palade bodies and release it in a delayed fashion (Wolff *et al.*, 1998).

As a result of proteolytic cleavage, IL-8 versions with a different NH$_2$ terminus and length can be produced (Baggiolini *et al.*, 1994). It has been suggested that EC release mainly a 77aa version of IL-8, which is less active in activating leukocytes than the most common 73-residue form (Gimbrone *et al.*, 1989; Hebert *et al.*, 1990). Proteolytic conversion to smaller versions of the molecule can be catalyzed by thrombin (Hebert *et al.*, 1990).

EC of postcapillary venules bind IL-8, possibly though heparin-like molecules (Rot, 1992). EC of postcapillary venules in kidney and other tissues expess the promiscuous chemokine receptor also present on erythrocytes, known as Duffy antigen (Hadley *et al.*, 1994; Peiper *et al.*, 1995). This receptor is seen on EC of both Duffy+ and Duffy– individuals and may serve to present chemokines to circulating leukocytes. Solid phase IL-8 elicits haptotactic migration (Wang *et al.*, 1990). Thus, locally produced IL-8 may be retained on the surface of EC and activate adhesive interactions and migration (Rot, 1992).

EC activated *in vitro* by inflammatory cytokines express groα, which, according to one report, may in turn act on EC (Wen *et al.*, 1989). EC-bound groα may promote monocyte adhesion (Schwartz *et al.*, 1994).

IP10, an ELR⁻ member of the CXC family, is expressed in certain endothelia of mice exposed *in vivo* to IFNγ or to LPS (Narumi *et al.*, 1992; Gómez-Chiarri *et al.*, 1993). There are no reports on its *in vitro* expression in EC.

EC produce substantial amounts of the C–C chemokine MCP-1 (Rollins *et al.*, 1990; Sica *et al.*, 1990b). The pro-inflammatory signals IL-1, TNF and, to a lesser extent, LPS are potent stimuli for MCP-1 production (Rollins *et al.*, 1990; Sica *et al.*, 1990b). Under the same conditions, MCP-2 was undetectable in EC supernatants (J. Van Damme, personal communication). IL-4 and IL-13 are active, though less potent inducers of MCP-1 expression (Howell *et al.*, 1991; Rollins and Pober, 1991; Colotta *et al.*, 1992). IFNγ induces MCP-1 in human microvascular EC (Brown *et al.*, 1994). M-CSF was reported to induce MCP-1, though we did not detect the M-CSF receptor c-fms in HUVEC by Northern analysis (Shyy *et al.*, 1993). Given the roles of lipids and monocytes in the natural history of atherosclerosis, it is of interest that minimally modified low density lipoproteins (MM-LDL) induce MCP-1 production in EC and smooth muscle cells (Cushing *et al.*, 1990). Thrombin induced expression of MCP-1 in monocytes and, less markedly, in EC (Colotta *et al.*, 1994). The C–C chemokine RANTES was produced by EC exposed to TNF and IFNγ (Marfaingkoka *et al.*, 1995).

The molecular basis of stimulation of chemokine expression in EC has been studied to a limited extent. Induction by inflammatory signals and thrombin is independent of protein synthesis in EC but, interestingly, not in monocytes (Colotta *et al.*, 1994). Enhanced gene transcription was demonstrated directly for MCP-1 and IL-8 by nuclear run-off analysis (Sica *et al.*, 1990a, 1990b).

Early studies on MCP-1 already reported that vascular smooth muscle cells (SMC) secreted a monocyte chemoattractant (Valente *et al.*, 1984, 1988), which resembled a similar factor produced by tumor lines (Bottazzi *et al.*, 1983). The SMC-derived factor was subsequently identified as MCP-1. Indeed, IL-1, TNF, and MM-LDL induce the expression of MCP-1 in SMC with mechanisms and kinetics resembling those in EC (Cushing *et al.*, 1990; Wang *et al.*, 1991). IL-1 and TNF also stimulate the expression and release of IL-8 in SMC (Wang *et al.*, 1991). Kidney mesangial cells may have an ontogenetic relationship with SMC. They express and release MCP-1 and IL-8 in response to IL-1 and TNF (Zoja *et al.*, 1991; Rovin *et al.*, 1992; Satriano *et al.*, 1993a, 1993b).

Of special importance in relation to pathology is the induction of MCP-1 and IP10 by aggregated immunoglobulins (Satriano *et al.*, 1993a, 1993b). Reactive oxygen intermediates act as second messengers in induction of MCP-1 by aggregated Ig (Satriano *et al.*, 1993a). These results may have considerable relevance in kidney pathology involving mononuclear phagocyte infiltration.

9.3 Role of platelets and coagulation factors

Platelets store a multiplicity of cytokines and growth factors in their α-granules and release them upon activation. Classically, platelets contain PDGF and TGFß, as well as other growth factors that affect connective tissue elements. They also contain IL-1ß and can activate EC by a justacrine release of this pro-inflammatory cytokine (Figs 9.2 and 9.4) (Kaplanski *et al.*, 1994).

Platelets contain chemokines or chemokine precursors as preformed proteins. These include the CC chemokine RANTES and CXC ß-thromboglobulin. Beta-thromboglobulin has long been known to be contained in the platelet granules and has been used as a marker for platelet activation. With proteolytic processing at the N-terminus, ß-thromboglobulin eventually gives rise to neutrophil activating protein 2 (NAP-2), an agonist for the chemokine receptor CXCR2. Proteolytic processing of NAP-2 is mediated by enzymes produced by monocytes, as well as by thrombin. Thrombin can also process the N-terminal part of IL-8, a CXC chemokine produced by a variety of cell types including EC. Finally, platelets contain platelet factor 4 (PF4), a member of the CXC family that lacks the ELR motif before the CXC motif. PF4 is not active on neutrophils and does not interact with known chemokine receptors. It plays a role in the negative regulation of angiogenesis.

As discussed above, activated EC can activate the coagulation cascade. The main product of the coagulation cascade, thrombin, can in turn act on EC. Thrombin rapidly induces the adhesion molecule P-selectin stored in the Weibel and Palade bodies of EC. Thrombin has now been shown to induce chemokine production in EC and in smooth muscle cells and mesangial cells, notably the CC chemokine monocyte chemotactic protein-1 (MCP-1). Thus, activated EC promote the coagulation cascade and their function is modulated in turn by platelets and coagulation factors (Fig. 9.4) (Colotta *et al.*, 1994).

9.4 EC heterogeneity

Vascular endothelia are remarkably heterogeneous in terms of morphology, marker expression (e.g. von Willebrand factor), and function. Heterogeneity is evident at multiple levels and emerges from analysis of macro- and microvascular EC, of the vascular bed

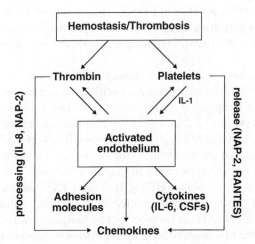

Fig. 9.4 Platelets, coagulation, and cytokines.

from different organs, and of EC from different compartments in the same organ. However, studies of EC heterogeneity in response to, and production of, cytokines are scanty and fragmentary. Unlike large vessel EC, microvascular EC express PDGF receptors (Beitz *et al.*, 1991) and respond to IL-4 with growth and uPA production (Strieter *et al.*, 1989; Wojta *et al.*, 1993). When EC from different levels of the lung—pulmonary artery and microvessels—were investigated for their responsiveness to TNF, only the former were damaged by this cytokine, which increased PGI_2 production in both (Meyrick *et al.*, 1991).

Human microvascular EC of dermal or brain origin have been amply studied. These differed from HUVEC in terms of expression of adhesion molecules in response to inflammatory cytokines or endothelins (Petzelbauer *et al.*, 1993; Rott *et al.*, 1993; McCarron *et al.*, 1995), antigen presentation regulated by IFNγ and IL-10 (Vora *et al.*, 1994), and tetrahydrobiopterin production regulated by various mediators (Schoedon *et al.*, 1993). As discussed above, production of chemokines may be regulated differently in different EC populations (Brown *et al.*, 1994). All in all, the question of EC heterogeneity is complex and its molecular and cellular basis, as well as the formulation of a conceptual framework for this descriptive phenomenology, remain elusive.

9.5 Pathology

Diseases involving a wide range of cellular and organ systems have vascular cells as targets or participants. Here we will focus on selected disorders in which the interplay between vascular cells and cytokines has a primary role.

9.5.1 Infectious diseases

Viral, bacterial, or protozoal infections directly or indirectly involve EC. Viruses infect or interact with EC and induce or modify cytokine production. For instance, Epstein-Barr virus (EBV) and cytomegalovirus (CMV) infect EC, and EBV cell lines induce IL-6 production (Almeida *et al.*, 1994; Jones *et al.*, 1995). High levels of MCP-1 were found in the cerebrospinal fluid of patients with HIV infection, specifically associated with CMV encephalitis (Bernasconi *et al.*, 1996); immunoreactive MCP-1 was detected in brain EC (L. Vago,. unpublished).

EC-cytokine networks have acquired importance in HIV-1 infection and associated clinical disorders, including Kaposi's sarcoma, bacillary angiomatosis, vasculitis, psoriasis, and non-Hodgkin lymphomas in the central nervous system. The interaction between infected monocytes and EC increases viral replication. This response appears to occur through cell contact and EC-derived cytokines (IL-6, GM-CSF and IL-1) (Fan *et al.*, 1994). An imbalance of inflammatory cytokine production has been described in AIDS patients and precedes the appearance of Kaposi's sarcoma (Fan *et al.*, 1993). A combination of inflammatory cytokines (IFNγ, IL-1, and TNF) induces EC *in vitro* to acquire phenotypic and functional features closely resembling cultured and *in situ* Kaposi's sarcoma spindle cells. These include spindle morphology, the responsiveness to HIV-Tat protein, and the neo-expression or up-regulation of adhesion molecules such as ICAM-1, VCAM, and E-selectin. Finally, these EC become angiogenic in nude mice

(Fiorelli *et al.*, 1995; Samaniego *et al.*, 1995). Thus, *in vivo* hyperplasia of EC observed in Kaposi's sarcoma and angiogenesis may be related to chronic exposure to inflammatory cytokines.

Rickettsia rickettsiae and *R.. conorii* cause spotted fevers characterized by generalized vascular inflammation. *Rickettsiae* enter and proliferate in EC. EC functions affected include permeability, expression of adhesion molecules, and release of von Willebrand factor. *Rickettsia. conorii* induced IL-1α in EC, and cell-associated IL-1α was responsible for induction of IL-8 and IL-6 (Kaplanski *et al.*, 1995). Therefore, a cytokine cascade triggered by rickettsial infection of EC may play an important role is spotted fever-associated vasculitis.

Gram-positive and gram-negative bacteria and their products interact with EC, inducing cytokine production, and this interaction accounts for some of the systemic manifestations of sepsis, as well as for located reactions. *Staphyllococcus aureus*, a gram-positive bacterium, interacts with EC and, after internalization, induces IL-1 and IL-6 production (Yao *et al.*, 1995). EC are a major determinant of systemic inflammatory response syndrome (SIRS)/toxic shock. Hypotension and coagulation abnormalities very likely primarily depend EC activation by LPS or LPS-induced IL-1 and TNF (Bradley *et al.*, 1994). Bacterial lipopolysaccharides (LPS) elicit a spectrum of EC responses similar to IL-1 and TNF (see above).

EC, which are CD14[-], interact with soluble CD14 and LPS-binding protein, both present in plasma (Haziot *et al.*, 1993; Pugin *et al.*, 1993a; Read *et al.*, 1993; von Asmuth *et al.*, 1993; Goldblum *et al.*, 1994). TLR-4 is expressed by EC and is probably essental for the formation of a signaling receptor complex, which recognizes LPS and possibly other microbial moieties (Zhang *et al.*, 1999). While direct activation of EC by LPS does occur, the indirect pathway, involving mononuclear phagocyte activation and production of inflammatory cytokines, is more effective in stimulation of EC by this bacterial product (Pugin *et al.*, 1993b).

Among parasitic disorders, vascular involvement is a prominent feature of cerebral malaria, a fatal complication of *Plasmodium falciparum* infection in humans. Circumstantial evidence in human and mouse models suggests that cytokines, particularly TNF, and alterations of endothelial cells play a pivotal role in the arrest of erythrocytes in the brain and subsequent vascular damage (Chirivi *et al.*, 1994; Willimann *et al.*, 1995). The glycosylphosphatidyl inositol toxin induces VCAM-1, ICAM-1, E-selectin, and NO synthase in EC via a tyrosine kinase and PKC-dependent mechanism (Schofield *et al.*, 1996; Tachado *et al.*, 1996). The mechanisms responsible for selective involvement of the brain vascular bed remain undefined.

Hemolytic uremic syndrome (HUS), the most common cause of acute renal failure in infants and small children, is caused by infection with verotoxin (VT, or Shiga-like toxin) producing *E. coli* (Remuzzi and Ruggenenti, 1995). VT is toxic for EC, activating them in a pro-inflammatory/prothrombotic sense, and synergizes with IL-1 and TNF (van de Kar *et al.*, 1992, 1995). These cytokines enhance galactosyltransferase and consequently surface expression of globotriaosylceramide (Gb3) (van de Kar *et al.*, 1995). The VT receptor is expressed in greater amounts on EC of certain vascular beds, such as the kidney. Therefore in increase of Gb3 underlies the synergism between inflammatory cytokines and VT and explains the selective organ involvement in HUS.

9.5.2 Neoplasia

Formation of new blood vessels is a limiting factor in tumor growth and progression. An analysis of pro- and anti-angiogenic factors is beyond the scope of this Chapter. IFN, IL-12, and chemokines were discussed above, and selected aspects of IL-1 and TNF, mainly related to hemorrhagic necrosis and the promotion of metastasis, will be discussed here (Chirivi *et al.*, 1994).

IL-1 and TNF regulate the lifespan of EC and angiogenesis with seemingly contradictory actions. Endogenous IL-1α appears to shorten the lifespan of EC by acting intracellularly and localizing in the nucleus (Maier *et al.*, 1990). IL-1 and TNF are not growth factors for EC, but TNF induces EC migration *in vitro* and angiogenesis *in vivo* (Mantovani *et al.*, 1992). These may be indirect effects. TNF (and IL-1) induce production of the secreted protein B.61, which serves as an EC chemo-attractant and angiogenic factor by acting as the ligand for the eck tyrosin receptor (Holzman *et al.*, 1990).

Other molecules cloned as IL-1/TNF inducible genes in EC may be relevant to vasculogenesis or angiogenesis. A20 is a zinc-finger transcription factor, which may help protect EC and other cell types against TNF toxicity. B24 is a gene of unknown function expressed in a complex way during vasculogenesis (Sarma *et al.*, 1992). IL-1 and TNF induce chemokines in EC, which act as pro- or anti-angiogenic factors (see above).

Some tumors at least use the same molecular pathways as leukocytes for interacting with EC and seeding at distant anatomical sites. Cytokines expressed constitutively by cancer cells, or produced locally, increase the expression of adhesion molecules recognized by tumor cell counter-receptors (e.g. VLA4-VCAM-1 in melanoma) (Chirivi *et al.*, 1994). In the same vein, EC-derived chemokines may play a role in cancer seeding at specific sites (Wakabayashi *et al.*, 1995).

The function of TNF shared by other inflammatory cytokines is to cause hemorragic necrosis of neoplastic or appropriately conditioned normal tissues (Schwartzman reaction). Involvement and damage of the vascular bed is a prominent feature of hemorrhagic necrosis (Mantovani *et al.*, 1992). TNF is not cytotoxic for confluent EC. It remains unclear exactly how TNF selectively damage the vasculature of murine and human (Lienard *et al.*, 1992) tumors.

9.5.3. Atherosclerosis and cardiovascular pathology

Monocyte recruitment is the first recognizable event in the natural history of atherosclerosis (Libby and Hansson, 1991). EC and SMC produce chemokines, MCP-1 in particular, in response to pathological or physiological stimuli (see above). MCP-1 expression has been detected in atheromatous lesions of rabbits, primates, and humans (Nelken *et al.*, 1991; Yla Herttuala *et al.*, 1991; Yu *et al.*, 1992; Takeya *et al.*, 1993). IL-8 and MCP-1 mRNA have been detected in increased amounts in aortic aneurysms (Koch *et al.*, 1993). Chemokine gene expression has been detected in various cellular elements, including SMC, EC, and mononuclear phagocytes, with somewhat different results in different studies. In the only study with mAb (Takeya *et al.*, 1993), cell populations positive for MCP-1 were different in lesions at different stages of the natural history of atherosclerosis. EC staining was prominent in diffuse intimal thickening and in fatty streaks, but weak in atheromatous lesions. Subendothelial macrophages were strongly positive for MCP-1 in fatty streak lesions and in atherosclerotic plaques. In plaques, a few intimal SMC stained for MCP-1. These results suggest that EC and macrophages are the main source of MCP-1 in early atherosclerotic lesions (Takeya *et al.*, 1993). Direct *in vivo* evidence of the importance of MCP-1 in atheroma formation was obtained recently using MCP-1 and CCR2 –/– mice (Boring *et al.*, 1998; Gu *et al.*, 1998).

Microbial infections localized in the vessel wall or elsewhere have been associated with atheromatous disease of the heart (Epstein *et al.*, 1996). There is increasing evidence that cytokines play an important role in the pathogenesis and eventual clinical manifestation of atherosclerosis, myocardial infarction, and stroke (Libby, 1996; Ross, 1993). These disorders are associated with high circulating levels of cytokines (TNF, IL-6, IL-8) and cytokine receptors (e.g. soluble TNF receptors) (Latini *et al.*, 1994). Recent results suggest that polymorphism at the IL-1 receptor antagonist locus affects coronary artery disease. Homozygous patients for the IL-1RN 2 allele have an odds ratio of 2.8 for single-vessel coronary disease, which is a risk factor higher than hypercholesterolemia (Francis *et al.*, 1999). Experimental findings indicate that anti-cytokine strategies have a beneficial effect on tissue damage following stroke or myocardial infarction. Most importantly, there is clinical evidence that C reactive protein, a pentraxin produced in the liver as the ultimate product of cytokine activation, is an important predictor of coronary events in patients with stable or unstable angina (Berk *et al.*, 1990; Liuzzo *et al.*, 1994; Heinrich *et al.*, 1995; Thompson *et al.*, 1995; Liuzzo *et al.*, 1996; Maseri *et al.*, 1996; Haverkate *et al.*, 1997).

Elevated levels of pro-inflammatory cytokines, particularly TNF, have been detected in severe congestive heart failure (Mann and Young, 1994; Aukrust *et al.*, 1998). Current views, which assign an important role to inflammatory cytokines as an amplification loop in ischemic heart disease, its sequelae, and stroke, call for an assessment of anticytokine strategies in these cardiovascular disorders (Meistrell *et al.*, 1997).

Inhibitors of cholesterol synthesis, which block HMH-CoA reductase (statins), reduce cholesterol levels and the risk of acute myocardial infarction. It has been argued that their therapeutic action cannot be explained solely on the basis of lowering cholesterol blood levels (Valantine and Schroeder, 1997). Lovastatin and mevastatin both inhibit cytokine and MCP-1 production in particular (Terkeltaub *et al.*, 1994; Kim *et al.*, 1995; Romano *et al.*, in press) and, given its established role in the pathogenesis of atherosclerosis (see above), these results raise the interesting possibility that inhibition of MCP-1 production is a component of the statins' therapeutic activity.

9.5.4 Transplantation and autoimmunity

EC are a major target for immune reactions directed against allo- or xenogeneic transplanted organs (Bach *et al.*, 1994) or self-antigens. Circulating anti-endothelial cell antibodies (AECA) have been detected in a variety of autoimmune diseases with vascular involvement. AECA are common in scleroderma, SLE, and Wegener granulomatosis. Antigens recognized include proteins (e.g. protease 3), phospholipids, and protein-PL complexes. AECA are frequently associated with severe clinical symptoms, notably thrombosis. These antibodies are generally not cytotoxic for EC, except in Kawasaki disease. AECA activate the expression of adhesion molecules, procoagulant activity, and cytokine production, and endogenous IL-1 is the ultimate mediator of at least some of these actions (Simantov *et al.*, 1995; Carvalho *et al.*, 1996; Del Papa *et al.*, 1996). Thus, EC activation is probably a major pathogenetic factor in the clinical manifestations associated with AECA.

9.6 Concluding remarks

Vascular cells, particularly EC, long considered a layer of nucleated cellophane, play an important active role in the onset and regulation of inflammatory and immune reactions. The varied spectrum of responses elicited by cytokines is a dramatic demonstration of vascular cell plasticity. The vast range of EC responses can be rationalized and represented in terms of cytokine-induced activation/differentiation programs. Work has now begun to unravel the molecular basis of EC activation by cytokines. However, many questions related to the mechanisms underlying expression restricted to EC and to EC heterogeneity remain unanswered. Information to date provides the basis for cytokine targeted therapies in certain human diseases, such as stroke and heart failure (Bristow, 1998; Giverts and Colucci, 1998).

References

Almeida, G. D., Porada, C. D., St Jeor, S., and Ascensao, J. L. (1994). Human cytomegalovirus alters interleukin-6 production by endothelial cells. *Blood*, **83**, 370–6.

Angiolillo, A. L., Sgadari, C., Taub, D. D., Liao, F., Farber, J. M., Maheshwari, S. *et al.* (1995). Human interferon-inducible protein 10 is a potent inhibitor of angiogenesis *in vivo*. *J. Exp. Med.*, **182**, 155–62.

Aukrust, P., Ueland, T., Muller, F., Andreassen, A. K., Nordoy, I., Kjekshus, J. *et al.* (1998). Elevated circulating levels of C-C chemokines in patients with congestive heart failure. *Circulation*, **97**, 1136–43.

Bach, F. H., Robson, S. C., Ferran, C., Winkler, H., Millan, M. T., Stuhlmeier, K. M. *et al.* (1994). Endothelial cell activation and thromboregulation during xenograft rejection. *Immunol. Rev.*, **141**, 5–30.

Baggiolini, M., Dewald, B., and Moser, B. (1994). Interleukin-8 and related chemotactic cytokines—CXC and CC chemokines. *Adv. Immunol.*, **55**, 99–179.

Balligand, J. L., Ungureanu Longrois, D., Simmons, W. W., Kobzik, L., Lowenstein, C. J., Lamas, S. *et al.* (1995). Induction of NO synthase in rat cardiac microvascular endothelial cells by IL-1 beta and IFN-gamma. *Am. J. Physiol.*, **268**, H1293-H303.

Beitz, J. G., Kim, I. S., Calabresi, P., and Frackelton, A. R. Jr. (1991). Human microvascular endothelial cells express receptors for platelet-derived growth factor. *Proc. Natl. Acad. Sci. USA.*, **88**, 2021–5.

Berk, B. C., Weintraub, W. S., and Alexander, R. W. (1990). Elevation of C-reactive protein in 'active' coronary artery disease. *Am. J. Cardiol.*, **65**, 168–72.

Bernasconi, S., Cinque, P., Peri, G., Sozzani, S., Crociati, A., Torri, W. *et al.* (1996). Selective elevation of monocyte chemotactic protein-1 in the cerebrospinal fluid of AIDS patients with cytomegalovirus encephalitis. *J. Infect. Dis.*, **174**, 1098–101.

Bertini, R., Sironi, M., Martin Padura, I., Colotta, F., Rambaldi, S., Bernasconi, S. *et al.* (1992). Inhibitory effect of recombinant intracellular interleukin 1 receptor antagonist on endothelial cell activation. *Cytokine*, **4**, 44–7.

Boring, L., Gosling, J., Cleary, M., and Charo, I. F. (1998). Decreased lesion formation in CCR2 –/– mice reveals a role for chemokines in the initiation of atherosclerosis. *Nature*, **394**, 894–7.

Bottazzi, B., Polentarutti, N., Acero, R., Balsari, A., Boraschi, D., Ghezzi, P. *et al.* (1983). Regulation of the macrophage content of neoplasms by chemoattractants. *Science*, **220**, 210–12.

Bottazzi, B., VouretCraviari, V., Bastone, A., DeGioia, L., Matteucci, C., Peri, G. *et al.* (1997). Multimer formation and ligand recognition by the long pentraxin PTX3—Similarities and differences with the short pentraxins C-reactive protein and serum amyloid P component. *J. Biol. Chem.*, **272**, 32817–23.

Bourdoulous, S., Bensaid, A., Martinez, D., Sheikboudou, C., Trap, I., Strosberg, A. D. *et al.* (1995). Infection of bovine brain microvessel endothelial cells with Cowdria ruminantium elicits IL-1 beta, -6, and -8 mRNA production and expression of an unusual MHC class II DQ alpha transcript. *J. Immunol.*, **154**, 4032–8.

Bradley, J. R., Wilks, D., and Rubenstein, D. (1994). The vascular endothelium in septic shock. *J. Infect.*, **28**, 1–10.

Breviario, F., d'Aniello, E. M., Golay, J., Peri, G., Bottazzi, B., Bairoch, A. *et al.* (1992). Interleukin-1-inducible genes in endothelial cells. Cloning of a new gene related to C-reactive protein and serum amyloid P component. *J. Biol. Chem.*, **267**, 22190–7.

Bristow, M. R. (1998). Tumor necrosis factor-α and cardiomyopathy. *Circulation*, **97**, 1340–1.

Brown, Z., Gerritsen, M. E., Carley, W. W., Strieter, R. M., Kunkel, S. L., and Westwick, J. (1994). Chemokine gene expression and secretion by cytokine- activated human microvascular endothelial cells—Differential regulation of monocyte chemoattractant protein-1 and interleukin-8 in response to interferon- gamma. *Am. J. Pathol.*, **145**, 913–21.

Bussolino, F., Arese, M., Silvestro, L., Soldi, R., Benfenati, E., Sanavio, F. *et al.* (1994a). Involvement of a serine protease in the synthesis of platelet-activating factor by endothelial cells stimulated by tumor necrosis factor-alpha or interleukin-1 alpha. *Eur. J. Immunol.*, **24**, 3131–9.

Bussolino, F., Bocchietto, E., Silvagno, F., Soldi, R., Arese, M., and Mantovani, A. (1994b). Actions of molecules which regulate hemopoiesis on endothelial cells: memoirs of common ancestors? *Pathol. Res. Pract.*, **190**, 834–9.

Bussolino, F., Silvagno, F., Garbarino, G., Costamagna, C., Sanavio, F., Arese, M. *et al.* (1994c). Human endothelial cells are targets for platelet-activating factor (PAF). Activation of alpha and beta protein kinase C isozymes in endothelial cells stimulated by PAF. *J. Biol. Chem.*, **269**, 2877–86.

Bussolino, F. and Camussi, G. (1995). Platelet-activating factor produced by endothelial cells. A molecule with autocrine and paracrine properties. *Eur. J. Biochem.*, **229**, 327–37.

Camacho, M., Godessart, N., Anton, R., Garcia, M., and Vila, L. (1995). Interleukin-1 enhances the ability of cultured human umbilical vein endothelial cells to oxidize linoleic acid. *J. Biol. Chem.*, **270**, 17279–86.

Cao, Y. H., Chen, C., Weatherbee, J. A., Tsang, M., and Folkman, J. (1995). gro-beta, a -C-X-C- chemokine, is an angiogenesis inhibitor that suppresses the growth of Lewis lung carcinoma in mice. *J. Exp. Med.*, **182**, 2069–77.

Carvalho, D., Savage, C. O. S., Blanck, C. M., and Pearson, J. D. (1996). IgG antiendothelial cell autoantibodies from scleroderma patients induce leukocyte adhesion to human vascular endothelial cells *in vitro*. *J. Clin. Invest.*, **97**, 111–9.

Chen, C. C. and Manning, A. M. (1996). TGF-beta 1, IL-10 and IL-4 differentially modulate the cytokine-induced expression of IL-6 AND IL-8 in human endothelial cells. *Cytokine*, **8**, 58–65.

Chirivi, R. G., Nicoletti, M. I., Remuzzi, A., and Giavazzi, R. (1994). Cytokines and cell adhesion molecules in tumor-endothelial cell interaction and metastasis. *Cell Adhes. Commun.*, **2**, 219–24.

Claria, J. and Serhan, C. N. (1995). Aspirin triggers previously undescribed bioactive eicosanoids by human endothelial cell-leukocyte interactions. *Proc. Natl. Acad. Sci. USA.*, **92**, 9475–9.

Clinton, S. K., Fleet, J. C., Loppnow, H., Salomon, R. N., Clark, B. D., Cannon, J. G. *et al.* (1991). Interleukin-1 gene expression in rabbit vascular tissue *in vivo*. *Am. J. Pathol.*, **138**, 1005–14.

Cobbs, C. S., Brenman, J. E., Aldape, K. D., Bredt, D. S., and Israel, M. A. (1995). Expression of nitric oxide synthase in human central nervous system tumors. *Cancer Res.*, **55**, 727–30.

Colotta, F., Sironi, M., Borre, A., Luini, W., Maddalena, F., and Mantovani, A. (1992). Interleukin 4 amplifies monocyte chemotactic protein and interleukin 6 production by endothelial cells. *Cytokine*, **4**, 24–8.

Colotta, F., Sciacca, F. L., Sironi, M., Luini, W., Rabiet, M. J., and Mantovani, A. (1994). Expression of monocyte chemotactic protein-1 by monocytes and endothelial cells exposed to thrombin. *Am. J. Pathol.*, **144**, 975–85.

Coulpier, M., Andreev, S., Lemercier, C., Dauchel, H., Lees, O., Fontaine, M. *et al.* (1995). Activation of the endothelium by IL-1 alpha and glucocorticoids results in major increase of complement C3 and factor B production and generation of C3a. *Clin. Exp. Immunol.*, **101**, 142–9.

Cushing, S. D., Berliner, J. A., Valente, A. J., Territo, M. C., Navab, M., Parhami, F. *et al.* (1990). Minimally modified low density lipoprotein induces monocyte chemotactic protein 1 in human endothelial cells and smooth muscle cells. *Proc. Natl. Acad. Sci. USA.*, **87**, 5134–8.

Debeaux, A. C., Maingay, J. P., Ross, J. A., Fearon, K. C. H., and Carter, D. C. (1995). Interleukin-4 and interleukin-10 increase endotoxin- stimulated human umbilical vein endothelial cell interleukin-8 release. *J. Interferon. Cytokine Res.*, **15**, 441–5.

De Caterina, R., Libby, P., Peng, H. B., Thannickal, V. J., Rajavashisth, T. B., Gimbrone, M. A. J. *et al.* (1995). Nitric oxide decreases cytokine-induced endothelial activation. Nitric oxide selectively reduces endothelial expression of adhesion molecules and proinflammatory cytokines. *J. Clin. Invest.*, **96**, 60–8.

Del Papa, N., Guidali, L., Sironi, M., Shoenfeld, Y., Mantovani, A., Tincani, A. *et al.* (1996). Anti-endothelial cell IgG antibodies from patients with Wegener's granulomatosis bind to human endothelial cells *in vitro* and induce adhesion molecule expression and cytokine secretion. *Arthritis Rheum.*, **39**, 758–66.

Dixit, V. M., Green, S., Sarma, V., Holzman, L. B., Wolf, F. W., O'Rourke, K. *et al.* (1990). Tumor necrosis factor-alpha induction of novel gene products in human endothelial cells including a macrophage-specific chemotaxin. *J. Biol. Chem.*, **265**, 2973–8.

Eissner, G., Kohlhuber, F., Grell, M., Ueffing, M., Scheurich, P., Hieke, A. *et al.* (1995). Critical involvement of transmembrane tumor necrosis factor-alpha in endothelial programmed cell death mediated by ionizing radiation and bacterial endoxin. *Blood*, **86**, 4184–93.

Epstein, S. E., Speir, E., Zhou, Y. F., Guetta, E., Leon, M., and Finkel, T. (1996). The role of infection in restenosis and atherosclerosis: focus on cytomegalovirus. *Lancet*, **348** (supplement 1), s13-s7.

Ezekowitz, R. A., Mulliken, J. B., and Folkman, J. (1992). Interferon alfa-2a therapy for life-threatening hemangiomas of infancy [see comments] [published errata appear in *New Engl. J. Med.* (1994) Jan 27; **330**(4), 300 and 1995 Aug 31; **333**(9), 595–6]. *N. Engl. J. Med.*, **326**, 1456–63.

Fan, J., Bass, H. Z., and Fahey, J. L. (1993). Elevated IFN-gamma and decreased IL-2 gene expression are associated with HIV infection. *J. Immunol.*, **151**, 5031–40.

Fan, S. T., Hsia, K., and Edgington, T. S. (1994). Upregulation of human immunodeficiency virus-1 in chronically infected monocytic cell line by both contact with endothelial cells and cytokines. *Blood*, **84**, 1567–72.

Fiorelli, V., Gendelman, R., Samaniego, F., Markham, P. D., and Ensoli, B. (1995). Cytokines from activated T cells induce normal endothelial cells to acquire the phenotypic and functional features of AIDS-Kaposi's sarcoma spindle cells. *J. Clin. Invest.*, **95**, 1723–34.

Fossiez, F., Djossou, O., Chomarat, P., Flores-Romo, L., Ait-Yahia, S., Maat, C. *et al.* (1996). T-cell IL-17 induces stromal cells to produce proinflammatory and hematopoietic cytokines. *J. Exp. Med.*, **183**, 2593–603.

Francis, S. E., Camp, N. J., Dewberry, R. M., Gunn, J., Syrris, P., Jeffery, S. *et al.* (1999). Interleukin-1 receptor antagonist gene polymorphism and coronary artery disease. *Circulation*, **99**, 861–6.

Fukuo, K., Inoue, T., Morimoto, S., Nakahashi, T., Yasuda, O., Kitano, S. *et al.* (1995). Nitric oxide mediates cytotoxicity and basic fibroblast growth factor release in cultured vascular smooth muscle cells. A possible mechanism of neovascularization in atherosclerotic plaques. *J. Clin. Invest.*, **95**, 669–76.

Gamble, J. R. and Vadas, M. A. (1991). Endothelial cell adhesiveness for human T lymphocytes is inhibited by transforming growth factor beta-1. *J. Immunol.*, **146**, 1149–54.

Gimbrone, M. A. J., Obin, M. S., Brock, A. F., Luis, E. A., Hass, P. E., Hebert, C. A. *et al.* (1989). Endothelial interleukin-8: a novel inhibitor of leukocyte-endothelial interactions. *Science*, **246**, 1601–3.

Givertz, M. M., and Colucci, W. S. (1998). New targets for heart-failure therapy: endothelin, inflammatory cytokines, and oxidative stress. *Lancet*, **352** (supplement 1), 34–38.

Goldblum, S. E., Brann, T. W., Ding, X., Pugin, J., and Tobias, P. S. (1994). Lipopolysaccharide (LPS)-binding protein and soluble CD14 function as accessory molecules for LPS-induced changes in endothelial barrier function, *in vitro. J. Clin. Invest.*, **93**, 692–702.

Gómez-Chiarri, M., Hamilton, T. A., Egido, J., and Emancipator, S. N. (1993). Expression of IP-10, a lipopolysaccharide- and interferon-gamma-inducible protein, in murine mesangial cells in culture. *Am. J. Pathol.*, **142**, 433–9.

Grosset, C., Jazwiec, B., Taupin, J. L., Liu, H., Richard, S., Mahon, F. X. *et al.* (1995). *In vitro* biosynthesis of leukemia inhibitory factor/human interleukin for DA cells by human endothelial cells: differential regulation by interleukin-1 alpha and glucocorticoids. *Blood*, **86**, 3763–70.

Gu, L., Okada, Y., Clinton, S. K., Gerard, C., Sukhova, G. K., Libby, P. *et al.* (1998). Absence of monocyte chemotactic protein-1 reduces atherosclerosis in low density lipoprotein receptor-deficient mice. *Mol. Cell*, **2**, 275–81.

Hadley, T. J., Lu, Z. H., Wasniowska, K., Martin, A. W., Peiper, S. C., Hesselgesser, J. *et al.* (1994). Postcapillary venule endothelial cells in kidney express a multispecific chemokine receptor that is structurally and functionally identical to the erythroid isoform, which is the Duffy blood group antigen. *J. Clin. Invest.*, **94**, 985–91.

Haverkate, F., Thompson, S. G., Pyke, S. D., Gallimore, J. R., and Pepys, M. B. (1997). Production of C-reactive protein and risk of coronary events in stable and unstable angina. European Concerted Action on Thrombosis and Disabilities Angina Pectoris Study Group. *Lancet*, **349**, 462–6.

Haziot, A., Rong, G. W., Silver, J., and Goyert, S. M. (1993). Recombinant soluble CD14 mediates the activation of endothelial cells by lipopolysaccharide. *J. Immunol.*, **151**, 1500–1507.

Hebert, C. A., Luscinskas, F. W., Kiely, J. M., Luis, E. A., Darbonne, W. C., Bennett, G. L. *et al.* (1990). Endothelial and leukocyte forms of IL-8. Conversion by thrombin and interactions with neutrophils. *J. Immunol.*, **145**, 3033–40.

Heinrich, J. N., Ryseck, R. P., Macdonald-Bravo, H., and Bravo, R. (1993). The product of a novel growth factor-activated gene, fic, is a biologically active C-C-type cytokine. *Mol. Cell Biol.*, **13**, 2020–30.

Heinrich, J., Schulte, H., Schonfeld, R., Kohler, E., and Assmann, G. (1995). Association of variables of coagulation, fibrinolysis and acute-phase with atherosclerosis in coronary and peripheral arteries and those arteries supplying the brain. *Thromb. Haemost.*, **73**, 374–9.

Heller, R., Bussolino, F., Ghigo, D., Garbarino, G., Pescarmona, G., Till, U. *et al.* (1992). Human endothelial cells are target for platelet-activating factor. II. Platelet-activating factor induces platelet-activating factor synthesis in human umbilical vein endothelial cells. *J. Immunol.*, **149**, 3682–8.

Hill, M. E., Bird, I. N., Daniels, R. H., Elmore, M. A., and Finnen, M. J. (1994). Endothelial cell-associated platelet-activating factor primes neutrophils for enhanced superoxide production and arachidonic acid release during adhesion to but not transmigration across IL-1 beta-treated endothelial monolayers. *J. Immunol.*, **153**, 3673–83.

Hollenbaugh, D., Mischel Petty, N., Edwards, C. P., Simon, J. C., Denfeld, R. W., Kiener, P. A. *et al.* (1995). Expression of functional CD40 by vascular endothelial cells. *J. Exp. Med.*, **182**, 33–40.

Holzman, L. B., Marks, R. M., and Dixit, V. M. (1990). A novel immediate-early response gene of endothelium is induced by cytokines and encodes a secreted protein. *Mol. Cell Biol.*, **10**, 5830–8.

Howell, G., Pham, P., Taylor, D., Foxwell, B., and Feldmann, M. (1991). Interleukin 4 induces interleukin 6 production by endothelial cells: synergy with interferon- gamma. *Eur. J. Immunol.*, **21**, 97–101.

Inoue, N., Venema, R. C., Sayegh, H. S., Ohara, Y., Murphy, T. J., and Harrison, D. G. (1995). Molecular regulation of the bovine endothelial cell nitric oxide synthase by transforming growth factor-beta 1. *Arterioscler. Thromb. Vasc. Biol.*, **15**, 1255–1261.

Introna, M., Vidal Alles, V., Castellano, M., Picardi, G., De Gioia, L., Bottazzi, B. *et al.* (1996). Cloning of mouse PTX3, a new member of the pentraxin gene family expressed at extrahepatic sites. *Blood*, **87**, 1862–1872.

Jackson, B. A., Goldstein, R. H., Roy, R., Cozzani, M., Taylor, L., and Polgar, P. (1993). Effects of transforming growth factor beta and interleukin-1 beta on expression of cyclooxygenase 1 and 2 and phospholipase A2 mRNA in lung fibroblasts and endothelial cells in culture. *Biochem. Biophys. Res. Commun.*, **197**, 1465–74.

Jeannin, P., Delneste, Y., Gosset, P., Molet, S., Lassalle, P., Hamid, Q. *et al.* (1994). Histamine induces interleukin-8 secretion by endothelial cells. *Blood*, **84**, 2229–33.

Jones, K., Rivera, C., Sgadari, C., Franklin, J., Max, E. E., Bhatia, K. *et al.* (1995). Infection of human endothelial cells with Epstein-Barr virus. *J. Exp. Med.*, **182**, 1213–21.

Kamijo, R., Harada, H., Matsuyama, T., Bosland, M., Gerecitano, J., Shapiro, D. *et al.* (1994). Requirement for transcription factor IRF-1 in NO synthase induction in macrophages. *Science*, **263**, 1612–5.

Kaplanski, G., Porat, R., Aiura, K., Erban, J. K., Gelfand, J. A., and Dinarello, C. A. (1993). Activated platelets induce endothelial secretion of interleukin-8 *in vitro* via an interleukin-1-mediated event. *Blood*, **81**, 2492–5.

Kaplanski, G., Farnarier, C., Kaplanski, S., Porat, R., Shapiro, L., Bongrand, P. *et al.* (1994). Interleukin-1 induces interleukin-8 secretion from endothelial cells by a juxtacrine mechanism. *Blood*, **84**, 4242–8.

Kaplanski, G., Teysseire, N., Farnarier, C., Kaplanski, S., Lissitzky, J. C., Durand, J. M. *et al.* (1995). IL-6 and IL-8 production from cultured human endothelial cells stimulated by infection with Rickettsia conorii a cell-associated IL-1alpha-dependent pathway. *J. Clin. Invest.*, **96**, 2839–44.

Karakurum, M., Shreeniwas, R., Chen, J., Pinsky, D., Yan, S. D., Anderson, M. *et al.* (1994). Hypoxic Induction of Interleukin-8 Gene Expression in Human Endothelial Cells. *J. Clin. Invest.*, **93**, 1564–70.

Karmann, K., Hughes, C. C., Schechner, J., Fanslow, W. C., and Pober, J. S. (1995). CD40 on human endothelial cells: inducibility by cytokines and functional regulation of adhesion molecule expression. *Proc. Natl. Acad. Sci. USA.*, **92**, 4342–6.

Kilgore, K. S., Shen, J. P., Miller, B. F., Ward, P. A., and Warren, J. S. (1995). Enhancement by the complement membrane attack complex of tumor necrosis factor-alpha-induced endothelial cell expression of E-selectin and ICAM-1. *J. Immunol.*, **155**, 1434–41.

Kim, S-Y., Guijarro, C., O'Donnel, M. P., Kasiske, B. L., Kim, Y., and Keane, W. F. (1995). Human mesangial cell production of monocyte chemoattractant protein-1: Modulation by lovastatin. *Kidney. Int.*, **48**, 363–71.

Koch, A. E., Polverini, P. J., Kunkel, S. L., Harlow, L. A., DiPietro, L. A., Elner, V. M. *et al.* (1992). Interleukin-8 as a macrophage-derived mediator of angiogenesis. *Science*, **258**, 1798–801.

Koch, A. E., Kunkel, S. L., Pearce, W. H., Shah, M. R., Parikh, D., Evanoff, H. L. *et al.* (1993). Enhanced production of the chemotactic cytokines interleukin-8 and monocyte chemoattractant protein-1 in human abdominal aortic aneurysms. *Am. J. Pathol.*, **142**, 1423–31.

Korpelainen, E. I., Gamble, J. R., Smith, W. B., Goodall, G. J., Qiyu, S., Woodcock, J. M. *et al.* (1993). The receptor for interleukin 3 is selectively induced in human endothelial cells by tumor necrosis factor alpha and potentiates interleukin 8 secretion and neutrophil transmigration. *Proc. Natl. Acad. Sci. USA.*, **90**, 11137–41.

Korpelainen, E. I., Gamble, J. R., Smith, W. B., Dottore, M., Vadas, M. A., and Lopez, A. F. (1995). Interferon-gamma upregulates interleukin-3 (IL-3) receptor expression in human endothelial cells and synergizes with IL-3 in stimulating major histocompatibility complex class II expression and cytokine production. *Blood*, **86**, 176–82.

Krakauer, T. (1995). IL-10 inhibits the adhesion of leukocytic cells to IL-1-activated human endothelial cells. *Immunol. Lett.*, **45**, 61–5.

Lamas, S., Michel, T., Collins, T., Brenner, B. M., and Marsden, P. A. (1992). Effects of interferon-gamma on nitric oxide synthase activity and endothelin-1 production by vascular endothelial cells. *J. Clin. Invest.*, **90**, 879–7.

Latini, R., Bianchi, M., Correale, E., Dinarello, C. A., Fantuzzi, G., Fresco, C. *et al.* (1994). Cytokines in acute myocardial infarction: selective increase in circulating tumor necrosis factor, its soluble receptor, and interleukin-1 receptor antagonist. *J. Cardiovasc. Pharmacol.*, **23**, 1–6.

Libby, P. (1996). Atheroma: more than mush. *Lancet*, **348** (supplement 1), s4-s7.

Libby, P. and Hansson, G. K. (1991). Biology of disease. Involvement of the immune system in human atherogenesis: current knowledge and unanswered questions. *Lab. Invest.*, **64**, 5–15.

Lienard, D., Ewalenko, P., Delmotte, J. J., Renard, N., and Lejeune, F. J. (1992). High-dose recombinant tumor necrosis factor alpha in combination with interferon gamma and melphalan in isolation perfusion of the limbs for melanoma and sarcoma. *J. Clin. Oncol.*, **10**, 52–60.

Liuzzo, G., Biasucci, L. M., Gallimore, J. R., Grillo, R. L., Rebuzzi, A. G., Pepys, M. B. *et al.* (1994). The prognostic value of C-reactive protein and serum amyloid a protein in severe unstable angina. *N. Engl. J. Med.*, **331**, 417–424.

Liuzzo, G., Biasucci, L. M., Rebuzzi, A. G., Gallimore, J. R., Caligiuri, G., Lanza, G. A. *et al.* (1996). Plasma protein acute-phase response in unstable angina is not induced by ischemic injury. *Circulation*, **94**, 2373–80.

Luster, A. D., Greenberg, S. M., and Leder, P. (1995). The IP-10 chemokine binds to a specific cell surface heparan sulfate site shared with platelet factor 4 and inhibits endothelial cell proliferation. *J. Exp. Med.*, **182**, 219–31.

Maier, J. A., Voulalas, P., Roeder, D., and Maciag, T. (1990). Extension of the life-span of human endothelial cells by an interleukin-1 alpha antisense oligomer. *Science*, **249**, 1570–4.

Maione, T. E., Gray, G. S., Petro, J., Hunt, A. J., Donner, A. L., Bauer, S. I. *et al.* (1990). Inhibition of angiogenesis by recombinant human platelet factor-4 and related peptides. *Science*, **247**, 77–9.

Mann, D. L. and Young, J. B. (1994). Basic mechanisms in congestive heart failure. Recognizing the role of proinflammatory cytokines. *Chest*, **105**, 897–904.

Mantovani, A. and Dejana, E. (1989). Cytokines as communication signals between leukocytes and endothelial cells. *Immunol. Today*, **10**, 370–5.

Mantovani, A., Bussolino, F., and Dejana, E. (1992). Cytokine regulation of endothelial cell function. *FASEB. J.*, **6**, 2591–9.

Mantovani A, Bussolino F, Introna M. (1997). Cytokine regulation of endothelial cell function: from molecular level to the bedside. *Immunol Today*, **18**, 231–40.

Mantovani, A., Allavena, P., Colotta, F., and Sozzani, S. (1996) Chemokines in vascular pathophysiology. In *Immune functions of the vessel wall* (ed. G. K. Hansson and P. Libby), pp. 65–76. Harwood Academic Publishers, Amsterdam.

Marfaingkoka, A., Devergne, O., Gorgone, G., Portier, A., Schall, T. J., Galanaud, P. *et al.* (1995). Regulation of the production of the RANTES chemokine by endothelial cells—Synergistic induction by IFN-gamma plus TNF-alpha and inhibition by IL-4 and IL-13. *J. Immunol.*, **154**, 1870–8.

Martin, E., Nathan, C., and Xie, Q. W. (1994). Role of interferon regulatory factor 1 in induction of nitric oxide synthase. *J. Exp. Med.*, **180**, 977–84.

Maseri, A., Biasucci, L. M., and Liuzzo, G. (1996). Inflammation in ischaemic heart disease. *Br. Med. J.*, **312**, 1049–50.

McCarron, R. M., Wang, L., Stanimirovic, D. B., and Spatz, M. (1995). Differential regulation of adhesion molecule expression by human cerebrovascular and umbilical vein entothelial cells. *Endothelium*, **2**, 339–46.

Meininger, C. J., Brightman, S. E., Kelly, K. A., and Zetter, B. R. (1995). Increased stem cell factor release by hemangioma-derived endothelial cells. *Lab. Invest.*, **72**, 166–73.

Meistrell, M. E., Botchkina, G. I., Wang, H., Di Santo, E., Cockroft, K. M., Bloom O. *et al.* (1997). Tumor necrosis factor is a brain damaging cytokine in cerebral ischemia. *Shock*, **8**, 341–8.

Meyrick, B., Christman, B., and Jesmok, G. (1991). Effects of recombinant tumor necrosis factor-alpha on cultured pulmonary artery and lung microvascular endothelial monolayers. *Am. J. Pathol.*, **138**, 93–101.

Modur, V., Li, Y. J., Zimmerman, G. A., Prescott, S. M., and McIntyre, T. M. (1997). Retrograde inflammatory signaling from neutrophils to endothelial cells by soluble interleukin-6 receptor alpha. *J. Clin. Invest.*, **100**, 2752–6.

Montrucchio, G., Lupia, E., Battaglia, E., Passerini, G., Bussolino, F., Emanuelli, G. *et al.* (1994). Tumor necrosis factor alpha-induced angiogenesis depends on *in situ* platelet-activating factor biosynthesis. *J. Exp. Med.*, **180**, 377–82.

Moyer, C. F., Sajuthi, D., Tulli, H., and Williams, J. K. (1991). Synthesis of IL-1alpha and IL-1 beta by arterial cells in atherosclerosis. *Am. J. Pathol.*, **138**, 951–60.

Murata, J., Corradin, S. B., Felley Bosco, E., and Juillerat Jeanneret, L. (1995). Involvement of a transforming-growth-factor-beta-like molecule in tumor-cell-derived inhibition of nitric-oxide synthesis in cerebral endothelial cells. *Int. J. Cancer*, **62**, 743–8.

Narumi, S., Wyner, L. M., Stoler, M. H., Tannenbaum, C. S., and Hamilton, T. A. (1992). Tissue-specific expression of murine IP-10 mRNA following systemic treatment with interferon-gamma. *J. Leukoc. Biol.*, **52**, 27–33.

Nathan, C. and Xie, Q. W. (1994). Nitric oxide synthases: roles, tolls, and controls. *Cell*, **78**, 915–8.

Nelken, N. A., Coughlin, S. R., Gordon, D., and Wilcox, J. N. (1991). Monocyte chemoattractant protein-1 in human atheromatous plaques. *J. Clin. Invest.*, **88**, 1121–7.

Niu, X. F., Smith, C. W., and Kubes, P. (1994). Intracellular oxidative stress induced by nitric oxide synthesis inhibition increases endothelial cell adhesion to neutrophils. *Circ. Res.*, **74**, 1133–40.

Oswald, I. P., Eltoum, I., Wynn, T. A., Schwartz, B., Caspar, P., Paulin, D. *et al.* (1994). Endothelial cells are activated by cytokine treatment to kill an intravascular parasite, Schistosoma mansoni, through the production of nitric oxide. *Proc. Natl. Acad. Sci. USA.*, **91**, 999–1003.

Patel, K. D., Modur, V., Zimmerman, G. A., Prescott, S. M., and McIntyre, T. M. (1994). The necrotic venom of the brown recluse spider induces dysregulated endothelial cell-dependent neutrophil activation—differential induction of GM-CSF, IL-8, and E- selectin expression. *J. Clin. Invest.*, **94**, 631–42.

Peiper, S. C., Wang, Z. X., Neote, K., Martin, A. W., Showell, H. J., Conklyn, M. J. *et al.* (1995). The Duffy antigen receptor for chemokines (DARC) is expressed in endothelial cells of Duffy negative individuals who lack the erythrocyte receptor. *J. Exp. Med.*, **181**, 1311–7.

Peng, H. B., Libby, P., and Liao, J. K. (1995a). Induction and stabilization of I kappa B alpha by nitric oxide mediates inhibition of NF-kappa B. *J. Biol. Chem.*, **270**, 14214–9.

Peng, H. B., Rajavashisth, T. B., Libby, P., and Liao, J. K. (1995b). Nitric oxide inhibits macrophage-colony stimulating factor gene transcription in vascular endothelial cells. *J. Biol. Chem.*, **270**, 17050–5.

Petzelbauer, P., Bender, J. R., Wilson, J., and Pober, J. S. (1993). Heterogeneity of dermal microvascular endothelial cell antigen expression and cytokine responsiveness in situ and in cell culture. *J. Immunol.*, **151**, 5062–72.

Petzelbauer, P., Watson, C. A., Pfau, S. E., and Pober, J. S. (1995). IL-8 and angiogenesis: Evidence that human endothelial cells lack receptors and do not respond to IL-8 *in vitro*. *Cytokine*, **7**, 267–72.

Pober, J. and Cotran, R. S. (1990). Cytokines and endothelial cell biology. *Physiol. Rev.*, **70**, 427–51.

Pugin, J., Schurer Maly, C. C., Leturcq, D., Moriarty, A., Ulevitch, R. J., and Tobias, P. S. (1993a). Lipopolysaccharide activation of human endothelial and epithelial cells is mediated by lipopolysaccharide-binding protein and soluble CD14. *Proc. Natl. Acad. Sci. USA.*, **90**, 2744–8.

Pugin, J., Ulevitch, R. J., and Tobias, P. S. (1993b). A critical role for monocytes and CD14 in endotoxin-induced endothelial cell activation. *J. Exp. Med.*, **178**, 2193–200.

Qi, J. F. and Kreutzer, D. L. (1995). Fibrin activation of vascular endothelial cells—induction of IL-8 expression. *J. Immunol.*, **155**, 867–76.

Radomski, M. W., Palmer, R. M., and Moncada, S. (1990). Glucocorticoids inhibit the expression of an inducible, but not the constitutive, nitric oxide synthase in vascular endothelial cells. *Proc. Natl. Acad. Sci. USA.*, **87**, 10043–7.

Rajavashisth, T. B., Andalibi, A., Territo, M. C., Berliner, J. A., Navab, M., Fogelman, A. M. *et al.* (1990). Induction of endothelial cell expression of granulocyte and macrophage colony-stimulating factors by modified low-density lipoproteins. *Nature*, **344**, 254–257.

Read, M. A., Cordle, S. R., Veach, R. A., Carlisle, C. D., and Hawiger, J. (1993). Cell-free pool of CD14 mediates activation of transcription factor NF-kappa B by lipopolysaccharide in human endothelial cells. *Proc. Natl. Acad. Sci. USA.*, **90**, 9887–91.

Remuzzi, G. and Ruggenenti, P. (1995). The hemolytic uremic syndrome. *Kidney. Int.*, **48**, 2–19.

Rollins, B. J., Yoshimura, T., Leonard, E. J., and Pober, J. S. (1990). Cytokine-activated human endothelial cells synthesize and secrete a monocyte chemoattractant, MCP-1/JE. *Am. J. Pathol.*, **136**, 1229–33.

Rollins, B. J. and Pober, J. S. (1991). Interleukin-4 induces the synthesis and secretion of MCP-1JE by human endothelial cells. *Am. J. Pathol.*, **138**, 1315–9.

Romano, M., Sironi, M., Toniatti, C., Polentarutti, N., Fruscella, P., Ghezzi, P. *et al.* (1997). Role of IL-6 and its soluble receptor in induction of chemokines and leukocyte recruitment. *Immunity*, **6**, 315–25.

Romano, M., Diomede, L., Sironi, M., Massimiliano, L., Sottocorno, M., Polentarutti, N. *et al.* (2000). Inihibition of monocyte chemotactic protein-1 synthesis by statins. *Lab. Invest.*, (In press).

Romer, L. H., McLean, N. V., Yan, H. C., Daise, M., Sun, J., and DeLisser, H. M. (1995). IFN-gamma and TNF-alpha induce redistribution of PECAM-1 (CD31) on human endothelial cells. *J. Immunol.*, **154**, 6582–92.

Rosenkranz Weiss, P., Sessa, W. C., Milstien, S., Kaufman, S., Watson, C. A., and Pober, J. S. (1994). Regulation of nitric oxide synthesis by proinflammatory cytokines in human umbilical vein endothelial cells. Elevations in tetrahydrobiopterin levels enhance endothelial nitric oxide synthase specific activity. *J. Clin. Invest.*, **93**, 2236–43.

Ross, R. (1993). The pathogenesis of atherosclerosis: a perspective for the 1990s. *Nature*, **362**, 801–9.

Rossi, V., Breviario, F., Ghezzi, P., Dejana, E., and Mantovani, A. (1985). Prostacyclin synthesis induced in vascular cells by interleukin-1. *Science*, **229**, 174–6.

Rot, A. (1992). Endothelial cell binding of NAP-1/IL-8: role in neutrophil emigration. *Immunol. Today*, **13**, 291–4.

Rott, O., Tontsch, U., Fleischer, B., and Cash, E. (1993). Interleukin-6 production in 'normal' and HTLV-1 tax-expressing brain-specific endothelial cells. *Eur. J. Immunol.*, **23**, 1987–91.

Rovin, B. H., Yoshimura, T., and Tan, L. (1992). Cytokine-induced production of monocyte chemoattractant protein-1 by cultured human mesangial cells. *J. Immunol.*, **148**, 2148–53.

Saadi, S., Holzknecht, R. A., Patte, C., Stern, D. M., and Platt, J. L. (1995). Complement-mediated regulation of tissue factor activity in endothelium. *J. Exp. Med.*, **182**, 1807–14.

Sakurai, H., Kohsaka, H., Liu, M. F., Higashiyama, H., Hirata, Y., Kanno, K. *et al.* (1995). Nitric oxide production and inducible nitric oxide synthase expression in inflammatory arthritides. *J. Clin. Invest.*, **96**, 2357–63.

Samaniego, F., Markham, P. D., Gallo, R. C., and Ensoli, B. (1995). Inflammatory cytokines induce AIDS-Kaposi's sarcoma-derived spindle cells to produce and release basic fibroblast growth factor and enhance Kaposi's sarcoma-like lesion formation in nude mice. *J. Immunol.*, **154**, 3582–92.

Sarma, V., Wolf, F. W., Marks, R. M., Shows, T. B., and Dixit, V. M. (1992). Cloning of a novel tumor necrosis factor-alpha-inducible primary response gene that is differentially expressed in development and capillary tube-like formation *in vitro*. *J. Immunol.*, **148**, 3302–12.

Sato, K., Miyakawa, K., Takeya, M., Hattori, R., Yui, Y., Sunamoto, M. *et al.* (1995). Immunohistochemical expression of inducible nitric oxide synthase (iNOS) in reversible endotoxic shock studied by a novel monoclonal antibody against rat iNOS. *J. Leukoc. Biol.*, **57**, 36–44.

Satriano, J. A., Hora, K., Shan, Z., Stanley, E. R., Mori, T., and Schlondorff, D. (1993a). Regulation of monocyte chemoattractant protein-1 and macrophage colony-stimulating factor-1 by IFN-gamma, tumor necrosis factor-alpha, IgG aggregates, and cAMP in mouse mesangial cells. *J. Immunol.*, **150**, 1971–8.

Satriano, J. A., Shuldiner, M., Hora, K., Xing, Y., Shan, Z., and Schlondorff, D. (1993b). Oxygen radicals as second messengers for expression of the monocyte chemoattractant protein, JE/MCP-1, and the monocyte colony-stimulating factor, CSF-1, in response to tumor necrosis factor-alpha and immunoglobulin-G—evidence for involvement of reduced nicotinamide adenine dinucleotide phosphate (NADPH)-dependent oxidase. *J. Clin. Invest.*, **92**, 1564–71.

Schoedon, G., Schneemann, M., Blau, N., Edgell, C. J., and Schaffner, A. (1993). Modulation of human endothelial cell tetrahydrobiopterin synthesis by activating and deactivating cytokines: new perspectives on endothelium-derived relaxing factor. *Biochem. Biophys. Res. Commun.*, **196**, 1343–8.

Schofield, L., Novakovic, S., Gerold, P., Schwarz, R. T., McConville, M. J., and Tachado, S. D. (1996). Glycosylphosphatidylinositol toxin of plasmodium upregulates intercellular adhesion molecule-1, vascular cell adhesion molecule-1, and E-selectin expression in vascular endothelial cells and increses leukocyte and parasite cytoadherence via tyrosine kinase-dependent signal transduction. *J. Immunol.*, **156**, 1886–96.

Schonbeck, U., Brandt, E., Petersen, F., Flad, H. D., and Loppnow, H. (1995). IL-8 specifically binds to endothelial but not to smooth muscle cells. *J. Immunol.*, **154**, 2375–83.

Schroder, J. M. and Christophers, E. (1989). Secretion of novel and homologous neutrophil-activating peptides by LPS-stimulated human endothelial cells. *J. Immunol.*, **142**, 244–251.

Schulz, R., Panas, D. L., Catena, R., Moncada, S., Olley, P. M., and Lopaschuk, G. D. (1995). The role of nitric oxide in cardiac depression induced by interleukin-1 beta and tumour necrosis factor-alpha. *Br. J. Pharmacol.*, **114**, 27–34.

Schwartz, D., Andalibi, A., Chaverrialmada, L., Berliner, J. A., Kirchgessner, T., Fang, Z. T. *et al.* (1994). Role of the GRO family of chemokines in monocyte adhesion to MM-LDL-stimulated endothelium. *J. Clin. Invest.*, **94**, 1968–73.

Shyy, Y. J., Wickham, L. L., Hagan, J. P., Hsieh, H. J., Hu, Y. L., Telian, S. H. *et al.* (1993). Human Monocyte Colony-Stimulating Factor Stimulates the Gene Expression of Monocyte Chemotactic Protein-1 and Increases the Adhesion of Monocytes to Endothelial Monolayers. *J. Clin. Invest.*, **92**, 1745–51.

Sica, A., Matsushima, K., Van Damme, J., Wang, J. M., Polentarutti, N., Dejana, E. *et al.* (1990a). IL-1 transcriptionally activates the neutrophil chemotactic factor/IL-8 gene in endothelial cells. *Immunology*, **69**, 548–53.

Sica, A., Wang, J. M., Colotta, F., Dejana, E., Mantovani, A., Oppenheim, J. J. *et al.* (1990b). Monocyte chemotactic and activating factor gene expression induced in endothelial cells by IL-1 and tumor necrosis factor. *J. Immunol.*, **144**, 3034–8.

Simantov, R., LaSala, J. M., Lo, S. K., Gharavi, A. E., Sammaritano, L. R., and Salmon, J. E. (1995). Activation of cultured vascular endothelial cells by antiphospholipid antibodies. *J. Clin. Invest.*, **96**, 2211–9.

Sironi, M., Breviario, F., Proserpio, P., Biondi, A., Vecchi, A., Van Damme, J. *et al.* (1989). IL-1 stimulates IL-6 production in endothelial cells. *J. Immunol.*, **142**, 549–53.

Sironi, M., Munoz, C., Pollicino, T., Siboni, A., Sciacca, F. L., Bernasconi, S. *et al.* (1993). Divergent effects of interleukin-10 on cytokine production by mononuclear phagocytes and endothelial cells. *Eur. J. Immunol.*, **23**, 2692–5.

Sironi, M., Sciacca, F. L., Matteucci, C., Conni, M., Vecchi, A., Bernasconi, S. *et al.* (1994). Regulation of endothelial and mesothelial cell function by interleukin-13: selective induction of vascular cell adhesion molecule-1 and amplification of interleukin-6 production. *Blood*, **84**, 1913–21.

Sporn, M. B., Roberts, A. B., Wakefield, L. M., and Crombrugghe, B. (1987). Some recent advances in the chemistry and biology of transforming growth factor-beta. *J. Cell Biol.*, **105**, 1039–45.

Strieter, R. M., Kunkel, S. L., Showell, H. J., Remick, D. G., Phan, S. H., Ward, P. A. *et al.* (1989). Endothelial cell gene expression of a neutrophil chemotactic factor by TNF-alpha, LPS, and IL-1 beta. *Science*, **243**, 1467–9.

Strieter, R. M., Kunkel, S. L., Elner, V. M., Martonyi, C. L., Koch, A. E., Polverini, P. J. *et al.* (1992). Interleukin-8. A corneal factor that induces neovascularization. *Am. J. Pathol.*, **141**, 1279–84.

Strieter, R. M., Polverini, P. J., Kunkel, S. L., Arenberg, D. A., Burdick, M. D., Kasper, J. *et al.* (1995). The functional role of the ELR motif in CXC chemokine-mediated angiogenesis. *J. Biol. Chem.*, **270**, 27348–57.

Suen, Y., Chang, M., Lee, S. M., Buzby, J. S., and Cairo, M. S. (1994). Regulation of interleukin-11 protein and mRNA expression in neonatal and adult fibroblasts and endothelial cells. *Blood*, **84**, 4125–34.

Suschek, C., Rothe, H., Fehsel, K., Enczmann, J., and Kolb Bachofen, V. (1993). Induction of a macrophage-like nitric oxide synthase in cultured rat aortic endothelial cells. IL-1 beta-mediated induction regulated by tumor necrosis factor-alpha and IFN-gamma. *J. Immunol.*, **151**, 3283–91.

Tachado, S. D., Gerold, P., McConville, M. J., Baldwin, T., Quilici, D., Schwarz, R. T. *et al.* (1996). Glycosylphosphatidylinositol toxin of plasmodium induces nitric oxide syntase expression in macrophages and vascular endothelial cells by a protein tyrosine kinase-dependent and protein kinase C-dependent signaling pathway. *J. Immunol.*, **156**, 1897–907.

Tachibana, K., Hirota, S., Lizasa, H., Yoshida, H., Kawabata, K., Kataoka, Y. *et al.* (1998). The chemokine receptor CXCR4 is essential for vascularization of the gastrointestinal tract. *Nature*, **393**, 591–4.

Takeya, M., Yoshimura, T., Leonard, E. J., and Takahashi, K. (1993). Detection of monocyte chemoattractant protein-1 in human atherosclerotic lesions by an anti-monocyte chemoattractant protein-1 monoclonal antibody. *Hum. Pathol.*, **24**, 534–9.

Tedesco, F., Pausa, M., Nardon, E., Introna, M., Mantovani, A., and Dobrina, A. (1997). The cytolytically inactive terminal complement complex activates endothelial cells to express adhesion molecules and tissue factor procoagulant activity. *J. Exp. Med.*, **185**, 1619–27.

Terkeltaub, R., Solan, J., Barry, M., Santoro, D., and Bokoch, G. M. (1994). Role of the mevalonate pathway of isoprenoid synthesis in IL-8 generation by activated monocytic cells. *J. Leukoc. Biol.*, **55**, 749–55.

Thompson, S. G., Kienast, J., Pyke, S. D., Haverkate, F., and van de Loo, J. C. (1995). Hemostatic factors and the risk of myocardial infarction or sudden death in patients with angina pectoris.

European Concerted Action on Thrombosis and Disabilities Angina Pectoris Study Group. *N. Engl. J. Med.*, **332**, 635–41.

Valantine, H. A. and Schroeder, J. S. (1997). HMG-CoA reductase inhibitors reduce transplant coronary artery disease and mortality. Evidence for antigen-indepentent mechanisms? *Circulation*, **96**, 1370–3.

Valente, A. J., Fowler, S. R., Sprague, E. A., Kelley, J. L., Suenram, C. A., and Schwartz, C. J. (1984). Initial characterization of a paripheral blood mononuclear cell chemoattractant derived from cultured arterial smooth muscle cells. *Am. J. Pathol.*, **117**, 409–17.

Valente, A. J., Graves, D. A., Vialle-Valentin, C. E., Delgado, R., and Schwartz, C. J. (1988). Purification of a monocyte chemotactic factor secreted by nonhuman primate vascular cells in culture. *Biochemistry*, **27**, 4162–8.

van de Kar, N. C., Monnens, L. A., Karmali, M. A., and van Hinsbergh, V. W. (1992). Tumor necrosis factor and interleukin-1 induce expression of the verocytotoxin receptor globotriaosylceramide on human endothelial cells: implications for the pathogenesis of the hemolytic uremic syndrome. *Blood*, **80**, 2755–64.

van de Kar, N. C., Kooistra, T., Vermeer, M., Lesslauer, W., Monnens, L. A., and van Hinsbergh, V. W. (1995). Tumor necrosis factor alpha induces endothelial galactosyl transferase activity and verocytotoxin receptors. Role of specific tumor necrosis factor receptors and protein kinase C. *Blood*, **85**, 734–43.

Villarete, L. H. and Remick, D. G. (1995). Nitric oxide regulation of IL-8 expression in human endothelial cells. *Biochem. Biophys. Res. Commun.*, **211**, 671–6.

Voest, E. E., Kenyon, B. M., O'Reilly, M. S., Truitt, G., D'Amato, R. J., and Folkman, J. (1995). Inhibition of angiogenesis *in vivo* by interleukin-12. *J. Natl. Cancer Inst.*, **87**, 581–6.

von Asmuth, E. J., Dentener, M. A., Bazil, V., Bouma, M. G., Leeuwenberg, J. F., and Buurman, W. A. (1993). Anti-CD14 antibodies reduce responses of cultured human endothelial cells to endotoxin. *Immunology*, **80**, 78–83.

von der Leyen, H. E., Gibbons, G. H., Morishita, R., Lewis, N. P., Zhang, L., Nakajima, M. *et al.* (1995). Gene therapy inhibiting neointimal vascular lesion: *in vivo* transfer of endothelial cell nitric oxide synthase gene. *Proc. Natl. Acad. Sci. USA.*, **92**, 1137–41.

Vora, M., Yssel, H., de Vries, J. E., and Karasek, M. A. (1994). Antigen presentation by human dermal microvascular endothelial cells. Immunoregulatory effect of IFN-gamma and IL-10. *J. Immunol.*, **152**, 5734–41.

Wakabayashi, H., Cavanaugh, P. G., and Nicolson, G. L. (1995). Purification and identification of mouse lung microvessel endothelial cell-derived chemoattractant for lung-metastasizing murine RAW117 large-cell lymphoma cells: identification as mouse monocyte chemotactic protein 1. *Cancer Res.*, **55**, 4458–64.

Wang, J. M., Taraboletti, G., Matsushima, K., Van Damme, J., and Mantovani, A. (1990). Induction of haptotactic migration of melanoma cells by neutrophil activating protein/interleukin-8. *Biochem. Biophys. Res. Commun.*, **169**, 165–70.

Wang, J. M., Sica, A., Peri, G., Walter, S., Padura, I. M., Libby, P. *et al.* (1991). Expression of monocyte chemotactic protein and interleukin-8 by cytokine-activated human vascular smooth muscle cells. *Arterioscler. Thromb.*, **11**, 1166–74.

Warner, S. J. and Libby, P. (1989). Human vascular smooth muscle cells. Target for and source of tumor necrosis factor. *J. Immunol.*, **142**, 100–9.

Wen, D., Rowland, A., and Derynck, R. (1989). Expression and secretion of *gro*/MGSA by stimulated human endothelial cells. *EMBO J.*, **8**, 1761–6.

Werner Felmayer, G., Werner, E. R., Fuchs, D., Hausen, A., Reibnegger, G., Schmidt, K. *et al.* (1993). Pteridine biosynthesis in human endothelial cells. Impact on nitric oxide-mediated formation of cyclic GMP. *J. Biol. Chem.*, **268**, 1842–6.

Willimann, K., Matile, H., Weiss, N. A., and Imhof, B. A. (1995). *In vivo* sequestration of Plasmodium falciparum-infected human erythrocytes: a severe combined immunodeficiency mouse model for cerebral malaria. *J. Exp. Med.*, **182**, 643–53.

Wojta, J., Gallicchio, M., Zoellner, H., Filonzi, E. L., Hamilton, J. A., and Mcgrath, K. (1993). Interleukin-4 stimulates expression of urokinase-type-plasminogen activator in cultured human foreskin microvascular endothelial cells. *Blood*, **81**, 3285–92.

Wolff, B., Burns, A. R., Middleton, J., and Roth, A. (1998). Endothelial cell 'memory' of inflammatory stimulation: human venular endothelial cells store interleukin 8 in Weibel-Palade bodies. *J. Exp. Med.*, **188**, 1757–62.

Woodroffe, S. B., Garnett, H. M., and Layton, J. E. (1994). Cytomegalovirus infection of vascular endothelial cells alters production of GM-CSF and G-CSF. *Immunol. Cell Biol.*, **72**, 187–90.

Yan, S. F., Tritto, I., Pinsky, D., Liao, H., Huang, J., Fuller, G. *et al.* (1995). Induction of interleukin 6 (IL-6) by hypoxia in vascular cells. Central role of the binding site for nuclear factor-IL-6. *J. Biol. Chem.*, **270**, 11463–71.

Yao, L., Bengualid, V., Lowy, F. D., Gibbons, J. J., Hatcher, V. B., and Berman, J. W. (1995). Internalization of *Staphylococcus aureus* by endothelial cells induces cytokine gene expression. *Infect. Immun.*, **63**, 1835–9.

Yellin, M. J., Brett, J., Baum, D., Matsushima, A., Szabolcs, A., Stern, D. *et al.* (1995). Functional interactions of T cells with endothelial cells: the role of CD40L-CD40-mediated signals. *J. Exp. Med.*, **182**, 1857–64.

Yla Herttuala, S., Lipton, B. A., Rosenfeld, M. E., Sarkioja, T., Yoshimura, T., Leonard, E. J. *et al.* (1991). Expression of monocyte chemoattractant protein 1 in macrophage-rich areas of human and rabbit atherosclerotic lesions. *Proc. Natl. Acad. Sci. USA.*, **88**, 5252–6.

Yoshizumi, M., Perrella, M. A., Burnett, J. C.,Jr., and Lee, M. E. (1993). Tumor necrosis factor downregulates an endothelial nitric oxide synthase mRNA by shortening its half-life. *Circ. Res.*, **73**, 205–9.

Yu, X., Dluz, S., Graves, D. T., Zhang, L., Antoniades, H. N., Hollander, W. *et al.* (1992). Elevated expression of monocyte chemoattractant protein 1 by vascular smooth muscle cells in hypercholesterolemic primates. *Proc. Natl. Acad. Sci. USA.*, **89**, 6953–7.

Zeiher, A. M., Fisslthaler, B., Schray Utz, B., and Busse, R. (1995). Nitric oxide modulates the expression of monocyte chemoattractant protein 1 in cultured human endothelial cells. *Circ. Res.*, **76**, 980–6.

Zhang F. X., Kirschning C. J., Mancinelli R., Jin Y., Faure E., Mantovani A. *et al.* (1999). Bacterial lipoppolysaccharide activates NF-kB through interleukin-1 signaling mediators in cultured human dermal endothelial cells and human mononuclear phagocytes. *J. Biol. Chem.*, **274**, 7611–4.

Zhang, R., Min, W., and Sessa, W. C. (1995). Functional analysis of the human endothelial nitric oxide synthase promoter. Sp1 and GATA factors are necessary for basal transcription in endothelial cells. *J. Biol. Chem.*, **270**, 15320–6.

Ziche, M., Morbidelli, L., Masini, E., Amerini, S., Granger, H. J., Maggi, C. A. *et al.* (1994). Nitric oxide mediates angiogenesis *in vivo* and endothelial cell growth and migration *in vitro* promoted by substance P. *J. Clin. Invest.*, **94**, 2036–44.

Zoja, C., Wang, J. M., Bettoni, S., Sironi, M., Renzi, D., Chiaffarino, F. *et al.* (1991). Interleukin-1 beta and tumor necrosis factor-alpha induce gene expression and production of leukocyte chemotactic factors, colony-stimulating factors, and interleukin-6 in human mesangial cells. *Am. J. Pathol.*, **138**, 991–1003.

10 *Cancer*

Tumor immunology has long been an area of descriptive phenomenology, wild speculation, and unfullfilled expectations. Attempts at activating host resistance to tumors go back to early in this century with Coley's toxin, a bacterial preparation with some anti-tumor activity. The only remnant of the 'bacterial era' of tumor immunotherapy in widespread clinical use, is probably intravesical Bacillus Calmette–Guérin in early bladder carcinoma. The latest tools, including molecularly defined tumor antigens, gene transfer techniques, and cytokines, have renewed interest in the possibility of exploiting host-immune responses in the treatment of neoplasia and are the basis for a renaissance of tumor immunology as a clinically important discipline.

Cytokines are part of the complex interplay between tumor and host. The most evident manifestation of this interplay is the formation of tumor stroma, which is dependent on the action of cytokines. The interplay between malignant cells and components of the stroma is essential not only for solid tumors but also for some hematological malignancies, such as malignant myeloma. Stroma and malignant cells are discrete but interdependent compartments, in that malignant cells elicit stroma formation, essential for neoplastic growth and progression, at least beyond a minimal size of 1–2 mm, as estimated in experimental systems. In tumors of epithelial origin, the malignant and stroma compartments are usually physically separated to a large extent by a basement membrane.

Components of the tumor stroma include new blood vessels, matrix components, and the cells responsible for their production, a fibrin–gel matrix, and inflammatory leukocytes (Dvorak, 1986). The most obvious role of cytokines in the immunobiology of neoplastic tissues is as messengers between malignant cells and stromal components. The pathophysiology of cytokines in neoplastic progression will be discussed, then the potential role of cytokines as future anti-tumor agents will be reviewed. Cytokines in current clinical use (IL-2, colony stimulating factors, interferon) will not be discussed.

10.1 Pathophysiology

10.1.1 Primary inflammatory cytokines and neoplastic progression

IL-1 and TNF have contradictory actions on tumor growth and neoplastic progression (Table 10.1). IL-1 and, most notably, TNF *in vitro* inhibit the proliferation of some tumor cells and cause apoptosis. When injected locally, they both cause hemorrhagic necrosis of neoplastic tissues, which largely depends on their actions on vascular cells (see Chapters

Table 10.1   Pro- and anti-tumor effects of inflammatory cytokines in neoplastic progression

A Anti-tumor effects	1. Direct antiproliferative activity 2. Activation of vessel wall cells and tissue necrosis (hemorrhagic necrosis) 3. Leukocyte activation
B Pro-tumor actions	1. Autocrine or paracrine growth factors (e.g. IL-1 in myeloid leukemias, TNF in ovarian carcinoma, IL-6 in multiple myeloma) 2. Progression factors (stimulation of metastasis by the hematic or peritoneal route; angiogenesis) 3. Mediators of the systemic manifestations of malignancies (e.g. acute-phase proteins, cachexia, systemic immunosuppression)

1 and 9). Recent clinical studies using infusion of TNF into the tumor vascular bed in the lower limbs suggest that this necrotic action can indeed occur in humans (Lejeune and Lienard, 1996).

While these properties should potentially inhibit tumor growth, in the absence of therapeutic intervention, IL-1, TNF, and IL-6 can, however, actually stimulate tumor growth and progression under pathophysiological conditions. Both act as growth factors for certain human tumors, such as ovarian carcinoma, stomach carcinoma, and hematopoietic malignancies. Direct *in vivo* evidence for a pro-tumor function of TNF was obtained in a skin carcinogenesis model using gene-targeted mice (Moore *et al.*, 1999). Recent results indicate that IL-1 polymorphisms are associated with increased risk of gastric cancer (El-Omar *et al.*, 2000). The pro-inflammatory haplotype *IL-1B-3IT* (IL-1β locus)/IL-1RN★2 (IL-1Ra locus) increases the likelihood of a chronic hypochlorhydric response to *H. pylori* infection and the risk of stomach carcinoma. IL-6 is a major growth factor in the regulation of the proliferation of myeloid cells. It may be part of an autocrine/paracrine circuit involving myeloma cells and stromal components. IL-6 also acts as a growth factor for chronic lymphocytic leukemia cells, as well as for lymphoid cells in Castelman's disease. IL-1 seems to play a major role in promoting the proliferation of myeloid leukemias, which produce IL-1. IL-1 may act as a growth factor in itself, or by inducing GM-CSF production. Therapeutic efforts have thus been made to block IL-1 and IL-6 in appropriate hematological malignancies, using antibodies, the IL-1ra, and, at least *in vitro*, IL-10.

Adult T-cell leukemia is associated with the retrovirus HTLV-1. Through the transactivating protein TAX, HTLV-1 activates expression of the IL-2 receptor and of IL-2, and this cytokine is involved in the pathogenesis of this disease.

Cachexia is a manifestation of advanced malignancy. Primary pro-inflammatory cytokines have obvious biological actions on metabolism and on the central nervous system, which may account for malignant cachexia. There is evidence that cytokines such as IL-6 are important chachectic mediators, at least in certain murine tumors.

IL-1 and TNF enhance metastasis formation in a variety of murine tumors and in human tumors transplanted in immunodeficient mice (Giavazzi *et al.*, 1990). As mentioned in Chapter 1, IL-1 and TNF induce the expression of adhesion molecules on vascular endothelium, which are recognized by leukocyte counter receptors. Pathogens, including neoplastic cells, employ the pathways used by the professional migrants—leukocyes—to disseminate and implant at distant anatomical sites. For instance, human melanomas express VLA4 and recognize VCAM-1 expressed on endothelial cells upon exposure to IL-1 and TNF. Colon carcinomas use the E-selectin-syalyl Lewis-X or syalyl Lewis-A pathways. There is evidence in human melanoma specimens that expression of VLA4 does indeed correlate with disease aggressiveness (Martin Padura *et al.*, 1991). Finally, primary pro-inflammatory cytokines account for, or contribute to, some of the systemic manifestations associated with malignancies. These mediators, most notably IL-6, produced by macrophages or by neoplastic cells, cause anorexia, cachexia, or production of acute phase proteins, manifestations commonly associated with advanced malignancies.

10.1.2 Secondary cytokines: chemokines

The leukocyte infiltrate

Ever since the first description by Virchow in 1863, histopathologists have recognized that host leukocytes are found in tumor tissues or at their periphery. Interestingly, Virchow felt that the frequent lymphoreticular infiltrate in human neoplasms reflected the origin of cancer at sites of previous chronic inflammation. In 1907, Hardley reported that normal cell infiltration in malignant melanoma indicated a 'regressive process' (discussed in Mantovani *et al.* 1992a). This observation marked a complete change in the general opinion on the significance of the 'lymphoreticular infiltrate', a change reflected by a number of reports on pathology and prognosis. These opposite views of the relationship between leukocyte infiltration and malignancy have polarized opinions in the field but do in fact reflect the pleiotropic, ambivalent functions of infiltrating cells.

Mononuclear phagocytes are an important component of the stroma of neoplastic tissues often underestimated in conventional histological sections (Evans, 1972; Mantovani *et al.*, 1992a; van Ravenswaay Claasen *et al.*, 1992). Solid tumors consist of malignant cells and stroma, which, as we said earlier, are discrete but interdependent, in that malignant cells elicit the stroma formation essential for neoplastic growth and progression. Tumor-associated macrophages (TAM) can interact with both the neoplastic and the stromal components of a tumor.

Interest in cells of the mononuclear phagocyte lineage in relation to neoplasia stemmed largely from the observation that these effector cells, when appropriately activated, are able to kill neoplastically transformed target cells *in vitro* and that normal cells are usually relatively resistant to this killing. The cytotoxic function of activated macrophages on transformed target cells led to the hypothesis, still not adequately tested, that they amount to a mechanism of non-specific surveillance against neoplasia (Hibbs, 1976; Adams and Snyderman, 1979; Cianciolo *et al.*, 1981). The spectrum of the cytotoxic action of activated mononuclear phagocytes encompasses tumor cells with various forms of resistance to chemotherapeutic agents, which has obvious implications for combined therapies (Allavena *et al.*, 1987).

The *in vivo* relevance of the *in vitro* cytotoxic interaction of activated macrophages with tumor cells has not been unequivocally demonstrated, even under conditions in which macrophages are likely to have anti-tumor activity. Tissue-destructive reactions centered on vascular elements (see Chapter 9), induced by mononuclear phagocytes through their secretory products (e.g. TNF), are likely to be an important mechanism of anti-tumor activity *in vivo* (Mantovani *et al.*, 1992b).

Macrophages have various functions essential for tissue remodelling, inflammation, and immunity. Analysis of TAM, using the tools of cellular and molecular biology, suggests that these pleiotropic cells affect diverse aspects of the immunobiology of neoplastic tissues, including vascularization, growth rate and metastasis, stroma formation and dissolution. As discussed below, in some neoplasms, including common human cancers, the protumor functions of TAM appear to prevail. In certain tumors, neutrophils have the same tumor-promoting function as TAM (Pekarek *et al.*, 1995). The 'macrophage balance' hypothesis (Mantovani *et al.*, 1992a) stresses the dual potential of TAM to influence neoplastic growth and progression in opposite directions, with a prevailing protumor activity in the absence of therapeutic intervention in many neoplasms.

The search for tumor-derived chemotactic factors (TDCF), which might explain the recruitment of mononuclear phagocytes in neoplastic tissues, was one path that led to the identification of the prototypic CC chemokine monocyte chemotactic protein-1 (MCP-1) (Bottazzi *et al.*, 1983a). Here we review the evidence that chemokines, particularly MCP-1, are important in regulating macrophage recruitment in tumors, and we look at how chemokines acting on activated NK cells, and on dendritic cells, can serve as tools to stimulate specific immunity against neoplasms.

Chemokines in murine tumors

The percentage of TAM for each tumor is usually maintained as a relatively stable 'individual' property during tumor growth and upon transplantation in syngeneic hosts. Transplant of xenogeneic human (but not allogeneic murine) tumors is associated with a different pattern of distribution of TAM within the lesion: peripheral rather than diffuse (Bucana *et al.*, 1992). Macrophages also infiltrate metastatic lesions, although TAM have been less extensively studied in secondary foci (Mantovani *et al.*, 1992a). Even at macrophage-rich sites, such as the liver, macrophage infiltration in metastasis depends largely on recruitment of monocytic precursors (Heuff *et al.*, 1993). Experiments in which tumors were transplanted in hosts with defective T or NK cell immunity suggest that, for many neoplasms, specific immunity is not a major determinant of macrophage infiltration, and that factors derived from the tumor itself play a pivotal role in the regulation of macrophage levels in poorly immunogenic metastatic tumors (Mantovani *et al.*, 1992a).

Analysis of the mechanisms of macrophage recruitment in tumors was one path that led to the identification of MCP-1 (Bottazzi *et al.*, 1983a; Graves *et al.*, 1989; Yoshimura *et al.*, 1989; Mantovani *et al.*, 1992a; Opdenakker and Van Damme, 1992b) (see Fig. 10.1). MCP-1 may be an important determinant of the levels of TAM (Mantovani *et al.*, 1992a; Opdenakker and Van Damme, 1992b). In early studies with murine tumors or human tumors in nude mice, a correlation was found between MCP-1 activity and the percentage of TAM, and this was confirmed in subsequent experiments with the MCP-1 probe (Walter *et al.*, 1991). Subcutaneous inoculation of tumor-derived human MCP-1, MCP-2, and MCP-3, led to macrophage infiltration (Zachariae *et al.*, 1990; Van Damme *et al.*, 1992; Hirose *et al.*, 1995). Conclusively, transfer of the mouse or human MCP-1 gene was associated with higher levels of macrophage infiltration (Rollins and Sunday, 1991; Bottazzi *et al.*, 1992). High expression of MCP-1 was associated with loss of tumorigenicity of CHO cells (Rollins and Sunday, 1991) but not of malignant mouse tumors (Bottazzi *et al.*, 1992). At low tumor inocula, MCP-1 gene transfer was associated with higher tumorigenicity and lung-colonizing ability, despite reduced growth of the resulting lesions (Bottazzi *et al.*, 1992; Mantovani *et al.*, 1993a). These findings were interpreted in the light of TAM's dual influence on tumor growth (Mantovani *et al.*, 1992a; Opdenakker and Van Damme, 1992b).

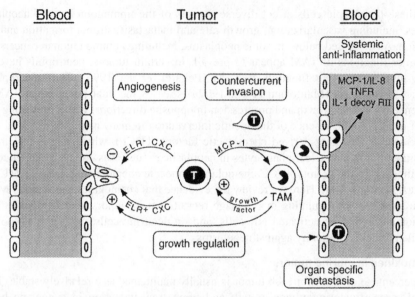

Fig. 10.1 Chemokines in the immunobiology of neoplastic tissues: a synopsis. Most tumors constitutively produce inducible chemokines, which in normal cells require stimuli for production. These act as autocrine growth and migration factors (e.g IL-8 and MGSA/gro in melanoma); they attract macrophages, which in turn affect growth and angiogenesis (e.g. MCP-1 produced by a variety of tumors); they positively or negatively regulate angiogenesis (e.g. IL-8, ELR+, and IP10, ELR-); they prepare the path for tumor invasion by attracting macrophages (e.g. MCP-1; countercurrent invasion).

Expression of MCP-1/JE was detected in various rat tumors (Yamashiro *et al.*, 1994). Using markers selective for monocyte-derived or tissue macrophages, MCP-1/JE gene transfer caused recruitment of mononuclear phagocytes from the blood compartment (Yamashiro *et al.*, 1994). Evidence of the role of MCP-1 in recruitment was obtained in human tumor xenografts (Melani *et al.*, 1995)

Leukocyte infiltration in murine tumors is associated with cytokines, such as interferons, IL-2, or IL-4, administered by conventional routes or following gene transfer. Interferon, IL-12, and IL-2 induce endogenous chemokines in renal and colon cancer models (Sonouchi *et al.*, 1994; Tannenbaum *et al.*, 1996). Thus, secondary induction of chemokines may be pivotal in leukocyte recruitment in tumors treated with cytokines other than chemokines.

Chemokines in human tumors

Various human tumor lines express MCP-1 *in vitro* spontaneously or after exposure to inflammatory signals, and some do so *in vivo*. The latter include gliomas, histiocytomas, sarcomas, and melanoma (Yoshimura *et al.*, 1989; Zachariae *et al.*, 1990; Takeya *et al.*, 1991; Graves *et al.*, 1992). Expression of MCP-1 was found in Kaposi's sarcoma (KS) *in vivo* and in KS-derived spindle cell cultures (Sciacca *et al.*, 1994). Since KS presents a conspicuous macrophage infiltrate and is believed to be a cytokine-propelled disease, the production of MCP-1 may be particularly significant. Interestingly, human herpes virus 8

(HHV8), very likely involved in the pathogenesis of KS, encodes a constitutively active chemokine receptor, which stimulates cell proliferation (Arvanitakis *et al.*, 1997), as well as chemokines (see Chapter 7 and below).

Human tumor lines of epithelial origin (breast, colon, ovary) (Bottazzi *et al.*, 1983a, 1985) release small molecular-weight chemo-attractant(s). For ovarian carcinoma, TDCF was identified as MCP-1 (Negus *et al.*, 1995; see below). RANTES is expressed in advanced breast carcinoma and correlates with disease stage (Luboshits *et al.*, 1999). Interestingly, certain chemokines, including RANTES, induce migration of mammary carcinoma cells (Teruya-Feldstein *et al.*, 1999). As in ovarian cancer, TAM recruited by chemokines may promote progression (Luboshits *et al.*, 1999) and references therein).

The expression of MCP-1 in relation to cervical cancer has been investigated by *in vitro* and *in vivo* approaches (Hirose *et al.*, 1995; Riethdorf *et al.*, 1996). Somatic cell hybrids were generated between human papillomavirus type 18 (HPV18) cells and normal cells. Only non-tumorigenic hybrids expressed MCP-1, which was undetectable in tumorigenic segregants and in HPV positive cervical carcinoma lines. By *in situ* hybridization, MCP-1 was detected in certain human cervical cancers. In high-grade squamous intra-epithelial lesions, MCP-1 expression was detected in normal, dysplastic and neoplastic epithelia, as well as in macrophages and endothelial cells. MCP-1 expression was most marked at the epithelial-mesenchymal junction and was associated with macrophage infiltration. In intra-epithelial lesions, expression of MCP-1 and of the human papilloma virus (HPV) oncogenes E6/E7 tended to be mutually exclusive, whereas in squamous cell carcinoma MCP-1 was also expressed in the presence of transcriptional activity of E6/E7.

HHV-8, also known as Kaposi's sarcoma virus (KSV), is involved in the pathogenesis of human KS and in some hematological malignancies. HHV-8 has been associated with body-cavity lymphomas and with malignant myeloma. The virus genome encodes cytokines and cytokine receptors. A receptor belonging to the chemokine receptor family (GPCR), which interacts with various chemokines, is constitutively activated and provides a proliferation signal. The virus also encodes CC chemokines and a cytokine related to IL-6. The latter may be involved in the pathogenesis of hematological malignancies.

The CC chemokines encoded by HHV-8 have certain particular properties, as discussed in Chapter 7. The HHV-8-encoded chemokine called vMIP-II (where v stands for viral) has agonist activity for CCR3 and CCR8 receptors, which are preferentially expressed on Th2 cells (Bonecchi *et al.*, 1998; Sozzani *et al.*, 1998b). vMIP-II also recognizes the CCR4 receptor, expressed on Th2 cells. A preferential attraction of Th2 cells was also demonstrated for vMIP-I and vMIP-III (Endres *et al.*, 1999; Stine *et al.*, 1999) and T cell infiltrating KS have a skewed Th2 phenotype (Sozzani *et al.*, 1998b). HHV-8 encoded chemokines might thus be a strategy to subvert immunity, by activating Th2 responses and diverting effective Th1 defense mechanisms.

Various human tumors express chemokines of the CXC family. Some neoplasms of the melanocyte lineage express groα, and the related molecule, IL-8, which induce proliferation and migration of melanoma cells (Wang *et al.*, 1990; Balentien *et al.*, 1991; Schadendorf *et al.*, 1993; Luan *et al.*, 1997). Transfer of the gro gene into an untransformed melanocytic line rendered it competent to form tumors in immunodeficient mice (Balentien *et al.*, 1991); this effect might be related to direct growth stimulation or to promotion of an inflammatory reaction, which would in turn favor tumor formation (see below). Inflammation and wound healing have, in fact, been implicated in the initial steps of melanocyte oncogenesis (Medrano *et al.*, 1993; Mintz and Silvers, 1993).

IL-8 is produced by various human tumor lines *in vitro*, particularly carcinomas and brain tumors, either spontaneously or after exposure to IL-1 and TNF (Sakamoto *et al.*, 1992; Van Meir *et al.*, 1992; Bellocq *et al.*, 1998; Kitadai *et al.*, 1998). IL-8 may contribute to lymphocytic infiltration in brain tumors (Van Meir *et al.*, 1992). In addition, IL-8 has angiogenic activity (Koch *et al.*, 1992), and could thus contribute to tumor angiogenesis. A member of the CXC family, granulocyte chemotactic protein-2 (GCP-2), was identified in supernatants of stimulated sarcoma cells (Proost *et al.*, 1993). Direct evidence that ELR+CXC chemokines play a positive role in tumor angiogenesis has been obtained in non-small cell lung cancer (Smith *et al.*, 1994; Arenberg *et al.*, 1996; Bellocq *et al.*, 1998; Kitadai *et al.*, 1998). In this human tumor, angiogenesis appears to be regulated by a balance between pro and anti-angiogenic (IP-10) chemokines (Arenberg *et al.*, 1996).

Constitutive production of chemokines has also been detected in hematologic malignancies. In B cell chronic lymphocytic leukemia, IL-8 is a survival factor for leukemia cells (di Celle *et al.*, 1994; Francia di Celle *et al.*, 1994). Chemokines are expressed in tissues involved by Hodgkin's disease and eotaxin correlates with eosinophil infiltration (Teruya-Feldstein *et al.*, 1999). Chemo-attractants are produced by HTLV-1 infected adult T cell leukemia cells (ATL) (Saggioro *et al.*, 1991; Bertini *et al.*, 1995). Constitutive chemokine production results in activation of adhesion molecules, binding to endothelium and tissue infiltration, which can occur massively in ATL and is associated with poor prognosis (Tanaka *et al.*, 1998).

Defective systemic immunity and inflammation in cancer patients: a role for chemokines?

In terms of immuno-inflammatory reactions, neoplastic disorders constitute, in a way, a paradox. As discussed above, many, if not all, tumors produce chemo-attractants and are infiltrated by leukocytes; yet it has long been known that neoplastic disorders are associated with immunosuppression and a defective capacity to mount inflammatory reactions at sites other than the tumor (Snyderman and Cianciolo, 1984). It has repeatedly been demonstrated that circulating monocytes from cancer patients are defective in their capacity to respond to chemo-attractants (Boechter and Leonard, 1974; Normann and Sorkin, 1976, 1977; Snyderman and Pike, 1976; Stevenson and Meltzer, 1976; Cianciolo *et al.*, 1981; Normann *et al.*, 1981).

We have speculated that tumor-derived chemokines may play a role in the two seemingly contradictory aspects of monocyte function in neoplasia (Table 10.2) (Mantovani, 1994). Chemokines released continuously from a growing tumor may, beyond a certain tumor size, leak into the systemic circulation. Chemo-attractants cause desensitization, which, depending on the exposure time, may be restricted to agents that use the same receptor (homologous) or involve other 7-transmembrane domain receptors. Therefore, continuous exposure to tumor-derived chemo-attractants may paralyze leukocytes. A more subtle anti-inflammatory action depends on the chemo-attractants' effect on the receptors of the primary cytokines IL-1 and TNF (Porteu and Nathan, 1990; Colotta *et al.*, 1995). Chemotactic agents cause rapid shedding of the TNF receptors, most efficiently RII/p75, and of the type II IL-1 'decoy' receptor.

Table 10.2   Chemokines as mediators of the systemic defective immunity and inflammation in cancer

1. Reverse gradient
2. Receptor desensitization
3. Release of the decoy IL-1 receptor and of the TNF receptor
4. Induction of IL-10

IL-8 was able to induce rapid decoy RII release, though less efficiently than FMLP or C5a (Colotta *et al.*, 1995). However, IL-8 had additive effects with other elements in the cascade of recruitment, such as platelet-activating factor (S. Orlando, unpublished data). Most likely, rapid shedding of the TNFR and of the IL-1 decoy R serves to buffer primary pro-inflammatory cytokines leaking from sites of inflammation. Consistent with the concept of an anti-inflammatory potential of chemokines, systemic IL-8 inhibits local inflammatory reactions, and transgenic mice over-expressing MCP-1 have impaired resistance to intracellular pathogens (Rutledge *et al.*, 1995). Thus, chemo-attractant-induced continuous release of these molecules, which can block IL-1 and TNF, may contribute to the defective capacity to mount an inflammatory response systemically, coexisting with continuous leukocyte recruitment at the tumor site.

Monocyte functions other than chemotaxis

CC chemokines, particularly MCP-1, affect several functions of mononuclear phagocytes related to recruitment or effector activity. Interaction and localized digestion of extracellular matrix components are essential for phagocyte extravasation and progression in tissues. MCP-1 induces production of gelatinase and of urokinase-type plasminogen activator (uPA) (Opdenakker and Van Damme, 1992a; Mantovani *et al.*, 1993b). Concomitantly, MCP-1 enhances the expression of the cell surface receptor for uPA (uPA-R). Induction of gelatinase was also observed with MCP-2 and -3 (Van Damme *et al.*, 1992). Thus, CC chemokines arm monocytes with the molecular tools for local and polarized digestion of extracellular matrix components during recruitment. In tumor tissues, the release of lytic enzymes by MCP-1-stimulated TAM may provide a ready-made pathway for tumor cell invasion (counter-current invasion), thus contributing to the augmented metastasis associated with inflammation (Opdenakker and Van Damme, 1992a, 1992b; Van Damme *et al.*, 1992; Mantovani *et al.*, 1993b; Opdenakker *et al.*, 1993). In one mouse model, MCP-1 gene transfer increased lung colony formation (Mantovani *et al.*, 1993a) and chemokines were involved in selective metastasis to the kidney in a mouse lymphoma (Wang *et al.*, 1998).

MCP-1 induces a respiratory burst in human monocytes, though it is a weak stimulus compared to other agonists (Zachariae *et al.*, 1990; Jiang *et al.*, 1992). Natural MCP-1 was reported to induce IL-1 and IL-6 but not TNF production (Jiang *et al.*, 1992). In another study, recombinant MCP-1 had little effect on IL-6 release (M. Sironi *et al.*, unpublished data). Human MCP-1 induced monocyte cytostasis for a tumor line (Zachariae *et al.*, 1990) or synergized with bacterial products (but not with interferonγ, IFNγ) in stimulation of mouse macrophage cytotoxicity (Singh *et al.*, 1993; Asano *et al.*, 1996). In one particularly intriguing study, human MCP-1 inhibited NO synthase induction in the macrophage cell line J774 (Rojas *et al.*, 1993). TAM have reduced NO synthase activity (DiNapoli *et al.*, 1996). If confirmed, this would suggest that MCP-1 could account for both recruitment and concomitant partial functional deactivation of TAM (see below).

10.1.3 Ovarian cancer as a paradigm of inflammatory cytokines in solid malignancy

Ovarian carcinoma is the one human tumor that has been extensively studied for cytokine circuits between tumor cells and infiltrating leukocytes (Burke *et al.*, 1996) (see Fig. 10.2). These studies have led to the design of therapeutic strategies targeted to TAM, which have given encouraging results (Allavena *et al.*, 1990; Colombo *et al.*, 1992). The role of chemokines in the ping-pong interaction between ovarian carcinoma cells and macrophages has been discussed. Freshly isolated ovarian carcinoma cells, primary cultures, and some established cell lines, released tumor-derived chemotactic factor (TDCF) activity in early studies (Bottazzi *et al.*, 1983a, 1983b, 1985). These observations were subsequently revisited (Negus *et al.*, 1995). Immunohistochemistry and *in situ* hybridization demonstrated that ovarian carcinoma cells, and, in some tumors, also stromal elements, express MCP-1. High levels of MCP-1 were measured in the ascites (but not in blood) of patients with ovarian cancer but not in the peritoneal fluid of patients with nonmalignant conditions. Production of MCP-1 and recruitment of TAM are likely to play an important role in the progression of this disease because macrophage-derived cytokines (mainly TNF) promote the growth of ovarian carcinoma and its secondary implantation in peritoneal organs (Mantovani, 1994; Negus *et al.*, 1995). Finally, the high levels of IL-10 in ovarian ascites fluid may be induced by MCP-1 and cause immunosuppression.

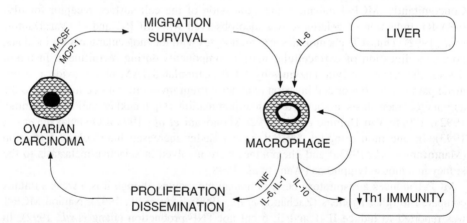

Fig. 10.2 Ovarian carcinoma as a paradigm for the role of inflammatory cytokines in tumor growth and progression. Ovarian tumor cells produce chemokines (MCP-1), which attract macrophages. These cancer cells respond to inflammatory cytokines, notably TNF, which can be produced by tumor cells themselves, with proliferation. Inflammatory cytokines promote the seeding of ovarian cancer on the peritoneal surface by enhancing the expression of adhesion molecules and chemokines in mesothelial cells. Cytokines also induce acute phase protein (e.g. fibrinogen) and subvert immunity.

10.2 Therapy

Cytokines are part of the pharmacological armamentarium of medical oncology. Colony-stimulating factors are used to protect the bone marrow from the side-effects of chemotherapy and to stimulate bone marrow precursor expansion and differentiation. Molecules such as interferons (see Appendix) and IL-2 are used as anti-tumor agents in diseases such as lymphomas, multiple myelomas (interferons), renal cell carcinoma, and melanoma. These agents have been used both as systemic therapies and by local inoculation. For instance, IL-2 has been given locally to patients with advanced head and neck squamous cell carcinoma using intra-lesional and perilymphatic infiltration (Musiani *et al.*, 1997; Nanni *et al.*, 1999).

The intraperitoneal route was used to treat patients with ovarian carcinoma with IL-2 or IFN (Allavena *et al.*, 1990; Colombo *et al.*, 1992). The 'local' approach has also been used for TNF. The development of TNF as a systemic anti-tumor agent in humans has been hampered by severe systemic side-effects. In an interesting trial, TNFα was studied in combination with IFNγ and melphalan in lymph perfusion for melanoma and sarcoma. Rapid, impressive, and lasting responses of melanoma metastasis and sarcoma recurrences were seen with high-dose TNF alone or combined with IFNγ and chemotherapy (Lejeune and Lienard, 1996). Morphological analysis revealed fast and specific destruction of the tumor vascular bed. This finding is reminiscent of observations in rodents, where TNF causes hemorrhagic necrosis, and is consistent with some of the effects of this cytokine on vascular endothelium, although the precise mechanism of action remains undefined.

New cytokines are frequently considered as potential anti-tumor agents. The pathway of clinical evaluation is a complex one, as exemplified recently by IL-12. The identification of IL-12 as a natural killer cells stimulatory factor (NKCF) raised the possibility to use it in cancer therapy. Given the roles of IL-12 in inflammation and in septic shock (Lamont and Adorini, 1996), one should not be surprised that IL-12 would have toxic effects. In fact, mice treated chronically with IL-12 develop pulmonary edema, macrophage infiltrates in tissues and show body weight loss, with induction of TNF and IFNγ synthesis (Car *et al.*, 1995; Orange *et al.*, 1995). Toxicity is partially mediated by IFNγ, as antibodies to IFNγ inhibit decrease in food intake and body weight induced by chronic IL-12 treatment in mice, and a partial protection was also observed with dexamethasone, an inhibitor of cytokine synthesis (Sacco *et al.*, 1997).

However, a peculiarity of IL-12 was revealed only by clinical trials. In 1995 some patients in a clinical trial with IL-12 had severe toxic effects and two died. This toxicity was not observed in an earlier safety trial. Interestingly, in those earlier studies, patients were first injected with a single dose of IL-12, to determine the maximum safe single dose, and given multiple doses only after a washout period of a few weeks (Cohen, 1995). This suggested that pretreatment with a single dose of IL-12 prevented the toxic effects of a multiple-dose cycle started 2 weeks later. This hypothesis was confirmed in mice and monkeys, showing that early pretreatment with IL-12 inhibited subsequent IL-12-induced IFN-γ, but the cellular mechanisms for this phenomenon have not been fully established yet (Leonard *et al.*, 1997; Sacco *et al.*, 1997).

A detailed discussion of the properties of cytokines already in clinical use is beyond the scope of this book, except for type I interferon, which is discussed as a prototype of a clinically useful cytokine in the Appendix. Here we will discuss efforts aimed at exploiting the gene transfer approach, to take maximum advantage of the cytokines' antineoplastic potential and new cellular targets, such as blood vessels and dendritic cells, as potential effectors of this anti-tumor activity.

10.2.1 Therapeutic potential of chemokines: antiangiogenesis

As discussed in Chapter 9 and above, endotelial cells express certain chemokine receptors (e.g. CXCR4 and CXCR2) and respond to chemokines. Work done with gene-targeted mice has unequivocally shown that CXCR4 and its ligand have a non-redundant function in the ontogeny of the vascular bed in the gastro-intestinal tract. Therefore, it is not surprising that chemokines have been shown to regulate angiogenesis in various tumors (Koch *et al.*, 1992; Angiolillo *et al.*, 1995; Strieter *et al.*, 1995), such as non-small cell lung cancer (Smith *et al.*, 1994; Arenberg *et al.*, 1996); for review see Keane and Strieter (1999). Moreover, chemokines regulate angiogenesis also indirectly, via TAM, in complex ways; for instance, by processing plasminogen using a metalloelastase, thus generating angiostatin (Dong *et al.*, 1997). CXC chemokines with an ELR motif (e.g. IL-8) have been shown to be pro-angiogenic, whereas ELR CXC chemokines (e.g. IP10) have anti-angiogenic activity (Keane and Strieter, 1999). Therefore, the balance between pro- and anti-angiogenic chemokines, rather than absolute amounts, regulates tumor angiogenesis (Arenberg *et al.*, 1996). Anti-angiogenic chemokines (e.g. IP10 or mutated ELR$^+$ molecules) are therefore candidate anti-tumor agents, as protelus or in gene transfer approach.

IP10 and related CXC chemokines are induced by IFNγ, which in turn is induced by IL-12. They may represent ultimate mediators of the anti-angiogenic activity of IL-12 (Voest *et al.*, 1995). Thus, certain chemokines, such as IP-10, have anti-angiogenic activity, and constitute the ultimate mediator in the anti-tumor action of a cytokine cascade involving IL-12 and IFNγ. After gene transfer in certain tumors, other cellular targets (e.g. T cells) may play a role in the IP-10's anti-tumor activity.

10.2.2 Therapeutic potential of chemokines: attraction of dendritic cells

Cytokine gene transfer into tumor cells has resulted in tumor rejection in experimental systems and is under evaluation in human tumors. The anti-tumor activity of cytokine gene transfer is associated with distinct patterns of leukocyte infiltration (for a review see: Musiani *et al.*, 1997). Although it is likely that chemokines play a pivotal role in determining the timing, type, and amount of infiltrate under these conditions, detailed analysis is at present lacking.

Chemokines have been used in gene transfer studies. Depending on the tumor type, MCP-1 gene transfer has been associated with abrogation of tumorigenicity, reduced growth rate, increased tumor takes or metastasis, or no effect (Clauss *et al.*, 1990; Bottazzi *et al.*, 1992; Mantovani *et al.*, 1993a; Hirose *et al.*, 1995; Pardoll, 1995). Anti-tumor activity and activation of specific immunity has been observed after gene transfer of IP-10, TCA3, RANTES, lymphotactin, and MCP-3 (Luster and Leder, 1993; Laning *et al.*, 1994; Mulé *et al.*, 1996; Musiani *et al.*, 1997; and see below).

A major goal of immunotherapeutic approaches for tumors is activation of specific anti-tumor immunity. Here, dendritic cells (DC) may be crucial to success or failure. Recent results suggest that DC express receptors for, and respond to, chemokines (Sozzani *et al.*, 1995; Godiska *et al.*, 1997). DC precursors originate in the bone marrow and migrate to peripheral tissues and primary lymphoid organs, where they efficiently take up and process soluble antigens. After capturing antigen in tissues, DC migrate through the afferent lymphatics to draining lymph nodes or in the blood to the spleen, where they stimulate T cells (Caux *et al.*, 1995). As the molecules controlling these events are unknown, the chemotactic factors that attract this cell population and regulate their trafficking in tissues have been investigated (Sozzani *et al.*, 1995, 1998a., 1999).

In a classical microwell chemotaxis assay these cells migrated in response to a selected set of CC chemokines, such as MDC, MCP-3, RANTES, and MIP1α, and to two prototypical chemotactic factors, fMLP and C5a (Sozzani *et al.*, 1995). MCP-1 and MCP-2, two other CC chemokines, and all of the CXC chemokines tested (IL-8, IP-10, and Groß), except SDF1, were inactive. Peak active concentrations and the percentage of cells migrating in response to CC chemokines were comparable to those with monocytes.

On exposure to immune or inflammatory stimuli, DC migrate from peripheral tissues to lymphoid organs, where they present antigen. The molecular basis for their peculiar trafficking properties is largely unknown. CC chemokines induce chemotactic and transendothelial migration of immature DC generated *in vitro*, either from circulating monocytes or from CD34+ cells. Maturation of DC by CD40 ligation, or culture in the presence of inflammatory agonists, such as bacterial lipopolysaccharide, IL-1 and TNF, induces down-regulation of the two main CC chemokine receptors expressed by these cells, CCR1 and CCR5, and abrogates the chemotactic response to their ligands, MIP-1α, MIP-1β, RANTES, and MCP-3. Inhibition of chemotaxis was rapid (<1 h), and included the unrelated agent fMLP. In the same experimental conditions, the expression of CCR7 and the migration to its ligand ELC/MIP-3ß, a chemokine expressed in lymphoid organs, were strongly up-regulated, though this took longer (24–48 h). Rapid inhibition of responsiveness to chemo-attractants present at sites of inflammation, and the immune reaction, may enable DC to leave peripheral tissues. Conversely, the slower acquisition of responsiveness to ELC/MIP-3β may guide the subsequent localization of DC in lymphoid organs (Sozzani *et al.*, 1995, 1997, 1998a; Hallmann *et al.*, 1995; Power *et al.*, 1997).

In the context of studies on chemokines and DC, tumor cells were transfected with MCP-3 (Fioretti *et al.*, 1998). After MCP-3 gene transfer, P815 mastocytoma cells grew and were rejected. This rejection was associated with resistance to subsequent challenge with parental cells and with profound changes of leukocyte infiltration. TAM—already copious—T cells, eosinophils, and neutrophils increased in tumor tissues after MCP-3 gene transfer. DC (e.g. Dec205+, high MHC class II+ cells) did not increase substantially in the tumor mass. However, in peritumoral tissues, DC accumulated in perivascular areas. MCP-3-transfected tumor cells grew normally in nude mice. Accumulation of macrophages and PMN were also increased in nude mice. Antibodies against CD4, CD8, and IFNγ, but not against IL-4, inhibited the rejection of MCP-3 transfected P815 cells. An anti-PMN mAb only slowed the tumor rejection. Thus, MCP-3 gene transfer elicits tumor rejection by activating type I T-cell-dependent immunity.

It is tempting to speculate that altered trafficking of antigen-presenting cells, which express receptors and respond to MCP-3, together with recruitment of activated T cells, underlie the activation of specific immunity by MCP-3 transfected cells. Whether chemokines can in fact be useful for 'piloting' the DC traffick and eliciting anti-tumor immunity in a clinically meaningful setting, remains to be seen.

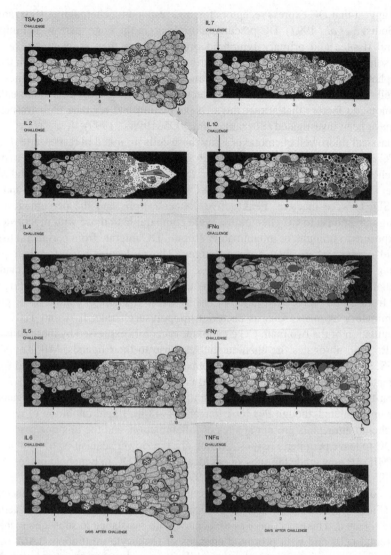

Fig. 10.3 A few reaction patterns elicited in a syngeneic host by a mouse mammary adenocarcinoma (TSA) engineered to release cytokines. Engineered tumor cells behave as biological minipumps, whose proliferation is controlled in a feedback fashion by the immune reaction they elicit. Speckled ovals, TSA cells; speckled ovals with black spots, damaged TSA cells; orange cells with a red nucleus, fibroblasts; red crescents around red spots, vessels and red cells; red crescents around red circles, thrombosed vessels; red crescents around an empty space, damaged vessels; red crescents around red spots and a speckled oval (IL-6 panel), vessels with a metastatizing tumor cell; hatched areas marked with a white arrow (IL-10 and IFNα panels), marked production of collagen fibres. Abbreviations: e, eosinophil (orange circle); IFNα, interferon α; Il-2, interleukin-2; L, lymphocyte (violet circle); M, macrophage (blue cell); n, neutrophil (green circle); nk, natural killer cell (mauve circle); TNFα, tumor necrosis factor α; TSA-pc, TSA-parental cell. Details and references in Musiani *et al.* (1997). (Modified from Musiani *et al.* (1997) *Immunol. Today*, **18**, 32, with permission of Elsevier Science.) See also colour plate.

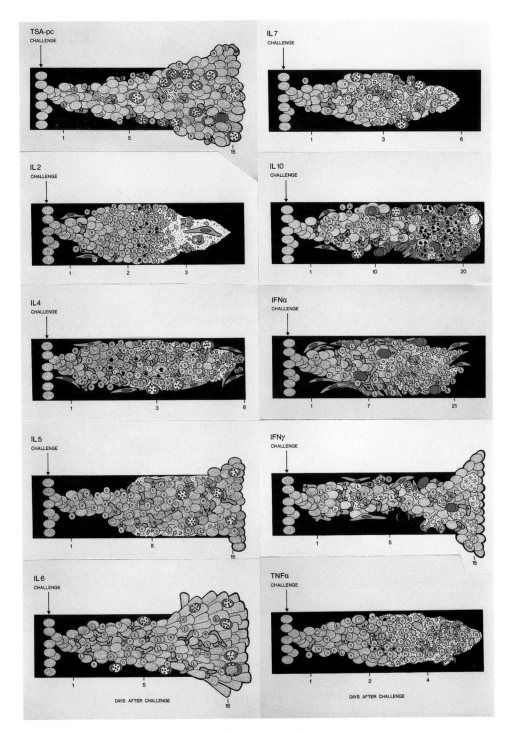

Fig. 10.3 A few reaction patterns elicited in a syngeneic host by a mouse mammary adenocarcinoma. See p. 236 for full caption.

10.2.3 Cytokine gene transfer

Development of cytokine gene therapy for cancer rests, on the one hand, on the molecular identification of cytokines and, on the other hand, on the molecular definition of the antigenicity of tumors (Disis and Cheever, 1996; Nanni *et al.*, 1999). Tumor-associated antigens range from mutated oncogene products to peptides abnormally expressed by tumor cells. In the absence of deliberate intervention, however, immune responses against these antigens are ineffective. Early studies found that cytokines, such as IL-2, sometimes elicited dramatic tumor regression. The same or even more striking results were obtained when minute amounts of cytokines, such as IL-2, were administered locally (Musiani *et al.*, 1997; Nanni *et al.*, 1999). Cytokine gene transfer resulted in even more dramatic rejection of transplanted tumor cells (Dranoff and Mulligan, 1995; Pardoll, 1995; Musiani *et al.*, 1997; Nanni *et al.*, 1999).

Virtually all cytokines have been tested in gene transfer approaches as anti-tumor agents. The effect in terms of anti-tumor activity and changes in the local microenvironment depended on the levels of production, the tumor type, the stage of the disease, etc. As summarized in Table 10.3, very few cytokine-transduced tumor cells have been used as vaccines in a realistic therapeutic context. Interestingly, as outlined in Fig. 10.3, different cytokines elicited distinct patterns of changes in the tumor micro-environment, to some extent consistently with the biology of the transduced mediator. Definite evidence of therapeutic activity was obtained under certain conditions.

Table 10.4 shows that vaccination with cytokine-engineered tumor cells has entered the clinical arena. In general, the approach is safe, but phase I studies indicate that objective

Table 10.3 Therapeutic efficacy of cytokine gene transfer against established, non-engineered rodent tumors[a]

Cytokine gene[b]	Number of studies	Number of protocols	Percentage of protocols reporting therapeutic efficacy[c]			
			Null	Low	Intermediate	High
IL-1	1	1		100%		
IL-2	17	31	29%	39%	10%	23%
IL-3	2	2	50%	50%		
IL-4	6	6	33%	67%		
IL-6	6	7	43%	43%	14%	
IL-7	2	3	67%	33%		
IL-10	1	1		100%		
IL-12	6	13	23%	8%	31%	38%
M-CSF	1	1	100%			
GM-CSF	12	22	18%	36%	18%	27%
TNFα	3	3	33%	33%	33%	
IFNα	5	7	14%	43%	29%	14%
IFNγ	9	11	9%	64%	18%	9%
Total	71	108	26%	40%	16%	18%

[b] The abbreviations used are: GM-CSF, granulocyte macrophage colony stimulating factor; IFN, interferon; IL, interleukin; M-CSF, macrophage colony stimulating factor; TNF. Tumor necrosis factor.

[c] Therapeutic efficacy was classified as: Low when <25% of mice mere tumor and metastasis free; Intermediate when tumor and metastasis free mice were between 25% and 50%; High when >50% of mice were tumor and metastasis free.

[a] Reproduced with permission from Nanni *et al.* (1999).

Table 10.4 Clinical trials involving cytokine gene transfera*

Cytokine gene	Number of clinical trials	In vitro gene transfer: cell target				In vivo gene transfer
		Cancer cells	Fibroblasts	Leukocytes	Cancer cells & leukocytes	
L-2	27 (49%)	16	4	1		6
IL-4	4 (7%)	2			1	1
IL-6	1 (2%)	1				
IL-7	3 (5%)	1	1	1		
IL-12	3 (5%)		1			2
GM-CSF	9 (16%)	6	1	1	1	
TNFα	2 (4%)	1		1		
IFNγ	2 (4%)	2				
Combined	4 (7%)	3				1
TOTAL	55	32 (58%)	7 (13%)	4 (7%)	1 (2%)	11 (20%)

* Reproduced with kind permission from Nanni P. *et al.*, (1999). Cytokine gene therapy: hopes and pitfalls. *Annals of Oncology*, **10**, 261-6.

responses are rare. Of course, based on preclinical models, it is expected that these therapeutic approaches will have maximal potential for benefit under conditions of minimal tumor burden, such as in patients with micrometastases.

References

Adams, D. O. and Snyderman, R. (1979). Do macrophages destroy nascent tumors?. *J. Natl. Cancer Inst.*, **62**, 1341–1745.

Allavena, P., Grandi, M., D'Incalci, M. *et al.* (1987). Human tumor cell lines with pleiotropic drug resistance are efficiently killed by interleukin-2 activated killer cells and by activated monocytes. *Int. J. Cancer*, **40**, 104–7.

Allavena, P., Peccatori, F., Maggioni, D. *et al.* (1990). Intraperitoneal recombinant gamma-interferon in patients with recurrent ascitic ovarian carcinoma: modulation of cytotoxicity and cytokine production in tumor-associated effectors and of major histocompatibility antigen expression on tumor cells. *Cancer Res.*, **50**, 7318–23.

Angiolillo, A. L., Sgadari, C., Taub, D. D. *et al.* (1995). Human interferon-inducible protein 10 is a potent inhibitor of angiogenesis *in vivo*. *J. Exp. Med.*, **182**, 155–62.

Arenberg, D. A., Kunkel, S. L., Polverini, P. J. *et al.* (1996). Interferon-gamma-inducible protein 10 (IP-10) is an angiostatic factor that inhibits human non-small cell lung cancer (NSCLC) tumorigenesis and spontaneous metastases. *J. Exp. Med.*, **184**, 981–92.

Arvanitakis, L., GerasRaaka, E., Varma, A. *et al.* (1997). Human herpesvirus KSHV encodes a constitutively active G-protein- coupled receptor linked to cell proliferation. *Nature*, **385**, 347–50.

Asano, T., An, T., Jia, S. F., and Kleinerman, E. S. (1996). Altered monocyte chemotactic and activating factor gene expression in human glioblastoma cell lines increased their susceptibility to cytotoxicity. *J. Leukocyte. Biol.*, **59**, 916–24.

Balentien, E., Mufson, B. E., Shattuck, R. L. *et al.* (1991). Effects of MGSA/GRO alpha on melanocyte transformation. *Oncogene*, **6**, 1115–24.

Bellocq, A., Antoine, M., Flahault, A. *et al.* (1998). Neutrophil alveolitis in Bronchioloalveolar carcinoma. Induction by tumor-derived interleukin-8 and relation to clinical outcome. *Am. J. Pathol.*, **152**, 83–92.

Bertini, R., Luini, W., Sozzani, S. *et al.* (1995). Identification of MIP-1 alpha/LD78 as a monocyte chemoattractant released by the HTLV-I-transformed cell line MT4. *AIDS Res. Hum. Retroviruses.*, **11**, 155–60.

Boechter, D. and Leonard, E. J. (1974). Abnormal monocyte chemotactic response in mice. *J. Natl. Cancer Inst.*, **52**, 1091–9.

Bonecchi, R., Bianchi, G., Bordignon, P. P. *et al.* (1998). Differential expression of chemokine receptors and chemotactic responsiveness of type 1 T helper cells (Th1) and Th2. *J. Exp. Med.*, **187**, 129–34.

Bottazzi, B., Polentarutti, N., Acero, R. *et al.* (1983a). Regulation of the macrophage content of neoplasms by chemoattractants. *Science*, **220**, 210–2.

Bottazzi, B., Polentarutti, N., Balsari, A. *et al.* (1983b). Chemotactic activity for mononuclear phagocytes of culture supernatants from murine and human tumor cells: evidence for a role in the regulation of the macrophage content of neoplastic tissues. *Int. J. Cancer*, **31**, 55–63.

Bottazzi, B., Ghezzi, P., Taraboletti, G. *et al.* (1985). Tumor-derived chemotactic factor(s) from human ovarian carcinoma: evidence for a role in the regulation of macrophage content of neoplastic tissues. *Int. J. Cancer*, **36**, 167–73.

Bottazzi, B., Walter, S., Govoni, D. *et al.* (1992). Monocyte chemotactic cytokine gene transfer modulates macrophage infiltration, growth, and susceptibility to IL-2 therapy of a murine melanoma. *J. Immunol.*, **148**, 1280–5.

Bucana, C. D., Fabra, A., Sanchez, R., and Fidler, I. J. (1992). Different patterns of macrophage infiltration into allogeneic-murine and xenogeneic-human neoplasms growing in nude mice. *Am. J. Pathol.*, **141**, 1225–36.

Burke, F., Relf, M., Negus, R., and Balkwill, F. (1996). A cytokine profile of normal and malignant ovary. *Cytokine*, **8**, 578–85.

Car, B. D., Eng, V. M., Schnyder, B. *et al.* (1995). Role of interferon-gamma in interleukin 12-induced pathology in mice [see comments]. *Am. J. Pathol.*, **147**, 1693–707.

Caux, C., Liu, Y. J., and Banchereau, J. (1995). Recent advances in the study of dendritic cells and follicular dendritic cells. *Immunol. Today*, **16**, 2–4.

Cianciolo, G. J., Hunter, J., Silva, J., Haskill, J. S., and Snyderman, R. (1981). Inhibitors of monocyte responses to chemotaxins are present in human cancerous effusions and react with monoclonal antibodies to the P15(E) structural protein of retroviruses. *J. Clin. Invest.*, **68**, 831–44.

Clauss, M., Gerlach, M., Gerlach, H. *et al.* (1990). Vascular permeability factor: a tumor-derived polypeptide that induces endothelial cell and monocyte procoagulant activity, and promotes monocyte migration. *J. Exp. Med.*, **172**, 1535–45.

Cohen, J. (1995). IL-12 deaths: explanation and a puzzle. *Science*, **270**, 908.

Colombo, N., Peccatori, F., Paganin, C. *et al.* (1992). Anti-tumor and immunomodulatory activity of intraperitoneal IFN-gamma in ovarian carcinoma patients with minimal residual tumor after chemotherapy. *Int. J. Cancer*, **51**, 42–6.

Colotta, F., Orlando, S., Fadlon, E. J. *et al.* (1995). Chemoattractants induce rapid release of the interleukin 1 type II decoy receptor in human polymorphonuclear cells. *J. Exp. Med.*, **181**, 2181–8.

di Celle, P. F., Carbone, A., Marchis, D. *et al.* (1994). Cytokine gene expression in B-cell chronic lymphocytic leukemia: evidence of constitutive interleukin-8 (IL-8) mRNA expression and secretion of biologically active IL-8 protein. *Blood*, **84**, 220–8.

DiNapoli, M. R., Calderon, C. L., and Lopez, D. M. (1996). The altered tumoricidal capacity of macrophages isolated from tumor-bearing mice is related to reduced expression of the inducible nitric oxide synthase gene. *J. Exp. Med.*, **183**, 1323–9.

Disis, M. L. and Cheever, M. A. (1996). Oncogenic proteins as tumor antigens. *Curr. Opin. Immunol.*, **8**, 637–42.

Dong, Z., Kumar, R., Yang, X., and Fidler, I. J. (1997). Macrophage-derived metalloelastase is responsible for the generation of agiostatin in Lewis lung carcinoma. *Cell*, **88**, 801–10.

Dranoff, G. and Mulligan, R. C. (1995). Gene transfer as cancer therapy. *Adv. Immunol.*, **58**, 417–54.

Dvorak, H. F. (1986). Tumors: wounds that do not heal. Similarities between tumor stroma generation and wound healing. *N. Engl. J. Med.*, **315**, 1650–9.

El-Omar, E. M., Carrington, M., Chow, W-H., *et al.* (2000). Interleukin-1 polymorphisms associated with increased risk of gastric cancer. *Nature*, **404**, 398–402.

Endres, M. J., Garlisi, C. G., Xiao, H. *et al.* (1999).The Kaposi's sarcoma-related herpesvirus (KSHV)-encoded chemokine vMIP-I is a specific agonist for the CC chemokine receptor (CCR)8. *J. Exp. Med.*, **189**, 1993–8.

Evans, R. (1972). Macrophages in syngeneic animal tumours. *Transplantation.*, **14**, 468–70.

Fioretti, F., Fradelizi, D., Stoppacciaro, A., Ruco, L., Minty, A., Sozzani, S. *et al.* (1998). Reduced tumorigenicity and augmented leukocyte infiltration after MCP-3 gene transfer: perivascular accumulation of dendritic cells in peritumoral tissue and neutrophil recruitment within the tumor. *J. Immunol.*, **161**, 342–6.

Francia di Celle, P., Carbone, A., Marchis, D. *et al.* (1994). Cytokine gene expression in B-cell chronic lymphocytic leukemia: evidence of constitutive interleukin-8 (IL-8) mRNA expression and secretion of biologically active IL-8 protein. *Blood*, **84**, 220–8.

Giavazzi, R., Garofalo, A., Bani, M. R. *et al.* (1990). Interleukin 1-induced augmentation of experimental metastases from a human melanoma in nude mice. *Cancer Res.*, **50**, 4771–5.

Godiska, R., Chantry, D., Raport, C. J. *et al.* (1997). Human macrophage derived chemokine (MDC) a novel chemoattractant for monocytes, monocyte derived dendritic cells, and natural killer cells. *J. Exp. Med.*, **185**, 1595–604.

Graves, D. T., Jiang, Y. L., Williamson, M. J., and Valente, A. J. (1989). Identfcation of monocyte chemotactic activity produced by malignant cells. *Science*, **245**, 1490–3.

Graves, D. T., Barnhill, R., Galanopoulos, T., and Antoniades, H. N. (1992). Expression of monocyte chemotactic protein-1 in human melanoma *in vivo. Am. J. Pathol.*, **140**, 9–14.

Hallmann, R., Mayer, D. N., Berg, E. L., Broermann, R., and Butcher, E. C. (1995). Novel mouse endothelial cell surface marker is suppressed during differentiation of the blood brain barrier. *Dev. Dyn.*, **202**, 325–32.

Heuff, G., van der Ende, M. B., Boutkan, H. *et al.* (1993). Macrophage populations in different stages of induced hepatic metastases in rats: an immunohistochemical analysis. *Scand. J. Immunol.*, **38**, 10–6.

Hibbs, J. B. (1976) The macrophage as a tumoricidal effector cell: a review of *in vivo* and *in vitro* studies on the mechanism of the activated macrophage nonspecific cytotoxicity reaction. In *The macrophage and neoplasia* (ed. M. A. Fink), pp. 83–98. Academic Press, New York.

Hirose, K., Hakozaki, M., Nyunoya, Y.. *et al.* (1995). Chemokine gene transfection into tumour cells reduced tumorigenicity in nude mice in association with neutrophilic infiltration. *Br. J. Cancer*, **72**, 708–14.

Jiang, Y., Beller, D. I., Frendl, G., and Graves, D. T. (1992). Monocyte chemoattractant protein-1 regulates adhesion molecule expression and cytokine production in human monocytes. *J. Immunol.*, **148**, 2423–8.

Keane, M. P. and Strieter, R. M. (1999). The role of CXC chemokines in the regulation of angiogenesis. In: *Chemokines—chemical immunology vol. 72* (ed. A. Mantovani), pp. 86–101. Karger, Basel.

Kitadai, Y., Haruma, K., Sumii, K. *et al.* (1998). Expression of Interleukin-8 correlates with vascularity in human gastric carcinomas. *Am. J. Pathol.*, **152**, 93–100.

Koch, A. E., Polverini, P. J., Kunkel, S. L. *et al.* (1992). Interleukin-8 as a macrophage-derived mediator of angiogenesis. *Science*, **258**, 1798–1801.

Lamont, A. G. and Adorini, L. (1996). IL-12: a key cytokine in immune regulation. *Immunol. Today*, **17**, 214–7.

Laning, J., Kawasaki, H., Tanaka, E., Luo, Y., and Dorf, M. E. (1994). Inhibition of *in vivo* tumor growth by the beta chemokine, TCA3. *J. Immunol.*, **153**, 4625–35.

Lejeune, F. J. and Lienard, D. (1996). TNF-α: shock-free cancer remission. *Nat. Biotechnol.*, **14**, 706–8.

Leonard, J. P., Sherman, M. L., Fisher, G. L. *et al.* (1997). Effects of single-dose interleukin-12 exposure on interleukin-12-associated toxicity and interferon-gamma production. *Blood*, **90**, 2541–8.

Luan, J., Shattuck-Brandt, R., Haghnegahdar, H. *et al.* (1997). Mechanism and biological significance of constitutive expression of MGSA/GRO chemokines in malignant melanoma tumor progression. *J. Leukoc. Biol.*, **62**, 588–97.

Luboshits, G., Shina, S., Kaplan, O. *et al.* (1999). Elevated expression of the CC chemokine RANTES in advanced breast carcinoma. *Cancer Res.*, (in press).

Luster, A. D. and Leder, P. (1993). IP-10, a -C-X-C- chemokine, elicits a potent thymus-dependent anti-tumor response *in vivo*. *J. Exp. Med.*, **178**, 1057–65.

Mantovani, A., Bottazzi, B., Colotta, F., Sozzani, S., and Ruco, L. (1992a). The origin and function of tumor-associated macrophages. *Immunol. Today*, **13**, 265–70.

Mantovani, A., Bussolino, F., and Dejana, E. (1992b). Cytokine regulation of endothelial cell function. *FASEB. J.*, **6**, 2591–9.

Mantovani, A., Bottazzi, B., Sozzani, S. *et al.* (1993a). Cytokine regulation of tumour-associated macrophages. *Res. Immunol.*, **144**, 280–3.

Mantovani, A., Sozzani, S., Bottazzi, B. *et al.* (1993b). Monocyte chemotactic protein-1 (MCP-1): signal transduction and involvement in the regulation of macrophage traffic in normal and neoplastic tissues. *Adv. Exp. Med. Biol.*, **351**, 47–54.

Mantovani, A. (1994). Tumor-associated macrophages in neoplastic progression: A paradigm for the *in vivo* function of chemokines. *Lab. Invest.*, **71**, 5–16.

Martin Padura, I., Mortarini, R., Lauri, D. *et al.* (1991). Heterogeneity in human melanoma cell adhesion to cytokine activated endothelial cells correlates with VLA-4 expression. *Cancer Res.*, **51**, 2239–41.

Medrano, E. E., Farooqui, J. Z., Boissy, R. E. *et al.* (1993). Chronic growth stimulation of human adult melanocytes by inflammatory mediators *in vitro*: implications for nevus formation and initial steps in melanocyte oncogenesis. *Proc. Natl. Acad. Sci. USA.*, **90**, 1790–4.

Melani, C., Pupa, S. M., Stoppacciaro, A. *et al.* (1995). An *in vivo* model to compare human leukocyte infiltration in carcinoma xenografts producing different chemokines. *Int. J. Cancer*, **62**, 572–8.

Mintz, B. and Silvers, W. K. (1993). Transgenic mouse model of malignant skin melanoma. *Proc. Natl. Acad. Sci. USA.*, **90**, 8817–21.

Moore, R. J., Owens, D. M., Stamp, G. *et al.* (1999). Mice deficient in tumor necrosis factor-α are resistant to skin carcinogenesis. *Nature Med.*, **5**, 828–31.

Mulé, J. J., Custer, M., Averbook, B. *et al.* (1996). RANTES secretion by gene-modified tumor cells results in loss of tumorigenicity *in vivo*: role of immune cell subpopulations. *Hum. Gene Ther.*, **7**, 1545–53.

Musiani, P., Modesti, A., Giovarelli, M. *et al.* (1997). Cytokines, tumor-cell death and immunogenicity: a question of choice. *Immunol. Today*, **18**, 32–6.

Nanni, P., Forni, G., and Lollini, P. L. (1999). Cytokine gene therapy: hopes and pitfalls. *Ann. Oncol.*, **10**, 261–6.

Negus, R. P., Stamp, G. W., Relf, M. G. *et al.* (1995). The detection and localization of monocyte chemoattractant protein-1 (MCP-1) in human ovarian cancer. *J. Clin. Invest.*, **95**, 2391–6.

Normann, S. J. and Sorkin, E. (1976). Cell-specific defect in monocyte function during tumor growth. *J. Natl. Cancer Inst.*, **57**, 135–40.

Normann, S. J. and Sorkin, E. (1977). Inhibition of macrophage chemotaxis by neoplastic and other rapidly proliferating cells *in vitro*. *Cancer Res.*, **37**, 705–11.

Normann, S. J., Schardt, M., and Sorkin, E. (1981). Biphasic depression of macrophage function after tumor transplantation. *Int. J. Cancer*, **28**, 185–90.

Opdenakker, G. and Van Damme, J. (1992a). Cytokines and proteases in invasive processes: molecular similarities between inflammation and cancer. *Cytokine*, **4**, 251–8.

Opdenakker, G. and Van Damme, J. (1992b). Chemotactic factors, passive invasion and metastasis of cancer cells. *Immunol. Today*, **13**, 463–4.

Opdenakker, G., Froyen, G., Fiten, P., Proost, P., and Van Damme, J. (1993). Human monocyte chemotactic protein-3 (MCP-3): molecular cloning of the cDNA and comparison with other chemokines. *Biochem. Biophys. Res. Commun.*, **191**, 535–42.

Orange, J. S., Salazar-Mather, T. P., Opal, S. M. *et al.* (1995). Mechanism of interleukin 12-mediated toxicities during experimental viral infections: role of tumor necrosis factor and glucocorticoids. *J. Exp. Med.*, **181**, 901–14.

Pardoll, D. M. (1995). Paracrine cytokine adjuvants in cancer immunotherapy. *Annu. Rev. Immunol.*, **13**, 399–415.

Pekarek, L. A., Starr, B. A., Toledano, A. Y., and Schreiber, H. (1995). Inhibition of tumor growth by elimination of granulocytes. *J. Exp. Med.*, **181**, 435–40.

Porteu, F. and Nathan, C. (1990). Shedding of tumor necrosis factor receptor by activated human neutrophils. *J. Exp. Med.*, **172**, 599–607.

Power, C. A., Church, D. J., Meyer, A. *et al.* (1997). Cloning and characterization of a specific receptor for the novel CC chemokine MIP-3 alpha from lung dendritic cells. *J. Exp. Med.*, **186**, 825–35.

Proost, P., De Wolf Peeters, C., Conings, R. *et al.* (1993). Identification of a novel granulocyte chemotactic protein (GCP-2) from human tumor cells. *In vitro* and *in vivo* comparison with natural forms of GRO, IP-10, and IL-8. *J. Immunol.*, **150**, 1000–10.

Riethdorf, L., Riethdorf, S., Gutzlaff, K., Prall, F., and Loning, T. (1996). Differential expression of the monocyte chemoattractant protein-1 gene in human papillomavirus-16-infected squamous intraepithelial lesions and squamous cell carcinomas of the cervix uteri. *Am. J. Pathol.*, **149**, 1469–76.

Rojas, A., Delgado, R., Glaria, L., and Palacios, M. (1993). Monocyte chemotactic protein-1 inhibits the induction of nitric oxide synthase in J774 cells. *Biochem. Biophys. Res. Commun.*, **196**, 274–9.

Rollins, B. J. and Sunday, M. E. (1991). Suppression of tumor formation *in vivo* by expression of the JE gene in malignant cells. *Mol. Cell Biol.*, **11**, 3125–31.

Rutledge, B. J., Rayburn, H., Rosenberg, R. *et al.* (1995). High level monocyte chemoattractant protein-1 expression in transgenic mice increases their susceptibility to intracellular pathogens. *J. Immunol.*, **155**, 4838–43.

Sacco, S., Heremans, H., Echtenacher, B. *et al.* (1997). Protective effect of a single interleukin-12 (IL-12) predose against the toxicity of subsequent chronic IL-12 in mice: role of cytokines and glucocorticoids. *Blood*, **90**, 4473–9.

Saggioro, D., Wang, J. M., Sironi, M., Luini, W., Mantovani, A., and Chieco Bianchi, L. (1991). Chemoattractant(s) in culture supernatants of HTLV-I-Infected T-cell lines. *AIDS Res. Hum. Retroviruses.*, **7**, 571–7.

Sakamoto, K., Masuda, T., Mita, S. *et al.* (1992). Interleukin-8 is constitutively and commonly produced by various human carcinoma cell lines. *Int. J. Clin. Lab. Res.*, **22**, 216–9.

Schadendorf, D., Moller, A., Algermissen, B. *et al.* (1993). IL-8 produced by human malignant melanoma cells *in vitro* is an essential autocrine growth factor. *J. Immunol.*, **151**, 2667–75.

Sciacca, F. L., Stürzl, M., Bussolino, F. *et al.* (1994). Expression of adhesion molecules, platelet-activating factor, and chemokines by Kaposi's sarcoma cells. *J. Immunol.*, **153**, 4816–25.

Singh, R. K., Berry, K., Matsushima, K., Yasumoto, K., and Fidler, I. J. (1993). Synergism between human monocyte chemotactic and activating factor and bacterial products for activation of tumoricidal properties in murine macrophages. *J. Immunol.*, **151**, 2786–93.

Smith, D. R., Polverini, P. J., Kunkel, S. L. *et al.* (1994). Inhibition of IL-8 attenuates angiogenesis in bronchogenic carcinoma. *J. Exp. Med.*, **179**, 1409–15.

Snyderman, R. and Pike, M. C. (1976). An inhibitor of macrophage chemotaxis produced by neoplasms. *Science*, **192**, 370–2.

Snyderman, R. and Cianciolo, G. J. (1984). Immunosuppressive activity of the retroviral envelope protein P15E and its possible relationship to neoplasia. *Immunol. Today*, **5**, 240–4.

Sonouchi, K., Hamilton, T. A., Tannenbaum, C. S. *et al.* (1994). Chemokine gene expression in the murine renal cell carcinoma, renca, following treatment *in vivo* with interferon-alpha and interleukin-2. *Am. J. Pathol.*, **144**, 747–55.

Sozzani, S., Sallusto, F., Luini, W. *et al.* (1995). Migration of dendritic cells in response to formyl peptides, C5a and a distinct set of chemokines. *J. Immunol.*, **155**, 3292–5.

Sozzani, S., Luini, W., Borsatti, A. *et al.* (1997). Receptor expression and responsiveness of human dendritic cells to a defined set of CC and CXC chemokines. *J. Immunol.*, **159**, 1993–2000.

Sozzani, S., Allavena, P., D'Amico, G. *et al.* (1998a). Cutting edge: Differential regulation of chemokine receptors during dendritic cell maturation: A model for their trafficking properties. *J. Immunol.*, **161**, 1083–6.

Sozzani, S., Luini, W., Bianchi, G. *et al.* (1998b). The viral chemokine macrophage inflammatory protein-II is a selective Th2 chemoattractant. *Blood*, **92**, 4036–9.

Sozzani, S., Allavena, P., Vecchi, A., and Mantovani, A. (1999). The role of chemokines in the regulation of dendritic cell trafficking. *J. Leukoc. Biol.*, **66**, 1–9.

Stevenson, M. M. and Meltzer, M. S. (1976). Depressed chemotactic responses *in vitro* of peritoneal macrophages from tumor-bearing mice. *J. Natl. Cancer Inst.*, **57**, 847–52.

Stine, J. T., Wood, C., Hill, M. *et al.* (1999). The KSHV-encoded CC chemokine vMIP-III is a CCR4 agonist, stimulates angiogenesis, and selectively chemoattracts TH2 cells. *Blood*, (in press).

Strieter, R. M., Polverini, P. J., Kunkel, S. L. *et al.* (1995). The functional role of the ELR motif in CXC chemokine-mediated angiogenesis. *J. Biol. Chem.*, **270**, 27348–57.

Takeya, M., Yoshimura, T., Leonard, E. J. *et al.* (1991). Production of monocyte chemoattractant protein-1 by malignant fibrous histiocytoma: relation to the origin of histiocyte-like cells. *Exp. Mol. Pathol.*, **54**, 61–71.

Tanaka, Y., Mine, S., Figdor, C. G. *et al.* (1998). Constitutive chemokine production results in activation of leukocyte function-associated antigen-1 on adult t-cell leukemia cells. *Blood*, **91**, 3909–19.

Tannenbaum, C. S., Wicker, N., Armstrong, D. *et al.* (1996). Cytokine and chemokine expression in tumors of mice receiving systemic therapy with IL-12. *J. Immunol.*, **156**, 693–9.

Teruya-Feldstein, J., Jaffe, E. S., Burd, P. R. *et al.* (1999). Differential chemokine expression in tissue involved by Hodgkin's disease: direct correlation of eotaxin expression and tissue eosinophila. *Blood*, **93**, 2463–70.

Van Damme, J., Proost, P., Lenaerts, J. P., and Opdenakker, G. (1992). Structural and functional identification of two human, tumor-derived monocyte chemotactic proteins (MCP-2 and MCP-3) belonging to the chemokine family. *J. Exp. Med.*, **176**, 59–65.

Van Meir, E., Ceska, M., Effenberger, F. *et al.* (1992). Interleukin-8 is produced in neoplastic and infectious diseases of the human central nervous system. *Cancer Res.*, **52**, 4297–4305.

van Ravenswaay Claasen, H. H., Kluin, P. M., and Fleuren, G. J. (1992). Tumor infiltrating cells in human cancer. On the possible role of CD16+ macrophages in anti-tumor cytotoxicity. *Lab. Invest.*, **67**, 166–74.

Voest, E. E., Kenyon, B. M., O'Reilly, M. S. *et al.* (1995). Inhibition of angiogenesis *in vivo* by interleukin-12. *J. Natl. Cancer Inst.*, **87**, 581–6.

Walter, S., Bottazzi, B., Govoni, D., Colotta, F., and Mantovani, A. (1991). Macrophage infiltration and growth of sarcoma clones expressing different amounts of monocyte chemotactic protein/JE. *Int. J. Cancer*, **49**, 431–5.

Wang, J. M., Taraboletti, G., Matsushima, K., Van Damme, J., and Mantovani, A. (1990). Induction of haptotactic migration of melanoma cells by neutrophil activating protein/interleukin-8. *Biochem. Biophys. Res. Commun.*, **169**, 165–70.

Wang, J-M., Chertov, P., Proost, P. *et al.* (1998). Purification and identification of chemokines potentially involved in kidney-specific metastasis by a murine lymphoma variant: induction of migration and NFkB activation. *Int. J. Cancer* **75**, 900–7.

Yamashiro, S., Takeya, M., Nishi, T. *et al.* (1994). Tumor-derived monocyte chemoattractant protein-1 induces intratumoral infiltration of monocyte-derived macrophage subpopulation in transplanted rat tumors. *Am. J. Pathol.*, **145**, 856–67.

Yoshimura, T., Robinson, E. A., Tanaka, S., Appella, E., Kuratsu, J., and Leonard, E. J. (1989). Purification and amino acid analysis of two human glioma-derived monocyte chemoattractants. *J. Exp. Med.*, **169**, 1449–59.

Zachariae, C. O., Anderson, A. O., Thompson, H. L. *et al.* (1990). Properties of monocyte chemotactic and activating factor (MCAF) purified from a human fibrosarcoma cell line. *J. Exp. Med.*, **171**, 2177–82.

11 Liver and lung

11.1 Liver

Cytokines are important mediators, not only of primary liver diseases such as hepatitis or chemical injury, but also in liver injury associated with sepsis and multiple-organ failure. The liver is the tissue that contains the largest mass of macrophages in the whole organism. Liver macrophages (Kupffer cells) have a key role in lipopolysaccharide (LPS) detoxification. Very early it was clear that Kupffer cells could play a role in hepatotoxicity through the release of soluble mediators that included 'pyrogens' and 'tumoricidal factors' (reviewed in: Nolan, 1975, 1981; Nolan and Camara, 1982). Although the most important effect of cytokines on the liver is probably the induction of acute-phase proteins, the liver is a target organ of the pathogenic action of cytokines.

11.1.1 Cytokines in acute and chronic hepatitis

One of the most widely used, and misnamed, models of 'endotoxic shock' consists of the injection of LPS in D-galactosamine-sensitized mice. In fact, galactosamine increases the lethality of LPS by several orders of magnitude (in terms of doses), so that a few micrograms of LPS are lethal in D-galactosamine-treated mice (while the lethal dose in normal mice is about one milligram) (Galanos et al., 1979; Lehmann et al., 1987). In fact, D-galactosamine sensitizes mice against the lethal effect of TNF (Lehmann et al., 1987). A similar effect was also reported with actinomycin D (Wallach et al., 1988; Gadina et al., 1991), which also sensitizes to the lethal effect of IL-1 (Bertini et al., 1989). These are actually models of fulminant hepatitis, as documented by elevation of transaminases (Tiegs et al., 1989; Shedlofsky and McClain, 1991). It is important to note that no elevation of transaminases is observed in models of lethality of LPS in the absence of galactosamine or actinomycin D sensitization (Gadina et al., 1991). It has been suggested that this model of fulminant hepatitis involves leukotriene D4 and reactive oxygen intermediates as terminal mediators, as the lipoxygenase inhibitor BW775C and the LTD4 receptor antagonist FPL55712 were protective against galactosamine/LPS (Tiegs et al., 1989). More importantly, this model is glucocorticoid-resistant, since dexamethasone is not protective against galactosamine/LPS or actinomycin D/LPS hepatotoxicity (Gadina et al., 1991). Another chemical that induces sensitization to LPS, by causing hepatic damage, is lead (Selye et al., 1966). Lead enhancement of LPS lethality and liver injury is associated with a marked increase in plasma TNF levels (Honchel et al., 1991; Shedlofsky and McClain, 1991).

Historically, it is also important to note that TNF was originally described as a tumoricidal factor released in the serum of mice that received an LPS treatment after they had been 'primed' with BCG or Corynebacteria (Carswell *et al.*, 1975). Interestingly, injection of LPS into BCG- or corynebacterium parvum-pretreated mice induces a fulminant hepatitis and death (Ferluga *et al.*, 1979; Ferluga, 1981), while no hepatitis (as detected by transaminase elevation) is observed with even lethal doses of LPS alone (Gadina *et al.*, 1991). TNF and IL-1 were also detected in patients with fulminant hepatitis, thus strengthening the importance of the results obtained in mice.

In a model of concanavalin A-induced, CD4+ T cell-dependent experimental hepatitis in mice, in which TNF is a central mediator of apoptotic and necrotic liver damage, Kusters *et al.* (1997) reported that transgenic mice deficient in wild-type soluble TNF, but expressing a mutated non-secretable form of TNF, developed hepatitis. These data, while showing the importance of TNF in this model, also indicate that drugs that inhibit the release of soluble TNF from the membrane form into its soluble form might not be effective in TNF-mediated liver diseases. In agreement with this hypothesis, a matrix metalloproteinase inhibitor, GM-6001, which has a protective effect against endotoxic shock (Solorzano *et al.*, 1997), did not protect against D-galactosamine/LPS-induced hepatitis and actually exacerbated concanavalin A-induced hepatitis. In models of T cell-mediated hepatitis which is induced in leptin-deficient mice by administration of Con A or of *Pseudomonas aeruginosa* exotoxin A, either soluble TNF receptors or an anti-IL-18 antiserum are protective (Faggioni *et al.*, 2000).

Finally, mice over-expressing IFN-gamma in the liver develop chronic hepatitis (Toyonaga *et al.*, 1994). Since these mice had increased TNFα expression in the liver, it was suggested that TNF might be the terminal mediator of liver injury in this model (Okamoto *et al.*, 1996).

11.1.2 Depression of liver metabolizing enzymes by cytokines

Another effect of cytokines on the liver that has been regarded as 'toxic' is the depression of liver cytochrome P-450 and related drug metabolizing enzymes. Various studies have shown that administration to mice or rats of several recombinant cytokines, including IL-1, TNF, IL-6, and IL-12, can depress liver cytochrome P-450. These studies were prompted by the first reports in 1976, by Renton and Mannering (Renton and Mannering, 1976), showing that administration of IFN inducers decreased cytochrome P-450 levels. These findings probably explain the decreased cytochrome P-450 content, or liver drug-metabolizing capacity, after administration of vaccines. Depression of cytochrome P-450, one of the major protein components of the liver, might be understandable in terms of protein synthesis economy. In fact, several cytokines induce the synthesis of a set of proteins (acute-phase proteins) normally expressed at much lower levels. Cytokines like IL-1 thus switch protein synthesis from normal liver proteins (e.g. cytochrome P-450 and albumin) to acute-phase proteins.

Some studies have aimed at reversing this effect with various drugs. For instance, pentoxifylline administration to LPS-treated rats prevented the decrease of some P-450 isoenzymes but not others (Monshouwer *et al.*, 1996). Other works have tried to revert LPS-induced depression of cytochrome P-450 by acting on secondary mediators, such as reactive oxygen or nitrogen intermediates. For instance, partial protection against LPS-induced decrease of cytochrome P-450 can be obtained with the antioxidant N-acetylcysteine (Ghezzi *et al.*, 1985, 1986). Inhibitors of NOS, like L-NAME, prevent LPS-induced down-regulation of some P-450 isoenzymes, but not all (Khatsenko and Kikkawa, 1997; Sewer and Morgan, 1997).

11.1.3 Hepatotoxicants and cytokines

In addition to the LPS- or bacteria-dependent models outlined above, TNF can be important in chemically-induced liver disease. Early studies by Nolan (Nolan and Ali, 1973) have shown that endotoxin-tolerant mice were protected against the toxicity of CCl_4, and protection was also achieved with the LPS-binding molecule, polymixin B (Nolan and Leibowitz, 1978). This led to the suggestion that Kupffer cell activation products might have a role in the hepatotoxicity of carbon tetrachloride (CCl_4) (Nolan, 1975; Nolan and Camara, 1982). More recently it has been shown that several hepatotoxins, including CCl_4, alpha-naphtyl-isothiocyanate, and D-galactosamine, induce TNF (Roy *et al.*, 1992), and that neutralization of TNF by soluble TNF receptor protected against CCl_4 toxicity. Also, the acute toxicity of 2,3,7,8-tetrachlorodibenzo-p-dioxin (TCDD) is associated with induction of TNF and prevented by anti-TNF antibodies or dexamethasone (Taylor *et al.*, 1992).

11.1.4 Protection of cytokine-mediated liver injury

Liver injury and mortality induced by combined administration of lead and LPS can be ameliorated by dexamethasone or PGE_1, probably through inhibition of TNF production (Shedlofsky and McClain, 1991). Also phosphodiesterase inhibitors rolipram and zardaverine, by inhibiting TNF production, are protective in this model (Fischer *et al.*, 1993). Protection was also afforded by increasing cAMP levels with the adenylate cyclase activator, forskolin (Fischer *et al.*, 1993). On the other hand, we observed that dexamethasone is not protective against actinomycin D/LPS hepatotoxicity (Gadina *et al.*, 1991). The hepatotoxicity of galactosamine/LPS and induction of plasma TNF in this model are also inhibited by various antioxidants including superoxide dismutase, catalase and allopurinol (Neihörster *et al.*, 1992).

11.2 Lung

The role of cytokines in lung inflammation and injury has been the subject of excellent reviews (e.g. Lukacs and Ward, 1996). Cytokine-mediated pulmonary pathologies include chemically-induced pulmonary fibrosis and lung injury secondary to sepsis or pathologies of other tissues (e.g. hepatic ischemia/reperfusion). Most studies have focused on sepsis-associated lung injury, particularly acute respiratory distress syndrome (ARDS). High doses of LPS, often very close to the lethal dose (Gatti *et al.*, 1993), are required to induce lung damage. Thus, in some models, LPS is administered intratracheally to induce lung injury and inflammatory cytokines (van Helden *et al.*, 1997; Ulich *et al.*, 1991). These models were used to show the efficacy of soluble IL-1 receptor, soluble TNF receptor or antisera against the CXC chemokine CINC in pulmonary inflammation (Ulich *et al.*, 1993, 1994, 1995).

Hepatic ischemia/reperfusion also induces neutrophilic infiltrate, edema, and intra-alveolar hemorrhage and up-regulation of ICAM-1 in the lung. Furthermore, these are prevented by anti-TNF antibodies (Colletti *et al.*, 1990, 1998), pointing at TNF produced by hypoxic tissues as an important mediator of ARDS. Hemorragic shock also induces pulmonary damage and PMN activation via cytokines and xanthine oxidase-generated reactive oxygen species (Shenkar and Abraham, 1999).

11.2.1 Inhibitors of TNF production

There is not a unanimous consensus about the efficacy of inhibition of TNF production against the pulmonary complications induced by LPS. In fact, soluble TNF receptor was reported to prevent pulmonary PMN accumulation following intratracheal LPS (Ulich *et al.*, 1993), and similar results were reported with anti-TNF antibodies in a porcine model of sepsis (Windsor *et al.*, 1993) and with dexamethasone it was shown to inhibit PMN infiltration induced by intratracheal LPS (Yi *et al.*, 1996).

However, we did not find inhibition of PMN infiltrate or amelioration of pulmonary edema induced by systemic LPS with anti-TNF antibodies or inhibitors of TNF production, including dexamethasone or chlorpromazine (Gatti *et al.*, 1993). Others have observed that, while dexamethasone inhibited lung TNF production and PMN infiltration, it did not protect from vascular leak (O'Leary *et al.*, 1996).

11.2.2 Cyclic AMP-elevating agents

Pentoxifylline, rolipram, and other phosphodiesterase inhibitors were also tested in models of LPS-induced pulmonary damage, in view of its inhibitory activity on TNF production (see Chapter 2), and a protective effect with these drugs has been reported (Turner *et al.*, 1993; Miotla *et al.*, 1998). However, it should be mentioned that these drugs, or at least pentoxifylline, can also protect against pulmonary damage directly induced by TNF (Lilly *et al.*, 1989; Riva *et al.*, 1990), confirming the data showing a protective effect on TNF-treated endothelial cells *in vitro* (Zheng *et al.*, 1990). On the other hand, the structurally-related compound lisofylline prevents vascular leak, but not PMN infiltration, in rats intratracheally injected with IL-1 (Hybertson *et al.*, 1997). Inhibition of lung injury and neutrophil adhesion to the endothelium was also observed with drugs that elevate cAMP by activation of adenylate cyclase, such as the prostacyclin analogue, iloprost (Riva *et al.*, 1990). As a further mechanism that adds to the direct protection of endothelial cells, pentoxifylline was also shown to reverse the inhibition of surfactant synthesis by TNF (Balibrea-Cantero *et al.*, 1994).

11.2.3 Antioxidants

Pulmonary edema induced in mice or rats by administration of LPS, TNF, or IL-1 was inhibited by the antioxidant N-acetylcysteine (NAC) (Leff *et al.*, 1993; Faggioni *et al.*, 1994). This adds to a long list of studies with NAC in lung diseases that led to clinical trials with this drug (Suter *et al.*, 1994; Bernard *et al.*, 1997; Domenighetti *et al.*, 1997). Along the same line, the antioxidant and NF-κB inhibitor, PDTC, also protects from LPS-induced lung injury (Nathens *et al.*, 1997).

11.2.4 Anti-inflammatory cytokines

Several cytokines, including IL-4, IL-10, and IL-13, known to inhibit the production of TNF, IL-1, and chemokines, were reported to be protective against immune complex-induced lung injury (Mullighan *et al.*, 1993, 1997). There is also evidence that the protective effect of IL-10 administration in a model of LPS-induced pulmonary inflammation might be mediated by increase of PMN apoptosis (Cox, 1996).

Administration of leukemia-inhibitory factor (LIF) ameliorates pulmonary inflammation induced by intratracheal LPS. A study where IL-6-deficient mice were exposed to aerosolized LPS has shown that these mice are more sensitive to pulmonary inflammation in terms of levels of TNF and MIP-2, and PMN infiltration (Xing *et al.*, 1998), in agreement with previous studies showing that IL-6-deficient mice produce more TNF when injected with LPS (Fattori *et al.*, 1994; Di Santo *et al.*, 1997).

11.2.5 Chemically-induced lung injury

While the role of cytokines in lung damage associated with septic or endotoxic shock is not surprising, it may be not so obvious that TNF is implicated in chemically-induced lung disease, particularly fibrosis (Goldstein and Fine, 1995). Furthermore, over-expression of TNF in the lung of transgenic mice induces fibrosis (Miyazaki *et al.*, 1995). In fact, early data have indicated that anti-TNF antibodies (Piguet *et al.*, 1989, 1990) or soluble TNF receptors (Piguet and Vesin, 1994) are protective against bleomycin- or silica-induced lung fibrosis. A protective effect of IL-1Ra was also observed in these models (Piguet *et al.*, 1993).

Tetrandrine, an alkaloid from the traditional Chinese medicine herb, *Stephania tetrandra*, has anti-fibrotic effects in animal models of silica-induced fibrosis (Huang *et al.*, 1981). Subsequent studies have shown that tetrandrine inhibits both IL-1 production in silica-stimulated alveolar macrophages, as well as IL-1 activity (thymocyte proliferation), suggesting a possible mechanism for its antifibrotic action (Kang *et al.*, 1992).

Interestingly, a study with silica has shown that the inflammatory response (vascular leak and inflammatory infiltrate) was increased, as expected, in IL-10-deficient animals but the fibrotic response, evaluated 30 days after silica, was decreased, suggesting that IL-10 protects from lung inflammation but contributes to fibrogenesis (Huaux *et al.*, 1998).

A role for the CXC chemokines MIP-2 and KC was also hypothesized in a rat model of sulfur dioxide-induced bronchitis on the basis of their mRNA expression and of the protective effect of dexamethasone (Farone *et al.*, 1995), and in vanadium-induced pulmonary inflammation based on chemokine (MIP-2 and KC) mRNA expression *in vivo* (Pierce *et al.*, 1996).

References

Balibrea-Cantero, J. L., Arias-Diaz, J., Garcia, C., Torres-Melero, J., Simon, C., Rodriguez, J. M. *et al.* (1994). Effect of pentoxifylline on the inhibition of surfactant synthesis induced by TNF-alpha in human type II pneumocytes. *Am. J. Respir. Crit. Care Med.*, **149**, 699–706.

Bernard, G. R., Wheeler, A. P., Arons, M. M., Morris, P. E., Paz, H. L., Russell, J. A. *et al.* (1997). A trial of antioxidants N-acetylcysteine and procysteine in ARDS. The Antioxidant in ARDS Study Group. *Chest*, **112**, 164–72.

Bertini, R., Bianchi, M., and Ghezzi, P. (1989). Protective effect of chloropromazine against the lethality of interleukin 1 in adrenalectomized or actinomicin D- sensitized mice. *Biochem. Biophys. Res. Commun.*, **165**, 942–6.

Carswell, E. A., Old, L. J., Kassel, R. L., Green, S., Fiore, N., and Williamson, B. (1975). An endo-toxin-induced serum factor that causes necrosis of tumors. *Proc. Natl. Acad. Sci.USA*, **72**, 3666.

Colletti, L. M., Remick, D. G., Burtch, G. D., Kunkel, S. L., Strieter, R. M., and Campbell, D. A., Jr. (1990). Role of tumor necrosis factor-alpha in the pathophysiologic alterations after hepatic ischemia/reperfusion injury in the rat. *J. Clin. Invest.*, **85**, 1936–43.

Colletti, L. M., Cortis, A., Lukacs, N., Kunkel, S. L., Green, M., and Strieter, R. M. (1998). Tumor necrosis factor up-regulates intercellular adhesion molecule 1, which is important in the neu-trophil-dependent lung and liver injury associated with hepatic ischemia and reperfusion in the rat. *Shock*, **10**, 182–91.

Cox, G. (1996). IL-10 enhances resolution of pulmonary inflammation *in vivo* by promoting apop-tosis of neutrophils. *Am. J. Physiol.*, **271**, L566-L71.

Di Santo, E., Alonzi, T., Poli, V., Fattori, E., Toniatti, C., Sironi, M. *et al.* (1997). Differential effects of IL-6 on systemic and central production of TNF. *Cytokine*, **9**, 300–6.

Domenighetti, G., Suter, P. M., Schaller, M. D., Ritz, R., and Perret, C. (1997). Treatment with N-acetylcysteine during acute respiratory distress syndrome: a randomized, double-blind, placebo-controlled clinical study. *J. Crit. Care Med.*, **12**, 177–82.

Faggioni, R., Gatti, S., Demitri, M. T., Delgado, R., Echtenacher, B., Gnocchi, P. *et al.* (1994). Role of xanthine oxidase and reactive oxygen intermediates in LPS- and TNF-induced pul-monary edema. *J. Lab. Clin. Med.*, **123**, 394–9.

Faggioni, R., Jones-Carson, J., Reed, D. A., Dinarello, C. A., Feingold, K. R., Grunfeld, C. and Fantuzzi, G. (2000). Leptin-deficient (ob/ob) mice are protected from T cell-mediated hepa-totoxicity: Role of tumor necrosis factor alpha and IL-18. *Proc. Natl. Acad. Sci. USA*, **97**, 2367–72.

Farone, A., Huang, S., Paulauskis, J., and Kobzik, L. (1995). Airway neutrophilia and chemokine mRNA expression in sulfur-dioxide-induced bronchitis. *ajrcmb*, **12**, 345–50.

Fattori, E., Cappelletti, M., Costa, P., Sellitto, C., Cantoni, L., Carelli, M. *et al.* (1994). Defective inflammatory response in IL-6 deficient mice. *J. Exp. Med.*, **180**, 1243–50.

Ferluga, J. (1981). Tuberculin hypersensitivity hepatitis in mice infected with Mycobacterium bovis (BCG). *Am. J. Pathol.*, **105**, 82–90.

Ferluga, J., Doenhoff, M. J., and Allison, A. C. (1979). Increased hepatotoxicity of bacterial lipopolysaccharide in mice infected with Schistosoma mansoni. *Parasite Immunol.*, **1**, 289–94.

Fischer, W., Schudt, C., and Wendel, A. (1993). Protection by phosphodiesterase inhibitors against endotoxin-induced liver injury in galactosamine-sensitized mice. *Biochem. Pharmacol.*, **45**, 2399–403.

Gadina, M., Bertini, R., Mengozzi, M., Zandalasini, M., Mantovani, A., and Ghezzi, P. (1991). Protective effect of chlorpromazine on endotoxin toxicity and TNF production in glucocorticoid-sensitive and glucocorticoid-resistant models of endotoxic shock. *J. Exp. Med.*, **173**, 1305–10.

Galanos, C., Freudenberg, M. A., and Reutter, W. (1979). Galactosamine-induced sensitization to the lethal effects of endotoxin. *Proc. Natl. Acad. Sci.USA*, **76**, 5939–43.

Gatti, S., Faggioni, R., Echtenacher, B., and Ghezzi, P. (1993). Role of tumor necrosis factor and reactive oxygen intermediates in lipopolysaccharide-induced pulmonary oedema and lethality. *Clin. Exp. Immunol.*, **91**, 456–61.

Ghezzi, P., Bianchi, M., Gianera, L., Landolfo, S., and Salmona, M. (1985). Role of reactive oxygen intermediates in the interferon-mediated depression of hepatic drug metabolism and pro-tective effect of N-acetylcysteine in mice. *Cancer Res.*, **45**, 3444–7.

Ghezzi, P., Saccardo, B., and Bianchi, M. (1986). Role of reactive oxygen intermediates in the hepatotoxicity of endotoxin. *Immunopharmacology*, **12**, 241–4.

Goldstein, R. H. and Fine, A. (1995). Potential therapeutic initiatives for fibrogenic lung diseases. *Chest*, **108**, 848–55.

Honchel, R., Marsano, L., Cohen, D., Shedlofsky, S. I., and McClain, C. J. (1991). Lead enhances lipopolysaccharide and tumor necrosis factor liver injury. *J. Lab. Clin. Med.*, **117**, 202–8.

Huang, T., Liu, Y., Zhao, S., and Li, Y. (1981). Changes of acid-soluble collagen from lungs of silicotic rats and tetrandrine-treated silicotic rats. *Acta Biochem. Biophys.*, **13**, 61–8.

Huaux, F., Louahed, J., Hudspith, B., Meredith, C., Delos, M., Renauld, J. C. *et al.* (1998). Role of interleukin-10 in the lung response to silica in mice. *Am. J. Respir. Cell Mol. Biol.*, **18**, 51–9.

Hybertson, B. M., Bursten, S. L., Leff, J. A., Lee, Y. M., Jepson, E. K., Dewitt, C. R. *et al.* (1997). Lisofylline prevents leaks, but not neutrophil accumulation, in lungs of rats given IL-1 intratracheally. *J. Appl. Physiol.*, **82**, 226–32.

Kang, J. H., Lewis, D. M., Castranova, V., Rojanasakul, Y., Banks, D. E., Ma, J. Y. C. *et al.* (1992). Inhibitory action of tentrandrine on macrophage production of interleukin-1 (IL-1)-like activity in thymocyte proliferation. *Experimental Lung Research*, **18**, 715–29.

Khatsenko, O. and Kikkawa, Y. (1997). Nitric oxide differentially affects constitutive cytochrome P450 isoforms in rat liver. *J. Pharmacol. Exp. Ther.*, **280**, 1463–70.

Kusters, S., Tiegs, G., Alexopoulou, L., Pasparakis, M., Douni, E., Kunstle, G. *et al.* (1997). *In vivo* evidence for a functional role of both tumor necrosis factor (TNF) receptors and transmembrane TNF in experimental hepatitis. *Eur. J. Immunol.*, **27**, 2870–5.

Leff, J. A., Wilke, C. P., Hybertson, B. M., Shanley, P. F., Beehler, C. J., and Repine, J. E. (1993). Postinsult treatment with N-acetyl-L-cysteine decreases IL-1-induced neutrophil influx and lung leak in rats. *Am. J. Physiol.*, **265**, L501-L6.

Lehmann, V., Freudenberg, M. A., and Galanos, C. (1987). Lethal toxicity of lipopolysaccharide and tumor necrosis factor in normal and D-galactosamine-treated mice. *J. Exp. Med.*, **165**, 657–61.

Lilly, C. M., Sandhu, J. S., Ishizaka, A., Harada, H., Yonemaru, M., Larrick, J. W. *et al.* (1989). Pentoxifylline prevents tumor necrosis factor-induced lung injury. *Am. Rev. Respir. Dis.*, **139**, 1361–8.

Lukacs, N. W. and Ward, P. A. (1996). Inflammatory mediators, cytokines, and adhesion molecules in pulmonary inflammation and injury. *Adv. Immunol.*, **62**, 257–304.

Miotla, J. M., Teixeira, M. M., and Hellewell, P. G. (1998). Suppression of acute lung injury in mice by an inhibitor of phosphodiesterase type 4. *Am. J. Respir. Cell Mol. Biol.*, **18**, 411–20.

Miyazaki, Y., Araki, K., Vesin, C., Garcia, I., Kapanci, Y., Whitsett, J. A. *et al.* (1995). Expression of a tumor necrosis factor-alpha transgene in murine lung causes lymphocytic and fibrosing alveolitis. A mouse model of progressive pulmonary fibrosis. *J..Clin..Invest.*, **96**, 250–9.

Monshouwer, M., McLellan, R. A., Delaporte, E., Witkamp, R. F., van Miert, A. S., and Renton, K. W. (1996). Differential effect of pentoxifylline on lipopolysaccharide-induced downregulation of cytochrome P450. *Biochem. Pharmacol.*, **52**, 1195–200.

Mullighan, M. S., Jones, M. L., Vaporicyan, A. A., Howard, M. C., and Ward, P. A. (1993). Protective effect of IL-4 and IL-10 against immune complex-induced lung injury. *J..Immunol.*, **151**, 5666–74.

Mulligan, M. S., Warner, R. L., Foreback, J. L., Shanley, T. P., and Ward, P. A. (1997). Protective effects of IL-4, IL-10, IL-12, and IL-13 in IgG immune complex-induced lung injury: role of endogenous IL-12. *J. Immunol.*, **159**, 3483–9.

Nathens, A. B., Bitar, R., Davreux, C., Bujard, M., Marshall, J. C., Dackiw, A. P. *et al.* (1997). Pyrrolidine dithiocarbamate attenuates endotoxin-induced acute lung injury. *Am. J. Respir. Cell Mol. Biol.*, **17**, 608–16.

Neihörster, M., Inoue, M., and Wendel, A. (1992). A link between extracellular reactive oxygen and endotoxin-induced release of tumour necrosis factor α *in vivo*. *Biochem. Pharmacol.*, **43**, 1151–4.

Nolan, J. P. (1975). The role of endotoxin in liver injury. *Gastroenterology*, **69**, 1346–56.

Nolan, J. P. (1981). Endotoxin, reticuloendothelial function and liver injury. *Hepatology*, **1**, 458–65.

Nolan, J. P. and Ali, M. V. (1973). Endotoxin and the liver. II. Effect of tolerance on carbon tetra-chloride-induced injury. *J. Med.*, **4**, 28–38.

Nolan, J. P. and Camara, D. S., 1982, Endotoxin, sinusoidal cells, and liver injury. In *Progress in liver diseases*, vol. VII, (ed. H. Popper and F. Schaffner), pp. 361–376. Grune & Stratton, Inc., New York.

Nolan, J. P. and Leibowitz, A. I. (1978). Endotoxin and the liver. III. Modification of acute carbon tetrachloride injury by polymixin B-an antiendotoxin. *Gastroenterology*, **75**, 445–9.

O'Leary, E. C., Marder, P., and Zuckerman, S. H. (1996). Glucocorticoid effects in an endotoxin-induced rat pulmonary inflammation model: differential effects on neutrophil influx, integrin expression, and inflammatory mediators. *Am. J. Respir. Cell Mol. Biol.*, **15**, 97–106.

Okamoto, T., Furuya, M., Yamakawa, T., Yamamura, K., and Hino, O. (1996). TNF-α gene expression in the liver of the IFN-g transgenic mouse with chronic active hepatitis. *Biochem. Biophys. Res. Commun.*, **226**, 762–8.

Pierce, L. M., Alessandrini, F., Godleski, J. J., and Paulauskis, J. D. (1996). Vanadium-induced chemokine mRNA expression and pulmonary inflammation. *Toxicology and Applied Pharmacology*, **138**, 1–11.

Piguet, P. F. and Vesin, C. (1994). Treatment by human recombinant soluble TNF receptor of pulmonary fibrosis induced by bleomycin or silica in mice. *European Respiratory Journal*, **7**, 515–8.

Piguet, P. F., Collart, M. A., Grau, G. E., Kapanci, Y., and Vassalli, P. F. (1989). Tumor necrosis factor/cachectin plays a key role in bleomycin-induced pneumopathy and fibrosis. *J. Exp. Med.*, **170**, 655–63.

Piguet, P. F., Collart, M. A., Grau, G. E., Sappino, A. P., and Vassalli, P. (1990). Requirement of tumor necrosis factor for development of silica-induced pulmonary fibrosis. *Nature*, **344**, 245–7.

Piguet, P., Vesin, C., Grau, G. E., and Thompson, R. C. (1993). Interleukin 1 receptor antagonist (IL-1Ra) prevents or cures pulmonary fibrosis elicited in mice by bleomycin or silica. *Cytokine*, **5**, 57–61.

Renton, K. W. and Mannering, G. J. (1976). Depression of hepatic cytochrome P-450-dependent monooxygenase systems with administered interferon inducing agents. *Biochem. Biophys. Res. Commun*, **73**, 343–8.

Riva, C. M., Morganroth, M. L., Ljungman, A. G., Schoeneich, S. O., Marks, R. M., Todd, R. F. *et al.* (1990). Iloprost inhibits neutrophil-induced lung injury and neutrophil adherence to endothelial monolayers. *Am. J. Respir. Cell. Mol. Biol.*, **3**, 301–9.

Roy, A., Soni, G. R., Kolhapure, R. M., Banerjee, K., and Patki, P. S. (1992). Induction of tumour necrosis factor alpha in experimental animals treated with hepatotoxicants. *Indian J. Exp. Biol.*, **30**, 696–700.

Selye, H., Tuchweber, B., and Bertok, L. (1966). Effect of lead acetate on the susceptibility of rats to bacterial endotoxins. *J. Bacteriol.*, **91**, 884–90.

Sewer, M. B. and Morgan, E. T. (1997). Nitric oxide-independent suppression of P450 2C11 expression by interleukin-1beta and endotoxin in primary rat hepatocytes. *Biochem. Pharmacol.*, **54**, 729–37.

Shedlofsky, S. I. and McClain, C. (1991) Hepatic dysfunction due to cytokines. In *Cytokines and inflammation.* (ed. E. S. Kimball), pp. 235–273. CRC Press, Boca Raton.

Shenkar, R. and Abraham, E. (1999). Mechanisms of lung neutrophil activation after hemorrhage or endotoxemia: roles of reactive oxygen intermediates, NFκB, and cyclic AMP response element binding protein. *J. Immunol., 163*, 954–62.

Solorzano, C. C., Ksontini, R., Pruitt, J. H., Auffenberg, T., Tannahill, C., Galardy, R. E. *et al.* (1997). A matrix metalloproteinase inhibitor prevents processing of tumor necrosis factor alpha (TNF alpha) and abrogates endotoxin-induced lethality. *Shock.*, **7**, 427–31.

Suter, P. M., Domenighetti, G., Schaller, M. D., Laverriere, M. C., Ritz, R., and Perret, C. (1994). N-acetylcysteine enhances recovery from acute lung injury in man. A randomized, double-blind, placebo-controlled clinical study. *Chest*, **105**, 190–4.

Taylor, M. J., Lucier, G. W., Mahler, J. F., Thompson, M., Lockhart, A. C., and Clark, G. C. (1992). Inhibition of acute TCDD toxicity by treatment with anti-tumor necrosis factor antibody or dexamethasone. *Toxicology and Applied Pharmacology*, **117**, 126–32.

Tiegs, G., Wolter, M., and Wendel, A. (1989). Tumor necrosis factor is a terminal mediator in galactosamine/endotoxin-induced hepatitis in mice. *Biochem. Pharmacol.*, **38**, 627–31.

Toyonaga, T., Hino, O., Sugai, S., Wakasugi, S., Abe, K., Shichiri, M. *et al.* (1994). Chronic active hepatitis in transgenic mice expressing interferon-gamma in the liver. *Proc. Natl. Acad. Sci.USA.*, **91**, 614–8.

Turner, C. R., Esser, K. M., and Wheeldon, E. B. (1993). Therapeutic intervention in a rat model of ARDS: IV. Phosphodiesterase IV inhibition. *Circ. Shock*, **39**, 237–45.

Ulich, T. R., Watson, L. R., Yin, S. M., Guo, K. Z., Wang, P., Thang, H. *et al.* (1991). The intratracheal administration of endotoxin and cytokines. I. Characterization of LPS-induced IL-1 and TNF mRNA expression and the LPS-, IL-1-, and TNF-induced inflammatory infiltrate. *Am. J. Pathol.*, **138**, 1485–96.

Ulich, T. R., Yin, S., Remick, D. G., Russell, D., Eisenberg, S. P., and Kohno, T. (1993). Intratracheal administration of endotoxin and cytokines. IV. The soluble tumor necrosis factor receptor type I inhibits acute inflammation. *Am. J. Pathol.*, **142**, 1335–8.

Ulich, T. R., Yi, E. S., Yin, S., Smith, C., and Remick, D. (1994). Intratracheal administration of endotoxin and cytokines. VII. The soluble interleukin-1 receptor and the soluble tumor necrosis factor receptor II (p80) inhibit acute inflammation. *Clin. Immunol. Immunopathol.*, **72**, 137–40.

Ulich, T. R., Howard, S. C., Remick, D. G., Wittwer, A., Yi, E. S., Yin, S. *et al.* (1995). Intratracheal administration of endotoxin and cytokines. VI. Antiserum to CINC inhibits acute inflammation. *Am. J. Physiol.*, **268**, L245–50.

van Helden, H. P., Kuijpers, W. C., Steenvoorden, D., Go, C., Bruijnzeel, P. L., van Eijk, M. *et al.* (1997). Intratracheal aerosolization of endotoxin (LPS) in the rat: a comprehensive animal model to study adult (acute) respiratory distress syndrome. *Exp. Lung Res.*, **23**, 297–316.

Wallach, D., Holtmann, H., Engelmann, H., and Nophar, Y. (1988). Sensitization and desensitization to the lethal effects of tumor necrosis factor and IL-1. *J. Immunol.*, **140**, 2994–9.

Windsor, A. C., Walsh, C. J., Mullen, P. G., Cook, D. J., Fisher, B. J., Blocher, C. R. *et al.* (1993). Tumor necrosis factor-alpha blockade prevents neutrophil CD18 receptor upregulation and attenuates acute lung injury in porcine sepsis without inhibition of neutrophil oxygen radical generation. *J. Clin. Invest.*, **91**, 1459–68.

Xing, Z., Gauldie, J., Cox, G., Baumann, H., Jordana, M., Lei, X. F. *et al.* (1998). IL-6 is an antiinflammatory cytokine required for controlling local or systemic acute inflammatory responses. *J. Clin. Invest.*, **101**, 311–20.

Yi, E. S., Remick, D. G., Lim, Y., Tang, W., Nadzienko, C. E., Bedoya, A. *et al.* (1996). The intra-tracheal administration of endotoxin: X. Dexamethasone downregulates neutrophil emigration and cytokine expression *in vivo*. *Inflammation*, **20**, 165–75.

Zheng, H., Crowley, J. J., Chan, J. C., Hoffmann, H., Hatherill, J. R., Ishizaka, A. *et al.* (1990). Attenuation of tumor necrosis factor-induced endothelial cell cytotoxicity and neutrophil chemi-luminescence. *Am. Rev. Respir. Dis.*, **142**, 1073–8.

12 *Skin*

Together with the mucosal surfaces, the human integument is a major interface between host and environment, and an active micro-environment for the generation and expression of immunological reactions (Kupper, 1989; Bos and Kapsenberg, 1993). Moreover, inflammatory and allergic responses often involve the skin as a major site. The skin consists of the epidermis, dermis, and subcutaneous fat. Its resident and blood-derived cellular constituents are differentially distributed among these compartments. In the epidermal compartment, the keratinocyte is the predominant cell type, but there are also melanocytes, Langerhans cells, macrophages, and T cells. In the dermal compartment there are fibroblasts, endothelial cells, mast cells, dermal dendritic cells, macrophages, T cells, some B cells, NK cells, polymorphonuclear leukocytes, neuronal, and glandular cells. The subcutis contains fat cells, some endothelial cells, and glandular cells. Here we will summarize selected immunological properties of the skin constituents, with the emphasis on cytokine production and action, and discuss how cytokines are involved in psoriasis, taken as a prototypical inflammatory disorder specifically affecting the skin.

12.1 Skin cells

Keratinocytes are a major constituent of the epidermal layer. These cells derive from stem cells in the basal area. The epidermal stem cells undergo transient proliferation and amplification before terminal differentiation. Basal keratinocytes express $\beta1$ and $\beta4$ integrins, and K5 and K14 cytokeratins; as they move upward they lose $\beta1$ and $\beta4$ integrins, and express different keratins (K1 and K10) and other terminal differentiation proteins. Though they express $\beta1$ and $\beta4$ integrins, they do not express differentiation antigens, such as cytokeratins (K1 and K10). The stem cells undergo proliferation and amplification before the terminal differentiation of cells, which lack $\beta1$ integrins and express terminal differentiation markers such as cytokeratins.

Keratinocytes are much more than just a physical barrier between the organism and the external world; they play an active role in the generation and expression of immunity by expressing MHC molecules, co-stimulatory molecules, and cytokines. Upon exposure to IFNγ, a product of activated T cells and NK cells, keratinocytes express MHC class II antigens, though they have been reported to express low levels of the non-polymorphic invariant chain. Keratinocytes do not express B7–1 (CD80) and B7–2 (CD86) co-stimulatory molecules, which act as counter-receptors for CD28 expressed on T cells. The CD28 co-stimulation pathway synergizes with T cell receptor-CD3 stimulation to

Table 12.1 Principal cytokines and chemokines produced by human keratinocytes

Constitutive	Induced	Stimuli
IL-1α	+	IL-1α, TNFα, LPS, UVB, IFN-γ, haptens
IL-1β	+	IL-1α, TNFα, LPS, UVB, haptens
IL-1ra	+	IL-1α, TNFα, LPS, UVB, IFN-γ
TNFα	+	IL-1α, LPS, UVB, haptens
IL-6	+	IL-1α, LPS, haptens
MIF	+	IL-1α, TNFα, LPS, corticosteroids
GM-CSF	+	IL-1α, UVB, LPS
	IL-7	IL-1α
–	α-MSH	UVB, IL-1α
–	IL-8	TNFα, IL-1α, IFN-γ, IL-17, haptens, UVB
–	RANTES	IFN-γ, TNFα
–	MCP-1	IFN-γ, TNFα
–	IP-10	IFN-γ
–	MIP-2	IFN-γ

produce maximum cell proliferation and cytokine secretion (Kupper, 1989; Bos and Kapsenberg, 1993).

Keratinocytes express receptors for, respond to, and produce cytokines (Table 12.1). These cells do not produce IL-12, a key cytokine for the induction of Th1 responses. Besides growth factors (e.g. TGFα), cytokines such as IL-1, IL-6, and IL-8 also elicit keratinocytes proliferation. Induction of keratinocyte proliferation by cytokines is probably involved in the formation of new skin tissue and repair of damaged integument.

An intriguing aspect of keratinocytes is that they store large amounts of preformed IL-1 under normal unstimulated conditions (Kupper, 1989; Kupper and Groves, 1995). This IL-1 is mainly of the α species and remains largely cell-associated (Hauser *et al.*, 1986; Kupper, 1989). The human epidermis contains 20–60 μg of IL-1, potentially a devastating amount.

Keratinocytes also express other components of the IL-1 system. These include the IL-1 receptor antagonist, both the soluble form and large amounts of the two intracellular forms (Haskill *et al.*, 1991; Hammerberg *et al.*, 1992; Muzio *et al.*, 1995, 1999). Keratinocytes express the type I receptor and the type II decoy receptor (Groves *et al.*, 1994). Expression of IL-1 receptors in keratinocytes is regulated by cytokines. IFNγ upregulates the expression and release of the type II decoy receptor (Groves *et al.*, 1995a). The type II receptor *in vivo* is found in the basal layer of the epithelium (Groves *et al.*, 1994). Storage of preformed cell-associated IL-1 may serve to trigger inflammation and tissue repair in response to damage to the epidermal surface.

The connective tissue matrix is produced and maintained by fibroblasts. Skin fibroblasts and endothelial cells produce cytokines, which are involved—not only in inflammatory reactions—but are also mitogenic (IL-1, IL-6, and IL-8) for epidermal cells.

Although several skin cells can present antigen, dendritic cells are the most effective antigen presenters. Langerhans cells are professional antigen-presenting cells located in the epidermal layer, characterized by a dendritic morphology and the presence of characteristic Birbeck granules (Ibrahim *et al.*, 1995; Steinman *et al.*, 1995; Banchereau and Steinman, 1998). An important antigen-presenting cell in the dermis is the dendrocyte, which in this location is characterized by expression of the clotting factor XIIIa. Langerhans cells express class II MHC antigen, CD1, CD40, B71, ICAM-1, and LFA3.

Dendritic cells are heterogeneous and their pathways of differentiation have not been completely defined. Monocytes can undergo differentiation to cells with the properties of dendritic cells upon exposure to GM-CSF and IL-4 or IL-13 (Sallusto and Lanzavecchia, 1994; Piemonti *et al.*, 1995). These cells do not completely resemble the Langerhans' cells from normal skin, but they may have a normal counterpart in certain pathological states. For example, monocyte-derived dendritic cells are similar to a subset of dendritic cells seen in skin with atopic dermatitis, a condition where resident skin cells or immigrant inflammatory cells tend to produce higher levels of GM-CSF and IL-4 (Pastore *et al.*, 1997).

Cells with a Langerhans cell phenotype can be obtained by *in vitro* culture of bone marrow cells or circulating CD34+ cells in the presence of cytokine cocktails, which include TGFβ. Langerhans' cells are sentinel dendrocytes whose function is to perceive local damage. After antigen capture, or exposure to inflammatory signals such as bacterial products, IL-1 or TNF, dendritic cells travel through the lymph as vailed cells to regional lymph nodes where they present antigen to naive T cells. As dendritic cells mature their capacity to capture antigen via receptors, such as the Fcγ receptor or the mannose receptor, or via fluid-phase macropinocytosis, decreases, and there is an increase in the expression of class II MHC antigens and of antigen-presenting capacity. Maturation of dendritic cells is triggered by cytokines, such as IL-1 and TNF. It is, therefore, likely that damage to keratinocytes causes release of IL-1α, which in turns promotes the full maturation and migration of dendritic cells.

A key property of Langerhans' cells, as of dendritic cells in general, is that they are recruited from the blood compartment in a first phase of their natural history and subsequently migrate to regional lymph nodes or to the spleen (Fig. 12.1). Dendritic cells express receptors for certain chemokines, for C5a and for formyl peptides (Sozzani *et al.*, 1995). The expression of certain receptors (CCR6) and, accordingly, their responsiveness to the appropriate ligands (MIP-3α/exodus/LARC), distinguishes CD34-derived dendritic cells, which are responsive, from monocyte-derived dendritic cells, which are unresponsive (Hallmann *et al.*, 1995; Power *et al.*, 1997; Sozzani *et al.*, 1997). Expression of receptors for chemokines that are produced constitutively, such as CCR4 (the receptor for the 'macrophage-derived chemokine', MDC) and CXCR4 (the receptor for a CXC chemokine known as SDF1, stem cell differentiation factor 1), is likely to be responsible for the basal migratory activity of circulating precursors of dendritic cells to appropriate tissue sites. Responsiveness to inducible factors, such as MCP-3 and MIP-1α, mediated by other chemokine receptors, such as CCR1 and CCR5, is most likely responsible for the increased recruitment of precursors associated with local inflammation. Changes in chemokine receptor expression are probably important for the subsequent traffic to lymphoid organs (for review see: Sozzani *et al.*, 1999).

Immune and inflammatory stimuli or microbial products induce maturation of dendritic cells with acquisition of full antigen presenting capacity (Steinman, 1991; Austyn, 1996; Cella *et al.*, 1997; Hart, 1997; Banchereau and Steinman, 1998). *In vivo*, the same signals induce dendritic cell traffic to lymph nodes or spleen, where they present antigen. IL-1, TNF, LPS, and CD40 ligation regulate expression of chemokine receptors and responsiveness to their respective ligands differently (Sozzani *et al.*, 1998). The same signals

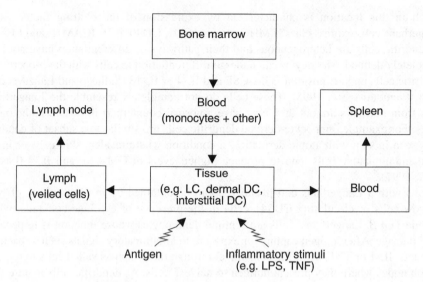

Fig. 12.1 Migratory capacity of dendritic cells.

abrogated the chemotactic response to CCR1 and CCR5 ligands, and reduced the mRNA expression of the two receptors. Inhibition of chemotaxis was almost maximal at times (<1 h), at which chemokine production (i.e. MIP-1α, RANTES, and MCP-1) was undetectable by sensitive ELISA, and also included the response to fMLP, an unrelated chemotactic factor of bacterial origin. Activation of dendritic cells with IL-1, TNF, LPS, and CD40L, strongly increased the chemotactic response to ELC and the expression of CCR7, the ELC receptor. This CC chemokine, previously considered lymphoid-specific, is at present the strongest agonist for chemotaxis and trans-endothelial migration for dendritic cells. Interestingly, the response to the inducible CCR1 and CCR5 agonists was inhibited before the ELC response increased.

These results are consistent with a 'weigh anchor/hoist the sail' model, based on changes in chemokine receptors, for the traffic of dendritic cells to lymphoid organs after antigen capture (see Fig. 12.2). Inhibition of the responsiveness to inducible chemokines, such as MIP1α, MIP-1β, or RANTES, would allow antigen-loaded DC to leave sites of infection and inflammation ('weigh anchor'). The slower induction of CCR7 expression would prepare the trafficking dendritic cells to respond to ELC ('hoist the sail'), which is constitutively expressed in lymphoid organs and would be instrumental to arrest and transmigration at these sites (Sozzani *et al.*, 1999).

The skin selectively recruits a unique set of skin homing T cells based on the interaction between cutaneous lymphocyte-associated antigen (CLA, a sialylated 223 carbohydrate) and E selectin on skin endothelial cells. Epiligrin is a basement membrane component of the epidermis and T cells, which expresses VLA3 and VLA4, preferentially home to the skin because of recognition of this component and of dermal fibronectin.

T cell-derived IFNγ is the key cytokine regulating the expression of inflammatory and immune responses in the skin, and keratinocytes are a primary target of IFNγ. Upon exposure to IFNγ, keratinocytes produce cytokines and chemokines (IL-8, MCP-1,

CHEMOKINES AND DC TRAFFICKING:
A 'WEIGH ANCHOR/HOIST THE SAIL' MODEL

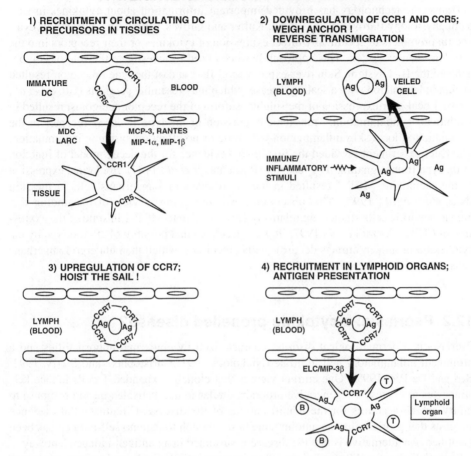

1) RECRUITMENT OF CIRCULATING DC PRECURSORS IN TISSUES

IMMATURE DC
BLOOD
CCR1
CCR5
MDC LARC
MCP-3, RANTES MIP-1α, MIP-1β
CCR1
TISSUE
CCR5

2) DOWNREGULATION OF CCR1 AND CCR5; WEIGH ANCHOR! REVERSE TRANSMIGRATION

LYMPH (BLOOD)
Ag Ag
VEILED CELL
IMMUNE/ INFLAMMATORY STIMULI
Ag Ag
Ag
Ag

3) UPREGULATION OF CCR7; HOIST THE SAIL!

LYMPH (BLOOD)
CCR7 CCR7
Ag Ag
CCR7 CCR7

4) RECRUITMENT IN LYMPHOID ORGANS; ANTIGEN PRESENTATION

LYMPH (BLOOD)
CCR7 CCR7
Ag Ag
CCR7 CCR7
ELC/MIP-3β
CCR7
T
B
Ag
Ag
Ag
CCR7
T
B
Lymphoid organ

Fig. 12.2 Role of chemokines in dendritic cell migration: a 'weigh anchor/hoist the sail' model. See text.

RANTES, IP-10, Mig), which attract and regulate the functions of T cells and other inflammatory cells. Also, IFNγ induces the expression of adhesion molecules (e.g. ICAM-1), which are important for retaining immigrating T cells in the epidermis. IFNγ-exposed keratinocytes can also express functional MHC class II antigens and stimulate effector T cells (Albanesi *et al.*, 1998). However, because keratinocytes do not express B7–1 (CD80) and B7–2 (CD86) co-stimulatory molecules, are inefficient at activating naive or resting T lymphocytes, which tend rather to undergo anergy. This mechanism may be important for the maintenance of peripheral tolerance to self antigens during skin immune responses associated with tissue necrosis.

Finally, IFNγ up-regulates the expression of *fas* by keratinocytes, which can undergo apoptosis upon interaction with the *fas* ligand expressed on activated T cells. However, keratinocytes can protect themselves from immune damage (and from pathogens) by expressing a variety of cytolytic proteins, such as granzyme B, perforin and *fas* ligand (Berthou *et al.*, 1997).

Transgenic technology has provided important information about cytokines in skin pathophysiology (Groves *et al.*, 1995a; Kuffer and Groves, 1995). The capacity of cytokeratin promoters to specifically direct expression of cytokines or their receptors into the skin has been exploited. This approach has been used to investigate the role of components of the IL-1 system. Skin over-expression of IL-1 and of the type I receptor, resulted in skin inflammation with a scaling disease, which may resemble psoriasis (Groves *et al.*, 1996). Local over-expression of the soluble isoform of the receptor antagonist resulted in inhibition of inflammation. Transgenic expression of the type II decoy receptor in the skin inhibited local skin inflammation with little or no effect on systemic inflammation. The latter experiment provided the first *in vivo* evidence for the decoy model of function of the type II nonsignaling IL-1 receptor (Rauschmayr *et al.*, 1997). Epidermal expression of the chemokine MCP-1 resulted in increased levels of Langerhans cells in the skin (Nakamura *et al.*, 1995). This observation was intriguing in view of the finding that human dendritic cells studied are relatively unresponsive to MCP-1 in spite of the expression of CCR2 (Sozzani *et al.*, 1997). It was speculated that possibly MCP-1, driven by the cytokeratin promoter, attracts dendritic cells precursors, which then undergo Langerhans cells maturation in the skin.

12.2 Psoriasis: a cytokine-propelled disease?

Psoriasis is a dermatological disorder characterized by epidermal abnormalities and a prominent inflammatory cell infiltrate (Nickoloff, 1991; Christophers and Sterry, 1993; Bos and De Rie, 1999). One current view is that clonally expanded T cells induce keratinocytes to express a regenerative program similar to that activated during response to injury, which accounts for the manifestations of the disease. Circumstantial evidence suggests that psoriasis has an autoimmune basis, though to date no self-antigen has been identified. An alternative is that the disease is sustained in an antigen-independent way.

Several lines of evidence indicate that immunopathological mechanisms trigger or mediate psoriatic lesions, including HLA associations (e.g. B13, B17, Cw6, and DR7); the appearance of skin-infiltrating mononuclear cells including T cells is one of the very first events, and psoriasis appears to be modulated by microbial agents, cytokine (IL-2 and IFNγ) therapy, or T cell selective immunosuppressive agents. Furthermore, T cells in psoriatic lesions are oligoclonal, suggesting they recognize an undefined specific antigen(s) (Shön, 1999; Micholoff, 1999).

Psoriasis involves dysregulation of cytokine networks at the site of the lesion and these alterations are likely to play a fundamental role. They may also account for changes in arachidonic acid-derived mediators, long known in psoriatic epidermis, and in alterations of mast cells and neuropeptides, given the actions of pleiotropic mediators such as IL-1. Finally, psoriatic lesions have served historically as a source of biological material for the identification of inflammatory mediators. For instance, one of the pathways that led to the identification of a certain number of CXC chemokines started with the recognition of neutrophil infiltration and neutrophil chemotactic activity in psoriatic epidermis (Schroder, 1992).

Alterations in psoriatic lesions encompass virtually all the elements present in the human tegument. Hyperproliferation of keratinocytes is a hallmark of psoriatic lesions. The stem cell population of B1+ B4+ keratin cells is responsible for hyperproliferation with accelerated terminal differentiation. Aberrant expression of *bcl2* has also been described in psoriatic epidermis, consistent with alterations in the apoptotic pathway for disposal of keratinocytes. All in all, the phenotype of keratinocytes is that of regenerative epidermal maturation similar, for instance, to wound healing.

Keratinocytes have high levels of MHC class I molecules, ICAM-1 and IP-10, a CXC chemokine without the ELR motif. All these alterations are indicative of exposure to IFNγ, presumably of T-cell origin. Psoriatic keratinocytes show alterations in the production of a variety of cytokines, including IL-6, IL-8, gro-α, MCP-1, TGFα, and vascular endothelium growth factor (VEGF). Psoriatic keratinocytes *in vitro* show altered response to chemokines with lower levels of inhibition in response to IFNγ, possibly dependent on lower levels of the relevant receptor.

Profound alterations in the IL-1 system have been detected in psoriatic skin (Gruaz *et al.*, 1989; Kupper, 1989; Cooper *et al.*, 1990; Hammerberg *et al.*, 1992; Groves *et al.*, 1994; Kupper and Groves, 1995). While the results are to some extent contradictory, depending on whether scale extracts, blister fluid, immunocytochemistry, or culture was used to investigate IL-1 related molecules, in general IL-1α was either decreased or unaffected, whereas levels of IL-1β mRNA and protein were high. The intracellular and the soluble isoforms of the IL-1 receptor antagonist are both increased in psoriatic lesions. Similarly, mRNA expression and protein levels of the IL-1 RII decoy receptor are raised in the lesions, whereas the signaling type I receptor is relatively unaffected.

These observations suggest the activation of inefficient loops of negative regulation of the IL-1 system in the local micro-environment. Consistent with the role of IL-1 in psoriatic skin disease is the observation that transgenic expression of IL-1β and the type I receptor in the skin results in pathological abnormalities resembling those found in psoriasis (see above).

Psoriatic fibroblasts are also hyperactive in terms of production of extracellular matrix proteins and proliferative response to serum factors. Transplantation experiments suggested that the interaction between psoriatic keratinocytes and the underlying dermis is essential to maintain epidermal hyperplasia *in vivo*.

Consistently, with the production of pro-inflammatory mediators, such as IFNγ and IL-1, papillary dermal microvascular endothelium was activated in psoriatic lesions and showed increased tortuosity, dilatation, and permeability, as well as angiogenesis. Expression of ICAM-1, E-selectin and VCAM-1 is up-regulated in the dermal endothelium. Active psoriasis is marked by the presence of intra-epidermal neutrophils, consistent with the production of peptide (e.g. IL-8 and related molecules) and lipid chemo-attractants. Mononuclear phagocytes and dendritic cells are also increased in psoriatic lesions. The dermis contains large numbers of Langerhans' cells, their morphology suggesting cell migration, and an increased number of factor XIIIa+ dendrocytes in contact with T cells. Macrophages in psoriatic skin are often located at the border between the epidermis and dermis, and peripheral blood monocytes have an increased capacity to produce proinflammatory cytokines such as TNFα and IL-6. Elevated serum levels of IL-6 have been detected in patients with severe psoriasis.

T cells are present in large amounts in psoriatic skin lesions and have an activated memory cell phenotye, with expression of CD45Ro, CLA, LFA1, and ICAM-1 at high

Table 12.2 Effect of anti-psoriasis agents on cytokines

Treatment	Effect	Selected references
Glucocorticoids	Inhibition of IL-1 and other cytokines Upregulation of decoy IL-1RII	(Colotta *et al.*, 1993) (Bos and Kapsenberg, 1993)
Vitamin D3 analogs	Inhibition of IL-8 Induction of IL-10	(Larsen *et al.*, 1991) (Michel *et al.*, 1997)
Retinoids	Induction of IL-1ra	(Schwarz *et al.*, 1987)
UV irradiation	Induction of IL-1ra	(Hammerberg *et al.*, 1992)

levels. CD4+ T cells predominate in florid lesions, whereas CD8+ T cells are more prominent in spontaneously resolving lesions. Vβ3 and Vβ13.1 are mainly used by intra-epidermal CD8+ T cells, whereas Vβ2 and Vβ6 dominate dermal T cell infiltrates. Sequence analysis of complementarity determining region 3 (CDR3) motifs found marked TCR oligoclonality in psoriatic lesions. T cell-derived cytokines in psoriatic plaques include IL-2, IFNγ and, intriguingly, IL-5, whereas IL-4 and IL-10 were not detected. Direct activation of keratinocyte stem cells by T cells has been suggested to play a central role in psoriasis (Bos and De Rie, 1999).

12.3 Anti-cytokine therapy for psoriasis

Therapeutic approaches for psoriasis include retinoids, glucocorticoid hormones, and ultraviolet radiation. These therapeutic approaches influence components of the IL-1 system, which may play a central role (Bos and Kapsenberg, 1993). For instance, glucocorticoids inhibit expression of IL-1 and up-regulate expression of the receptor antagonists and of the decoy receptor in keratinocytes (Lee *et al.*, 1991; see Chapter 1); retinoids inhibit production of IL-1 in keratinocytes, and ultraviolet radiation induces expression of the receptor antagonist (Schwarz *et al.*, 1987; Hammerberg *et al.*, 1992) (Table 12.2).

In a recent phase II study, IL-10 was administered i.v. to patients with psoriasis. There was objective and subjective evidence of therapeutic efficacy (Asadullah *et al.*, 1998). There was also evidence of immunosuppression and of a shift towards Th2-type responses. IL-10 raised IL-10 mRNA in the skin. Therefore, psoriasis, like inflammatory bowel disease and rheumatoid arthritis, may be a privileged disease for anti-cytokine strategies.

References

Albanesi, C., Cavani, A., and Girolomoni, G. (1998). Interferon-gamma-stimulated human keratinocytes express the genes necessary for the production of peptide-loaded MHC class II molecules. *J. Invest. Dermatol.*, **110**, 138–42.

Asadullah, K., Sterry, W., Stephanek, K., Jasulaitis, D., Audring, H., Volk, H. D. *et al.* (1998). IL-10 is a key cytokine in psoriasis. Proof of principle by IL-10 therapy: a new therapeutic approach. *J. Clin. Invest.*, **101**, 783–94.

Austyn, J. M. (1996). New insights into the mobilization and phagocytic activity of dendritic cells. *J. Exp. Med.*, **183**, 1287–92.

Banchereau, J. and Steinman, R. M. (1998). Dendritic cells and the control of immunity. *Nature*, **392**, 245–52.

Berthou, C., Michel, L., Soulie, A., Jean-Louis, F., Flageul, B., Sigaux, F. *et al.* (1997). Acquisition of granzyme B and Fas ligand proteins by human keratinocytes contributes to epidermal cell defense. *J. Immunol.*, **159**, 5293–300.

Bos, J. D. and De Rie, M. A. (1999). The pathogenesis of psoriasis: immunological facts and speculations. *Immunol. Today.*, **20**, 40–6.

Bos, J. D. and Kapsenberg, M. L. (1993). The skin immune system: progress in cutaneous biology. *Immunol. Today.*, **14**, 75–8.

Cella, M., Sallusto, F., and Lanzavecchia, A. (1997). Origin, maturation and antigen presenting function of dendritic cells. *Curr. Opin. Immunol.*, **9**, 10–6.

Christophers, E. and Sterry, W. (1993) Psoriasis. In *Dermatology in general medicine* (ed. T. B. Fitzpatric, A. Z. Eisen, K. Wolff, I. M. Freedberg, and K. F. Austen), pp. 489–515, McGraw-Hill, New York.

Colotta, F., Re, F., Muzio, M., Bertini, R., Polentarutti, N., Sironi, M. *et al.* (1993). Interleukin-1 type II receptor: a decoy target for IL-1 that is regulated by IL-4. *Science*, **261**, 472–5.

Cooper, K. D., Hammerberg, C., Baadsgaard, O., Elder, J. T., Chan, L. S., Sauder, D. N. *et al.* (1990). IL-1 activity is reduced in psoriatic skin. Decreased IL-1 alfa and increased nonfunctional IL-1beta_. *J. Immunol.*, **144**, 4593–603.

Groves, R. W., Sherman, L., Mizutani, H., Dower, S. K., and Kupper, T. S. (1994). Detection of interleukin-1 receptors in human epidermis. Induction of the type II receptor after organ culture and in psoriasis. *Am. J. Pathol.*, **145**, 1048–56.

Groves, R. W., Giri, J., Sims, J., Dower, S. K., and Kupper, T. S. (1995a). Inducible expression of type 2 IL-1 receptors by cultured human keratinocytes. Implication for IL-1-mediated processes in epidermis. *J. Immunol.*, **154**, 4065–72.

Groves, R. W., Mizutani, H., Kieffer, J. D., and Kupper, T. S. (1995b). Inflammatory skin disease in transgenic mice that express high levels of interleukin-1α in basal epidermis. *Proc. Natl. Acad. Sci. USA.*, **92**, 11874–8.

Groves, R. W., Rauschmayr, T., Nakamura, K., Sarkar, S., Williams, I. R., and Kupper, T. S. (1996). Inflammatory and hyperproliferative skin disease in mice that express elevated levels of the IL-1 receptor (Type I) on epidermal keratinocytes. *J. Clin. Invest.*, **98**, 336–44.

Gruaz, D., Didierjean, L., Grassi, J., Frobert, Y., Dayer, J. M., and Saurat, J. H. (1989). Interleukin 1 alpha and beta in psoriatic skin: enzymoimmunoassay, immunoblot studies and effect of systemic retinoids. *Dermatologica*, **179**, 202–6.

Hallmann, R., Mayer, D. N., Berg, E. L., Broermann, R., and Butcher, E. C. (1995). Novel mouse endothelial cell surface marker is suppressed during differentiation of the blood brain barrier. *Dev. Dyn.*, **202**, 325–32.

Hammerberg, C., Arend, W. P., Fisher, G. J., Chan, L. S., Berger, A. E., Haskill, S. J. *et al.* (1992). Interleukin-1 receptor antagonist in normal and psoriatic epidermis. *J. Clin. Invest.*, **90**, 571–83.

Hart, D. N. J. (1997). Dendritic cells: unique leukocyte populations which control the primary immune response. *Blood*, **90**, 3245–86.

Haskill, S., Martin, G., Van Le, L., Morris, J., Peace, A., Bigler, C. F. *et al.* (1991). cDNA cloning of an intracellular form of the human interleukin 1 receptor antagonist associated with epithelium. *Proc. Natl. Acad. Sci. USA.*, **88**, 3681–5.

Hauser, C., Saurat, J. H., Schmitt, A., Jaunin, F., and Dayer, J. M. (1986). Interleukin-1 is present in normal human epidermis. *J. Immunol.*, **136**, 3317–23.

Ibrahim, M. A. A., Chain, B. M., and Katz, D. R. (1995). The injured cell: the role of the dendritic cell system as a sentinel receptor pathway. *Immunol. Today.*, **16**, 181–6.

Kupper, T. S. (1989). Mechanisms of cutaneous inflammation. Interactions between epidermal cytokines, adhesion molecules, and leukocytes. *Arch. Dermatol.*, **125**, 1406–12.

Kupper, T. S. and Groves, R. W. (1995). The interleukin-1 axis and cutaneous inflammation. *J. Invest. Dermatol.*, **105** (Supplement 1), 62S–6S.

Larsen, C. G., Kristensen, M., Paludan, K., Deleuran, B., Thomsen, M. K., Zachariae, C. *et al.* (1991). 1,25(OH)2-D3 is a potent regulator of interleukin-1 induced interleukin-8 expression and production. *Biochem. Biophys. Res. Commun.*, **176**, 1020–6.

Lee, S. W., Morhenn, V. B., Ilnicka, M., Eugui, E. M., and Allison, A. C. (1991). Autocrine stimulation of interleukin-1alfa and transforming growth factor alfa production in human keratinocytes and its antagonism by glucocorticoids. *J. Invest. Dermatol.*, **97**, 106–10.

Michel, G., Gailis, A., Jarzebska-Deussen, B., Muschen, A., and Ruzicka, T. (1997). 1,25-(OH)2-vitamin D3 and calcipotriol induce IL-10 receptor gene expression in human epidermal cells. *Inflamm. Res.*, **46**, 32–4.

Muzio, M., Polentarutti, N., Sironi, M., Poli, G., De Gioia, L., Introna, M., *et al.* (1995). Cloning and characterization of a new isoform of the interleukin 1 receptor antagonist. *J. Exp. Med.*, **182**, 623–8.

Muzio M., Polentarutti N., Facchetti F., Peri G., Doni A., Sironi M. *et al.* (1999). Characterization of type II intracellular interleukin-1 receptor antagonist (IL-1ra3): a depot IL-1ra. *Eur. J. Immunol.*, **29**, 781–8.

Nakamura, K., Williams, I. R., and Kupper, T. S. (1995). Keratinocyte-derived monocyte chemoattractant protein 1 (MCP-1): Analysis in a transgenic model demonstrates MCP-1 can recruit dendritic and Langerhan's cells to skin. *J. Invest. Dermatol.*, **105**, 635–43.

Nickoloff, B. J. (1991). The cytokine network in psoriasis. *Arch. Dermatol.*, **127**, 871–84.

Nickoloff, B. J. (1999). Skin innate immune system in psoriasis: friend or foe? *J. Clin. Invest.* **104**, 1161–4.

Pastore, S., Fanale-Belasio, E., Albanesi, C., Chinni, L. M., Giannetti, A., and Girolomoni, G. (1997). Granulocyte macrophage colony-stimulating factor is overproduced by keratinocytes in atopic dermatitis. Implications for sustained dendritic cell activation in the skin. *J. Clin. Invest.*, **99**, 3009–17.

Piemonti, L., Bernasconi, S., Luini, W., Trobonjaca, Z., Minty, A., Allavena, P. *et al.* (1995). IL-13 supports differentiation of dendritic cells from circulating precursors in concert with GM-CSF. *Eur. Cytokine Netw.*, **6**, 245–52.

Power, C. A., Church, D. J., Meyer, A., Alouani, S., Proudfoot, A. E. I., Clark-Lewis, I. *et al.* (1997). Cloning and characterization of a specific receptor for the novel CC chemokine MIP-3 alpha from lung dendritic cells. *J. Exp. Med.*, **186**, 825–35.

Rauschmayr, T., Groves, R. W., and Kupper, T. S. (1997). Keratinocyte expression of the type 2 interleukin 1 receptor mediates local and specific inhibition of interleukin 1-mediated inflammation. *Proc. Natl. Acad. Sci. USA.*, **94**, 5814–9.

Sallusto, F. and Lanzavecchia, A. (1994). Efficient presentation of soluble antigen by cultured human dendritic cells is maintained by granulocyte/macrophage colony-stimulating factor plus interleukin-4 and downregulated by tumor necrosis factor-alpha. *J. Exp. Med.*, **179**, 1109–18.

Schön, M. P. (1999). Animal models of psoriasis – what can we learn from them? *J. Invest. Dermatol.*, **112**, 405–10.

Schroder, J. M. (1992). Generation of NAP-1 and related peptides in psoriasis and other inflammatory skin diseases. *Cytokines*, **4**, 54–76.

Schwarz, T., Urbanska, A., Gschnait, F., and Luger, T. A. (1987). UV-irradiated epidermal cells produce a specific inhibitor of interleukin 1 activity. *J. Immunol.*, **138**, 1457–63.

Sozzani, S., Sallusto, F., Luini, W., Zhou, D., Piemonti, L., Allavena, P. *et al.* (1995). Migration of dendritic cells in response to formyl peptides, C5a and a distinct set of chemokines. *J. Immunol.*, **155**, 3292–5.

Sozzani, S., Luini, W., Borsatti, A., Polentarutti, N., Zhou, D., Piemonti, L. *et al.* (1997). Receptor expression and responsiveness of human dendritic cells to a defined set of CC and CXC chemokines. *J. Immunol.*, **159**, 1993–2000.

Sozzani, S., Allavena, P., D'Amico, G., Luini, W., Bianchi, G., Kataura, M. *et al.* (1998). Cutting edge: Differential regulation of chemokine receptors during dendritic cell maturation: A model for their trafficking properties. *J. Immunol.*, **161**, 1083–6.

Sozzani, S., Allavena, P., Vecchi, A., and Mantovani, A. (1999). The role of chemokines in the regulation of dendritic cell trafficking. *J. Leukoc. Biol.*, **66**, 1–9.

Steinman, R., Hoffman, L., and Pope, M. (1995). Maturation and migration of cutaneous dendritic cells. *J. Invest. Dermatol.*, **105**, S2-S7.

Steinman, R. M. (1991). The dendritic cell system and its role in immunogenicity. *Annu. Rev. Immunol.*, **9**, 271–96.

13 *Septic shock*

13.1 The physiological catastrophe of septic shock

The diagnosis of sepsis syndrome or septic shock is based on a constellation of physiologic, metabolic, and hematologic abnormalities, most commonly occurring in patients with a known infection. In most cases, the patient is already hospitalized with an antecedent illness or has experienced recent surgery. Many patients, but not all, are being treated with appropriate antibiotics for a suspected infection. Approximately 25% of patients with sepsis syndrome are in hemodynamic shock at the time of presentation (Sands *et al.*, 1997). Characteristic of septic shock, the hypotension is unresponsive to rapid fluid replacement. In most circumstances, when blood pressure falls relative to the patient's normotensive level (a 25–35% reduction), 500 ml of saline infusion is rapidly administered. If there is no response (increase in mean arterial pressure), a diagnosis of hemodynamic shock is made. In the context of an on-going infection or suspected new infection, the patient is thought to be in septic shock. There is another disease that mimics the rapid evolution of septic shock, that is, acute pancreatitis, in which there is no associated infection but rather systemic inflammation. Clinically, it is often difficult to distinguish between these two. However, the vast majority of patients with hemodynamic shock have an infection as the cause.

If the hypotension is not corrected, progressive reduction in organ perfusion and increasing acidosis leads to tissue hypoxia and results in organ failure. Although the hypotension is initially treated with pressor drugs and antibiotics are either changed or new ones added, a downhill course can rapidly take place, resulting in death. In some patients, this rapid downhill course can be very dramatic. This physiologic cascade is illustrated in Fig. 13.1. Renal failure is an early sign that the hypotension and acidosis have been of sufficient magnitude and duration. Liver failure can also be rapid. However, increasing loss of cardiac function is of major concern, since there is no 'hold-over' therapy, such as hemodialysis, for renal failure.

In the past 5 years, the 28-day mortality in patients with sepsis syndrome has decreased somewhat but still ranges from 20 to 50%; mortality in those with septic shock and multiple-organ failure is higher despite aggressive intensive care. Intensive care units deliver hemodynamic, metabolic, ventilatory, and renal support, and critical care has become a recognized medical subspecialty. Clearly some patients survive the ordeal but it remains frustrating for the intensivist who cannot halt and reverse the downhill course leading to multiple-organ failure and death. New therapies have been sought and tested in these

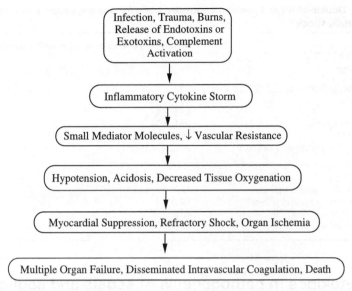

Fig. 13.1 Physiologic events associated with the development of septic shock.

patients. Ideally, the therapy should be able to 'rescue' the patient who continues to deteriorate in the face of considerable support efforts. Unfortunately, there is still no therapeutic agent or combination of treatments that have significantly reduced the mortality of this disease over that acheived with up-to-date intensive-care strategies (Abraham, 1997).

There is little question that the major advance in treating patients with septic shock was the avalability of broad-spectrum antibiotics. In fact, the sooner broad-spectrum antibiotics are administered, mortality decreases (Kreger *et al.*, 1980; Dunn, 1994). The testing of non-antibiotic-based, novel therapies is based on 50 years of research on how microorganisms trigger the cascade of events in septic shock. Although microbial products, such as endotoxins, are still targets for therapy, a fundamental concept is that the constellation of abnormalities in these patients is not due to the direct effect of the infectious agent or its products, but rather results from the patient's own response to the infection (or in some cases, response to massive trauma and blood loss). Initially, activation of complement was considered causal, particularly the fifth component of complement, which is a potent neutrophil activator and produces a capillary-leak syndrome. The release of platelet activating factor (PAF) was also thought to be responsible, particularly since PAF is a potent hypotensive agent. Using specific inhibitors of PAF, animals given lethal bacterial toxins survive. Similar results were obtained when cyclo-oxygenase inhibitors were administered to animals lethally challenged with endotoxin or bacteria; hence those experiments implicated cylo-oxygenase products as a contributing cause to septic shock. Numerous animal studies also demonstrated the protective effects of corticosteroids, and several large clinical trials using these potent anti-inflammatory agents were undertaken. Clinical trials of PAF antagonists, cyclo-oxygenase inhibitors, bradykinin antagonists, and corticosteroids have each failed to significantly reduce the 28-day mortality in septic shock patients (Table 13.1).

Table 13.1 Double-blind and placebo-controlled trials for treating patients with sepsis syndrome or septic shock

Agent	Number of patients enrolled in each trial of the agent
Corticosteroids	75, 223, 59, 382, 60, 48, 172, 85, 194
Anti-endotoxin antibodies:	
HA-1A	543, 2199
E5	448, 847
Bradykinin antagonist	251, 504
PAF antagonists	262, 668
Ibuprofen (cyclo-oxygenase inhibitor)	29, 30, 455
Anti-TNFα:	
Murine anti-TNFα	971, 564, 1879
Murine anti-TNFα Fab2' fragment	122, 39, 446
p75 TNF Receptor Fusion Protein	141
p55 TNF Receptor Fusion Protein	498
IL-1 receptor antagonist	99, 893, 696

13.2 Cytokines in pathogenesis of sepsis and septic shock

The field entered a new era when it was shown that neutralizing antibodies to the inflammatory cytokine tumor necrosis factor (TNF) prevented death in mice (Beutler *et al.*, 1985), rabbits (Mathison *et al.*, 1988), or baboons (Tracey *et al.*, 1987) given a lethal injection of *E. coli* or endotoxin. In the absence of any infection, high doses of TNF in animals induced circulatory collapse and organ necrosis, which were very similar to those observed in humans with septic shock. Similar results were observed with high doses of IL-1 in animals. Injecting a combination of low doses of IL-1 plus TNF revealed that these two cytokines acted synergistically in inducing a shock-like state (Okusawa *et al.*, 1988). Similar to neutralizing TNF activity, blocking IL-1 receptors were also effective in preventing death in animal models of lethal bacteremia or endotoxemia (Ohlsson *et al.*, 1990; Wakabayashi *et al.*, 1991). Since TNF induces IL-1, and IL-1 induces TNF, these animal studies showing synergism between the two cytokines made sense. Although a few studies revealed that, for some intracellular infections, blocking IL-1 or TNF would worsen disease, blocking these cytokines was considered of primary importance compared to loss of host defense function. For the patient without overt infection, for example, multiple trauma, the preclinical data demonstrated that the systemic injection of either IL-1 or TNF into experimental animals induced physiologic, hematologic, and pathological changes, which were nearly identical to that observed during bacteremia or multiple trauma.

Animal studies were confirmed when humans were injected with either IL-1 or TNF. The most impressive physiologic event following the intravenous injection of either cytokine in humans is the fall in blood pressure. Frank hypotension has been reported with doses of IL-1 or TNF as low as 50 ng/kg (Chapman *et al.*, 1987; Smith *et al.*, 1993). The hypotension is dose-dependent and despite a short plasma half-life of less than 10 min, the biological consequences can be observed for days. In studies in which IL-1 was administered as adjunct therapy for bone marrow transplant recovery, nearly all patients required pressor therapy (Smith *et al.*, 1992, 1993). In the few patients where the dose of

IL-1 was increased to 1 μg/kg, a shock-like state developed. In the case of TNF, an increase in the coagulation parameters and an early leukopenia occurred (van der Poll *et al.*, 1990, 1991). The logical clinical conclusion from a vast amount of data was that reducing the biological effects of systemic TNF or IL-1 would reduce the risk of dying from septic shock, in that these cytokines are essential for the manifestation of the disease.

13.3 The rationale for anti-cytokine therapy

The biological basis for the development of a shock-like state following systemic IL-1 or TNF has been established at the molecular level. Both cytokines activate the transcription of genes that increase the production of small, potent mediator molecules. For example, IL-1 and TNF increase gene expression and synthesis for phospholipase A$_2$ type II leading to increased PAF synthesis. Similarly, an increase in cyclo-oxygenase type II (COX-2) by IL-1 and TNF, results in elevated levels of PGE$_2$ (reviewed in: Dinarello, 1996). On a molar basis, nitric oxide (NO) is perhaps the most potent vasodilator and is thought to be primarily responsible for the hypotension and myocardial suppression in septic shock (Moncada *et al.*, 1991). Whereas constitutive NO production is part of homeostasis, increased production of NO in inflammation takes place when NO is the product of inducible nitric oxide synthase (Fang, 1997). IL-1, TNF, and IFNγ, particularly the combination of the three, activate gene expression and synthesis of inducible nitric oxide synthase.

Therefore, trials were carried out in which TNF was neutralized either with monoclonal anti-TNF or soluble TNF receptors, and IL-1 activity was blocked with the IL-1 receptor antagonist (Fisher *et al.*, 1994a, 1994b, 1996; Abraham *et al.*, 1995, 1997; Abraham, 1997). Although we discuss below some of the reasons why we believe these trials failed to significantly improve 28-day mortality, nevertheless, the results of trials based on reducing IL-1 or TNF activity have been disappointing. The most recent and largest trial, treating 1879 septic shock patients with murine monoclonal antibodies to TNF, improved 28-day mortality by only 2.5% (40.3 for anti-TNF versus 42.8% for the placebo).

13.4 Meta-analysis of septic shock intervention trials

In order to examine the outcomes in terms of safety and efficacy of the many trials in septic shock patients, a meta-analysis was performed (Zeni *et al.*, 1997). The analysis included 39 trials conducted over the past 30 years. There were 20 trials of non-glucocorticoids, such as interleukin-1 receptor antagonist, antibodies to TNF, and bradykinin and PAF antagonists. There were 10 trials for testing anti-endotoxin antibodies. There were several conclusions to the analysis:

(1) the mortality of the control arm (placebo) for the entire group of 39 trials was consistently 35–40%;

(2) high-dose glucocorticoids showed a harmful effect on survival;

(3) anti-mediator trials resulted in a small but significant survival benefit;

(4) anti-endotoxin trials showed no effect.

It is important to note that the anti-cytokine therapy trials did not increase mortality but rather 28-day mortality was decreased. This latter result is in contrast to predictions that blocking the biological effects of IL-1 or TNF would reduce host defense systems. In these highly vulnerable patients with severe infection, blocking IL-1 activity or neutralizing TNF had no harmful effect.

Compared to IL-1 and TNF, there is no other cytokine to date that reproduces the dramatic hypotension and physiologic parameters of septic shock in animals or in humans. That does not mean other cytokines do not particpate in the pathogenesis of the event. For example, animals treated with neutralizing antibodies to IFNγ, are protected against lethal endotoxemia (Heremans *et al.*, 1990). Similar data have been reported for mice lacking the receptor for IFNγ (Huang *et al.*, 1993). IFNγ is a potent macrophage activator and increases the production of, and response to, TNF. In contrast to the pro-inflammatory properties of IFNγ, the administration of IFNγ to certain patients with septic shock appears to be beneficial (Doecke *et al.*, 1997), although those data need confirmation in placebo-controlled, blinded trials. Nevertheless, the data in animals for blocking IFNγ, and the ability of IFNγ to increase gene expression for inducible nitric oxide, are compelling arguments for testing anti-IFNγ in humans. The issue of blocking IFNγ is clouded, since this cytokine has been injected into several thousand humans (some with infections) without producing hypotension or similar sepsis-like effects.

Other therapeutic approaches in septic patients target the chemokines and adhesion molecules. Although administration of large doses of IL-8 to primates does not result in hypotension, neutralizing antibodies to IL-8 in models of inflammation reduce neutrophil infiltration in the lung, joint, kidney, skin, and myocardium (Harada *et al.*, 1996). In particular, anti-IL-8 reduces neutrophil accumulation in the lung and myocardium following ischemia-reperfusion injury. If tested in humans, anti-IL-8 therapy would most likely be used in patients with ARDS. IL-8 is increased in bronchoalveolar lavage specimens from patients with ARDS and, in most patients at risk for ARDS, elevated bronchoalveolar lavage IL-8 levels have been predictive of the subsequent development of ARDS (Donnelly *et al.*, 1993). Blocking IL-8 reduces the entrance of neutrophils into inflammatory sites (Harada *et al.*, 1996). Although IL-8 is a sensible target in septic shock patients, particularly in halting the progress of ARDS, the production of IL-8 (and other chemokines) is markedly reduced by the combination of anti-IL-1 and anti-TNF agents. As shown in Fig. 13.2, blocking the biological activities of IL-1 and TNF is an upstream strategy for reducing the cascade of secondary mediators of systemic inflammation. A recent meta-analysis of anti-inflammatory agents, and anti-IL-1 and anti-TNF based therapies in septic patients, concluded that a consistent, although marginal, survival benefit has been observed in non-glucocorticoid trials (Zeni *et al.*, 1997). However, the survival benefit for monotherapy using any of these agents never reaches a level of significance that would allow approval by regulatory agencies.

Is there anything wrong with the concept of anti-cytokine based therapies for disease? Anti-TNF and anti-IL-1-based therapies have been used in patients with rheumatoid arthritis with clear and often dramatic clinical benefits, demonstrating that blocking either cytokine in humans is do-able and effective (Elliott *et al.*, 1994; Elliott and Maini, 1995; Watt and Cobby, 1996; Bresnihan *et al.*, 1998). Anti-TNF is also very effective when used to pretreat patients with a high risk of the Jarisch–Herxheimer reaction (Fekade *et al.*, 1996) and on a chronic basis in Crohn's disease (van Dullemen *et al.*, 1995);

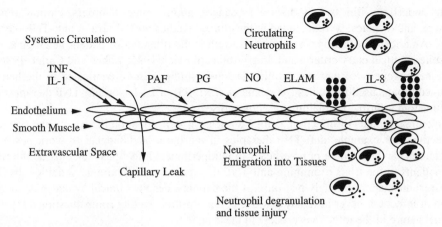

Fig. 13.2 Effect of IL-1 and TNF on endothelium. TNF and IL-1 activate endothelial cells and trigger the cascade of pro-inflammatory small molecule mediators. Increased gene expression for phospholipase A_2 type II, cyclo-oxygenase type-2 (COX-2) and inducible nitric oxide synthase (iNOS) results in elevated production of their products: PAF, PGE_2, and NO. Alone or in combination, these mediators decrease the tone of vascular smooth muscle, and systemic vascular resistance takes place. IL-1 and TNF also cause increased capillary leak. The up-regulation of endothelial leukocyte adhesion molecules results in adherence of circulating neutrophils to the endothelium, and increased production of chemokines, such as IL-8, facilitates the emigration of neutrophils into the tissues. Chemokines also activate degranulation of neutrophils. Activated neutrophils lead to tissue destruction, particularly in the lung.

IL-1Ra has reduced the severity of graft versus host disease in steroid-resistant patients (Antin *et al.*, 1994). Moreover, long-term (over one year) use of these anti-cytokine strategies has not been associated with any obvious impairment of host defense, even in patient populations with a well-established risk of increased infections. In fact, in a recent meta-analysis of the anti-cytokine therapy trials in septic patients, the authors conclude that the consistent survival benefit, although not statistically significant, supports the view that anti-cytokine treatment in sepsis is not harmful (Zeni *et al.*, 1997). If there is no harm, then why are the results using these very same agents in patients with septic shock without a significant reduction in mortality in the 'total' sepsis population?

13.5 A closer look at the patient population entering sepsis trials

Almost all of the clinical trials investigating new therapies for sepsis have determined patient entry using a broad definition of the 'sepsis syndrome', based on clinical criteria including the presence of tachycardia, hyper- or hypothermia, and elevated or decreased peripheral white blood cell counts. These are coupled with the presence of organ system dysfunction, such as lactic acidosis, disseminated intravascular coagulation, hypoxemia, hypotension, or decreased urine output. These entry criteria have permitted patients with a wide range of underlying illnesses and sources of infection to be treated. For example, patients with clinical evidence of urinary tract, respiratory, or intra-abdominal infection, with underlying illnesses as diverse as cancer, autoimmune disorders, chronic renal failure, and diabetes, were included in the clinical studies with IL-1ra or anti-TNF therapies. American and European studies also reflect the dilemma of patient heterogeneity, despite identical entry criteria and drug (Abraham *et al.*, 1995; Cohen and Carlet, 1996). The heterogeneity of patients enrolled in sepsis studies can be contrasted to the better defined groups used in studies (Abraham *et al.*, 1995) of IL-1ra or anti-TNF therapies in rheumatoid arthritis or inflammatory bowel disease.

In animal models of infection, cytokine release is dependent on the source and type of infection. For example, anti-TNF therapies in murine models appear to work best for bacteremia and have poor or no efficacy in intraperitoneal infections. Yet, only a minority of patients in the trials examining anti-TNF therapies were bacteremic. Additionally, in most studies, approximately one-third of the patients, despite clinical evidence or suspicion of infection, never have any positive culture results, leaving some question as to the actual nature of the infectious process in these patients.

With the exception of one study, none of the clinical trials has used a measure of enhanced cytokine release as an entry criterion. In that trial, employing murine anti-TNF Fab2′ fragments, a single circulating IL-6 level greater than 1000 pg/ml was utilized to identify a target patient group for this therapy (Reinhart *et al.*, 1996). Although IL-6 levels consistently corrrelate with disease severity in most patients with sepsis, patients with infectious and non-infectious diseases show remarkably variable circulating and tissue cytokine levels, and a single measurement can be misleading. Since circulating levels of endogenously produced IL-1ra and TNF soluble receptors are elevated in sepsis, the net biologically active IL-1 or TNF remains unclear. It would appear more useful to identify for enrollment those patients with increased generation of biologically active cytokine(s), which is the target of blocking therapy. Unfortunately, such identification is difficult because TNF and IL-1 are released at their greatest concentrations at the tissue sites, and rarely do the circulating levels correlate with the levels of local production. Therefore, clinical criteria will probably be required to identify patients with increased tissue IL-1 and TNF. These patients appear to be those with a rapidly occurring onset of organ system dysfunction secondary to infection, without major underlying and pre-existent medical problems. An example would be the young patient with acute onset of meningococcemia, in whom circulating and tissue levels of TNFα are dramatically elevated. In this setting, the greatest survival benefit from anti-cytokine therapy would be expected when the agent(s) is given very soon after diagnosis, and would be observed in the period immediately following therapy, as a direct result of reversal of pro-inflammatory cytokine driven organ dysfunction.

13.6 Is there a genetic predisposition to surviving septic shock?

Humans injected intravenously with either IL-1α or IL-1β also develop hypotension at doses above 50 ng/kg and frank hemodynamic shock at doses above 300 ng/kg (Smith *et al.*, 1992, 1993). These studies formed the rational basis for treating patients with sepsis and septic shock with IL-1ra. Although the overall results of the clinical trials with IL-1ra were not sufficient to warrant further development in all patients with severe sepsis, some patients during subgroup analyses did receive a survival benefit from receiving IL-1ra (Fisher *et al.*, 1994a, 1994b; Opal *et al.*, 1997). In recently published studies, targeted deletion of the IL-1ra gene in mice (also known as IL-1ra knock-out mice) has resulted in a phenotype highly vulnerable to endotoxin-induced lethality, whereas mice over-expressing IL-1ra, appear to be protected against lethal endotoxemia (Hirsch *et al.*, 1996). These latter experiments suggest that endogenous levels of IL-1ra may contribute to disease outcome, at least in the case of septic shock.

The working hypothesis is that those individuals with the genetic make-up to produce large amounts of IL-1ra when septic, are afforded a greater level of protection than another subject producing lower levels. The parallel working hypothesis is that those individuals with the genetic make-up to produce less bioactive IL-1β when septic, are less likely to die during septic shock compared to those subjects producing larger amounts of IL-1β. Although the ultimate proof of these two hypotheses is to measure the concentrations of IL-1ra and IL-1β in patients surviving and compare those levels with those patients dying of septic shock, such measurements in the context of the acute setting are affected by nutritional and non-genetic mechanisms present at the time of infection. Hence, an investigation into the genetic determinants that may result in high or low IL-1ra or IL-1β production should shed light in answering that question.

Messenger RNA does not cause disease. Even if the promoters for IL-1ra and the cleavage site for IL-1β are genetically different, unless these differences result in different levels of the gene product, any polymorphisms are of questionable importance to the outcome of disease. Nevertheless, there are lessons to be learned from examination of polymorphisms in cytokine genes. For example, persons homozygous for the TNFB2 allele of the NcoI site in the TNF locus is associated with non-survival in patients with severe sepsis (Stüber *et al.*, 1996). These patients also have elevated TNFα levels in the circulation and higher organ failure scores. Although there is increased mortality with the homozygous TNFB2 allele, there is no difference between the frquency of this polymorphism in the general population and the group of patients in the intensive care unit with a diagnosis of severe sepsis. It appears that if one develops severe sepsis, inheriting the TNFB2 allele makes one particularly at risk for death compared to heterozygotes or patients homozygous for the TNFB1 allele (Stüber *et al.*, 1996).

Another study (Fang *et al.*, 1999) examined two well-described genetic polymorphisms in the IL-1 family: the A1–5 allele in intron 2 of the IL-1ra gene; and the Taq1 site in exon 5 of the IL-1β gene. They compared the frequency of these alleles in 93 consecutive patients admitted to the surgical intensive care unit with 261 local blood donors in apparent health. The results were surprising in that there was a high allele frequency of the IL-1raA2 in the cohort with severe sepsis compared to the healthy cohort ($P<0.01$). Although there was no association with outcome (survival at 28 days), the conclusion of the study suggests that persons with this allele are more likely to find themselves in a surgical intensive care unit with severe sepsis that those without the allele. The internal control for this study was the lack of the Taq1 allele associated with this cohort of 93 patients compared to the population of 261 persons. In addition, these studies confirmed that the TNFB2 allele was again associated with non-survival in this cohort. However, there was no linkage between these two polymorphisms in the study. Yet, in eight individuals who were born homozygous for both the IL-1raA2 and TNFB2 alleles, all developed multiple organ failure with fatal outcome.

Can we believe that this allele in IL-1ra makes us more likely to be a patient with severe sepsis? What is known about this allele and IL-1ra production? In one study, the amount of IL-1ra produced from patients with insulin-dependent diabetes mellitus was reduced (Mandrup-Poulsen *et al.*, 1994). In another study, granulocyte-macrophage colony stimulating factor was used to stimulate IL-1ra production and persons with the IL-1raA2 allele exhibited increased production compared to those without this allele (Danis *et al.*, 1995a). In addition, in that study, there was reduced production of IL-1α in these subjects. Clearly, these results need to be confirmed but the concept that a gene polymorphism is associated with a measurable difference in the amount of the gene product and an outcome to disease may help resolve the problems encountered in new therapeutic clinical trials in septic shock patients. As it now stands, it seems that persons with the IL-1raA2 allele make more IL-1ra, which is a risk factor for developing severe sepsis following a surgical procedure.

Linkage of a particular cytokine gene polymorphism to disease is not always found in each population studied. For example, a predisposition to develop severe systemic lupus erythematosus was linked to the IL-1raA2 allele in a cohort of persons in the United Kingdom (Blakemore *et al.*, 1994). In a cohort living in Australia, this association was not found (Danis *et al.*, 1995b). Similarly, the association of the IL-1ra allele and ulcerative colitis in England (Mansfield *et al.*, 1994) was not observed in a cohort of patients living in Southern Germany (Hacker *et al.*, 1997). Therefore, the genetic studies in German patients need to be confirmed in another population.

13.7 New approaches to therapy

Although specific and successful monotherapy for a particular disease is a desirable goal in therapeutics, there are increasing examples where treatment is most effective when two or more agents are used. The obvious examples are cancer, autoimmune diseases, and HIV-1, where treatment with a single anti-tumor drug or immunosuppressive regimen or anti-viral agent has been replaced with the use of several agents, each targeting a somewhat different mechanism. If more than one agent would benefit the patient with septic shock, there are several possible combinations. In sepsis, involving a gram-negative organism, endotoxin itself acts like a cytokine in that it activates nearly the same genes as does IL-1 and TNFα. A combination of neutralizing antibodies to endotoxin, as well as blocking TNF and/or IL-1, may offer the patient with gram-negative septic shock the greatest chance of rescue. Administration of anti-IL-8 with either anti-TNF or anti-IL-1 may be effective for patients with a high risk of developing ARDS. The concept of combining more than one anti-cytokine agent has sound experimental basis. For example, in animals, a combination of anti-TNF plus anti-IL-1 treatment has increased survival over that using either agent as monotherapy.

Is the failure to rescue patients with anti-TNF or IL-1 blockade due to a delay in intervention? In many patients (75%) with sepsis syndrome, blood pressure and organ perfusion are unimpaired; however, when septic shock develops, circulatory collapse within a few hours is thought to coincide with the onset of a new bacteremia or endotoxemia. In addition, a 'cytokine storm' is thought to be responsible for triggering the shock. It has been the wisdom of anti-cytokine therapy that these patients also stand the greatest chance of a 'rescue' by blocking further cytokine receptor triggering. In other patients with similarly serious infections, a fall in blood pressure or the development of organ failure is slower (over days), and cytokine receptors may have already been engaged before circulatory collapse reaches the level of entry criteria into a trial. In those patients, the administration of anti-cytokine therapy may be too late to provide a successful rescue. Whereas animal studies have provided a compelling argument that blocking TNF or IL-1 would be a therapeutic success in treating septic shock, in animals the window of time for reversing the events of lethal sepsis is rather small. Does that mean that by the time the patient has overt signs of septic shock that it is too late for rescue with anti-cytokine therapy? In most of the anti-cytokine trials, the time that passes before a patient actually receives therapy can be 12–24 h after the early indications of altered mental status or blood pressure instability. What can be done to shorten the time between overt evidence of a life-threatening process and initiation of anti-cytokine therapy?

As noted above, the heterogeneity of the acute infectious and underlying chronic disease processes in the patients who were enrolled into sepsis studies may have prevented demonstration of efficacy for anti-cytokine therapies. Additionally, large numbers of patients with low risk of mortality were enrolled in these clinical trials. Such patients often do not have markedly accelerated pro-inflammatory responses amenable to anti-cytokine therapy, and their inclusion in the clinical studies may have diluted-out any survival benefit associated with the use of anti-cytokine therapy for sepsis. Therefore, an important advance for future trials would be to reduce patient heterogeneity. It has been received wisdom that larger patient cohorts, similar to the 20 000 patients used to evaluate thrombolytic therapy in acute myocardial infarction, would compensate for the 'background noise' of patient heterogeneity in the sepsis trials. However, increasing the number of patients and the number of participating hospitals has yielded the same patient heterogeneity.

During post-trial, retrospective analyses, many sepsis trials have uncovered a subgroup within the entire group, in which a survival benefit using the new therapy was present. In some of these analyses, this subgroup benefit was statistically significant. However, when prospectively studied in follow-up larger trials, the survival benefit was no longer demonstrable. It has been proposed that large patient heterogeneity in the expanded follow-up trials prevented the benefit from being statistically significant. Hence, anti-cytokine therapy for sepsis still awaits identification of the patient who can be rescued in a timely fashion from the downhill cascade caused by inflammatory cytokines.

References

Abraham, E. (1997). Therapies for sepsis. Emerging therapies for sepsis and septic shock. *West. J. Med.*, **166**, 195–200.

Abraham, E., Glauser, M. P., Butler, T., Garbino, J., Gelmont, D., Laterre, P. F. *et al.* (1997). p55 Tumor necrosis factor receptor fusion protein in the treatment of patients with severe sepsis and septic shock. A randomized controlled multicenter trial. Ro 45–2081 Study Group. *JAMA*, **277**, 1531–8.

Abraham, E., Wunderink, R., Silverman, H., Perl, T. M., Nasraway, S., Levy, H. *et al.* (1995). Efficacy and safety of monoclonal antibody to human tumor necrosis factor-α in patients with sepsis syndrome. *JAMA*, **273**, 934–41.

Antin, J. H., Weinstein, H. J., Guinan, E. C., McCarthy, P., Bierer, B. E., Gilliland, D. G. *et al.* (1994). Recombinant human interleukin-1 receptor antagonist in the treatment of steroid-resistant graft-versus-host disease. *Blood*, **84**, 1342–8.

Beutler, B., Milsark, I. W. and Cerami, A. (1985). Passive immunization against cachetin/tumor necrosis factor protects mice from lethal effect of endotoxin. *Science*, **229**, 869–71.

Blakemore, A. I., Tarlow, J. K., Cork, M. J., Gordon, C., Emery, P., and Duff, G. W. (1994). Interleukin-1 receptor antagonist gene polymorphism as a disease severity factor in systemic lupus erythematosus. *Arthritis Rheum.*, **37**, 1380–5.

Bresnihan, B., Alvaro-Gracia, J. M., Cobby, M., Doherty, M., Domljan, Z., Emery, P *et al.* (1998). Treatment of rheumatoid arthritis with recombinant human interleukin-1 receptor antagonist. *Arthritis Rheum.*, **41**, 2196–204.

Chapman, P. B., Lester, T. J., Casper, E. S., Gabrilove, J. L., Wong, G. Y., Kempin, S. J. *et al.* (1987). Clinical pharmacology of recombinant human tumor necrosis factor in patients with advanced cancer. *J. Clin. Oncol.*, **5**, 1942–51.

Cohen, J. and Carlet, J. (1996). Intersept: an international, multicenter, placebo-controled trial of monoclonal antibody to human tumor necrosis factor-alpha in patients with sepsis. *Crit. Care Med.*, **24**, 1431–40.

Danis, V. A., Millington, M., Huang, Q., Hyland, V., and Grennan, D. (1995a). Lack of association between an interleukin-1 receptor antagonist gene polymorphism and systemic lupus erythematosus. *Dis. Markers*, **12**, 135–9.

Danis, V. A., Millington, M., Hyland, V., and Grennan, D. (1995b). Cytokine production by normal human monocytes: inter-subject variation and relationship to an IL-1 receptor antagonist (IL-1Ra) gene polymorphism. *Clin. Exp. Immunol.*, **99**, 303–10.

Dinarello, C. A. (1996). Biological basis for interleukin-1 in disease. *Blood*, **87**, 2095–147.

Doecke, W. D., Randow, F., Syrbe, U., Krausch, D., Asadullah, K., Reinke, P. *et al.* (1997). Monocyte deactivation in septic patients: restoration by IFN-gamma treatment. *Nat. Med.*, **3**, 678–81.

Donnelly, S. C., Strieter, R. M., Kunkel, S. L., Walz, A., Robertson, C. R., Carter, D. C. *et al.* (1993). Interleukin-8 and development of adult respiratory distress syndrome in at-risk patient groups. *Lancet*, **341**, 643–7.

Dunn, D. L. (1994). Gram-negative bacterial sepsis and sepsis syndrome. *Surg. Clin. North Am.*, **74**, 621–35.

Elliott, M. J. and Maini, R. N. (1995). Anti-cytokine therapy in rheumatoid arthritis. *Baillieres Clin. Rheumatol.*, **9**, 633–52.

Elliott, M. J., Maini, R. N., Feldmann, M., Kalden, J. R., Antoni, C., Smolen, J. S *et al.* (1994). Randomised double-blind comparison of chimeric monoclonal antibody to tumour necrosis factor alpha (cA2) versus placebo in rheumatoid arthritis. *Lancet*, **344**, 1105–10.

Fang, F. C. (1997). Mechanisms of nitric oxide-related antimicrobial activity. *J. Clin. Invest.*, **99**, 2818–25.

Fang, X.-M., Schröder, S., Hoeft, A., and Stüber, F. (1999). Comparison of two polymorphisms of the interleukin-1 gene family: interleukin-1 receptor antagonist polymorphism contributyes to susceptibility to severe sepsis. *Crit. Care Med.*, **27**, 1330–4.

Fekade, D., Knox, K., Hussein, K., Melka, A., Lalloo, D. G., Coxon, R. E. *et al.* (1996). Prevention of Jarisch-Herxheimer reactions by treatment with antibodies against tumor necrosis factor alpha. *New Engl. J. Med.*, **335**, 311–5.

Fisher, C. J. J., Dhainaut, J. F., Opal, S. M., Pribble, J. P., Balk, R. A., Slotman, G. J. *et al.* (1994a). Recombinant human interleukin-1 receptor antagonist in the treatment of patients with sepsis syndrome. Results from a randomized, double blind, placebo-controlled trial. *JAMA,* **271,** 1836–43.

Fisher, C. J. J., Slotman, G. J., Opal, S. M., Pribble, J., Bone, R. C., Emmanuel, G. *et al.* (1994b). Initial evaluation of human recombinant interleukin-1 receptor antagonist in the treatment of sepsis syndrome: a randomized, open-label, placebo-controlled multicenter trial. *Crit. Care Med.,* **22,** 12–21.

Fisher, C., Jr., Agosti, J. M., Opal, S. M., Lowry, S. F., Balk, R. A., Sadoff, J. C. *et al.* (1996). Treatment of septic shock with the tumor necrosis factor receptor:Fc fusion protein. *New Engl. J. Med.,* **334,** 1697–702.

Hacker, U. T., Gomolka, M., Keller, E., Eigler, A., Folwaczny, C., Fricke, H. *et al.* (1997). Lack of association betwen an interleukin-1 receptor antagonist gene polymorphism and ulcerative colitis. *Gut,* **40,** 623–7.

Harada, A., Mukaida, N., and Matsushima, K. (1996). Interleukin-8 as a novel target for intervention therapy in acute inflammatory diseases. *Mol. Med. Today,* **2,** 482–9.

Heremans, H., van Damme, J., Dillen, C., Dikman, R., and Billiau, A. (1990). Interferon-γ, a mediator of lethal lipopolysaccharide-induced Shwartzman-like shock in mice. *J. Exp. Med.,* **171,** 1853–61.

Hirsch, E., Irikura, V. M., Paul, S. M., and Hirsh, D. (1996). Functions of interleukin-1 receptor antagonist in gene knockout and overproducing mice. *Proc. Natl. Acad. Sci. USA,* **93,** 11008–13.

Huang, S., Hendriks, W., Althage, A., Hemmi, S., Bluethmann, H., Kamijo, R. *et al.* (1993). Immune response in mice that lack the interferon-gamma receptor. *Science,* **259,** 1742–5.

Kreger, B. E., Craven, D. E., and McCabe, W. R. (1980). Gram-negative bacteremia. IV. reevaluation of clinical features and treatment in 612 patients. *Am. J. Med.,* **68,** 344–55.

Mandrup-Poulsen, T., Pociot, F., Mølvig, J., Shapiro, L., Nilsson, P., Emdal, T. *et al.* (1994). Monokine antagonism is reduced in patients with insulin-dependent diabetes melitus. *Diabetes,* **43,** 1242–7.

Mansfield, J. C., Holden, H., Tarlow, J. K., Di Giovine, F. S., McDowell, T. L., Wilson, A. G. *et al.* (1994). Novel genetic association between ulcerative colitis and the anti-inflammatory cytokine interleukin-1 receptor antagonist. *Gastroenterology,* **106,** 637–42.

Mathison, J. C., Wolfson, E., and Ulevitch, R. J. (1988). Participation of tumor necrosis factor in the mediation of gram negative bacterial lipopolysaccharide-induced injury in rabbits. *J. Clin. Invest.,* **81,** 1925–37.

Moncada, S., Palmer, R. M. J., and Higgs, E. A. (1991). Nitric oxide: physiology, pathophysiology, and pharmacology. *Pharmacol. Rev.,* **43,** 109–142.

Ohlsson, K., Bjork, P., Bergenfeldt, M., Hageman, R., and Thompson, R. C. (1990). Interleukin-1 receptor antagonist reduces mortality from endotoxin shock. *Nature,* **348,** 550–2.

Okusawa, S., Gelfand, J. A., Ikejima, T., Connolly, R. J., and Dinarello, C. A. (1988). Interleukin 1 induces a shock-like state in rabbits. Synergism with tumor necrosis factor and the effect of cyclooxygenase inhibition. *J. Clin. Invest.,* **81,** 1162–72.

Opal, S. M., Fisher, C. J. J., Dhainaut, J. F., Vincent, J.-L., Brase, R., Lowry, S. F. *et al.* (1997). Confirmatory interleukin-1 receptor antagonist trial in severe sepsis: a phase III, randomized, double-blind, placebo-controlled, multicenter trial. *Crit. Care Med.,* **25,** 1115–24.

Reinhart, K., Wiegand-Lohnert, C., Grimminger, F., Kaul, M., Withington, S., Treacher, D. *et al.* (1996). Assessment of the safety and efficacy of the monoclonal anti-tumor necrosis factor antibody-fragment, MAK 195F, in patients with sepsis and septic shock: a multicenter, randomized, placebo-controlled, dose- ranging study. *Crit. Care Med.*, **24**, 733–42.

Sands, K. E., Bates, D. W., Lanken, P. N., Graman, P. S., Hibberd, P. L., Kahn, K. L. *et al.* (1997). Epidemiology of sepsis syndrome in 8 academic centers. *JAMA*, **278**, 234–0.

Smith, J. W., Longo, D., Alford, W. G., Janik, J. E., Sharfman, W. H., Gause, B. L *et al.* (1993). The effects of treatment with interleukin-1α on platelet recovery after high-dose carboplatin. *New Engl. J. Med.*, **328**, 756–61.

Smith, J. W., Urba, W. J., Curti, B. D., Elwood, L. J., Steis, R. G., Janik, J. E. *et al.* (1992). The toxic and hematologic effects of interleukin-1 alpha administered in a phase I trial to patients with advanced malignancies. *J. Clin. Oncol.*, **10**, 1141–52.

Stüber, F., Petersen, M., Bokelmann, F., and Schade, U. (1996). A genomic polymorphism within the tumor necrosis factor locus influences plasma tumor necrosis factor alpha concentrations and outcome of patients with severe sepsis. *Crit. Care Med.*, **24**, 381–4.

Tracey, K., Fong, Y., Hesse, D. G., Manogue, K. R., Lee, A. T., Kuo, G. C *et al.* (1987). Anti-cachectin/TNF monoclonal antibodies prevent septic shock during lethal bacteremia. *Nature*, **330**, 662–4.

van der Poll, T., Bueller, H. R., ten Cate, H., Wortel, C. H., Bauer, K. A., van Deventer, S. J. H. *et al.* (1990). Activation of coagulation after administration of tumor necrosis factor to normal subjects. *New Engl. J. Med.*, **322**, 1622–7.

van der Poll, T., van Deventer, S. J. H., Hack, C. E., Wolbink, G. J., Aarden, L. A., Büller, H. R. *et al.* (1991). Effects of leukocytes following injection of tumor necrosis factor into healthy humans. *Blood*, **79**, 693–8.

van Dullemen, H. M., van Deventer, S. J. H., Hommes, D. W., Bijl, H. A., Jansen, J., Tytgat, G. N *et al.* (1995). Treatment of Crohn's disease with anti-tumor necrosis factor chimeric monoclonal antibody (cA2). *Gastroenterology*, **109**, 129–35.

Wakabayashi, G., Gelfand, J. A., Burke, J. F., Thompson, R. C., and Dinarello, C. A. (1991). A specific receptor antagonist for interleukin-1 prevents *Escherichia coli*-induced shock. *FASEB J*, **5**, 338–43.

Watt, I. and Cobby, M. (1996). Recombinant human interleukin-1 receptor antagonist reduces the rate of joint erosion in rheumatoid arthritis. *Arthrit. Rheumat.*, **39**, S123.

Zeni, F., Freeman, B., and Natanson, C. (1997). Anti-inflammatory therapies to treat sepsis and septic shock: a reassessment. *Crit. Care Med.*, **25**, 1095–00

Appendix
Mechanisms of action and clinical uses of Type I interferons

E. J. Bartholomé,[1] F. E. Roufosse,[2] and M. Goldman[3]
Departments of Neurology,[1] Internal Medicine,[2] and Immunology,[3] Hopital Erasme, and Laboratory of Experimental Immunology,[1] Université, Libre de Bruxelles, B-1070 Brussels, Belgium

1 Introduction

Interferons (IFNs) were discovered by two independent groups (Isaacs and Lindenmann, 1957; Nagano and Kojima, 1958) in the late fifties. This was the result of years of studies over the mechanism involved in resistance to viral infection. Infected cells are able to induce resistance in uninfected cells through the paracrine secretion of proteic factors. These proteins have been isolated and called interferons because of their ability to interfere with the viral infections of cells. Besides their anti-viral properties, IFNs have been demonstrated to elicit two other broad categories of biological actions, namely anti-proliferative and immuno-modulatory effects (Langer and Pestka, 1985; Pestka *et al.*, 1987). The most recently discovered IFN, trophoblast-IFN (τ-IFN), seems to have a significant role in maternal recognition of pregnancy and preparation of the endometrium for implantation (Martal *et al.*, 1979; Cross and Roberts, 1991).

Since the initial descriptions, more than 25 different IFNs have been isolated and characterized (Allen and Diaz, 1994). Some of them have been purified and cloned. Thus, purified preparations and recombinant products have become available for clinical use. The anti-viral and anti-proliferative properties of the Type I-IFNs were the first to be extensively studied and used for the therapy of human diseases (Sen and Ransohoff, 1993; Gutterman, 1994). Although long neglected, the immuno-modulatory effects of Type I-IFNs are now exploited for the treatment of human inflammatory diseases (Tilg, 1997). Moreover, the immuno-modulatory properties of Type I-IFNs probably participate to their anti-viral and anti-proliferative effects (Gutterman, 1994). It is likely that the understanding of the mechanisms underlying the contrasting effects of Type I-IFN will help to develop more effective drug regimens for various viral, proliferative or inflammatory diseases.

2 Classification of interferons

The current nomenclature for IFNs was determined by sequence analysis of the IFN genes (Sen and Ransohoff, 1993; Allen and Diaz, 1994; Arnason and Reder, 1994). IFNs were divided into two major classes (see Table A.1). α-IFNs (formerly α1), β-IFN, ω-IFN (formerly α2), and τ-IFN subtypes are designated as Type I-IFNs. There are at least 18 α-IFN non-allelic genes and 6 ω-IFN genes but only one β-IFN gene. Analysis of gene sequences suggests that at least four of the α-IFN genes and five of the ω-IFN genes are pseudo-genes. The α-IFN, ω-IFN, and β-IFN genes have all evolved from the same common ancestor. They have clustered on the short arm of chromosome 9 and are characterized by an unusual intronless structure (Pestka *et al.*, 1987).

All IFNs have secretory peptide sequences, which are cleaved off prior to secretion (Sen and Lengyel, 1992). Mature α-IFNs contain from 165 to 187 amino acids (AA) and there is extensive homology among them. Only some subtypes of α-IFNs are glycosylated. Mature β-IFN has 166 AA and is glycosylated. α-IFNs and β-IFN are 20–40% homologous in terms of nucleic acid and amino acid (AA) sequences. ω-IFN contains 166 AA and shares 57–63% homology with α-IFNs (Adolf, 1987; Mitsui *et al.*, 1993). Mature τ-IFNs contain 172 AA and the predicted AA sequence of the several isoforms reported to date are 45–55% homologous with α-IFNs (Imakawa *et al.*, 1987; Stewart *et al.*, 1987, 1989; Klemann *et al.*, 1990; Charlier *et al.*, 1991; Jarpe *et al.*, 1994).

The only Type II IFN is γ-IFN, which is encoded in a single-copy gene with three introns located on chromosome 12. γ-IFN has 143 amino acids, is glycosylated, and forms a homodimer. There is only slight similarity between segments of β-IFN and γ-IFN. Whereas IFNs-α and β-IFN share most of their biological effects, γ-IFN has a clearly different activity profile. Indeed, the effects of Type I and Type II-IFNs are mediated by different pathways and it is now proposed that the anti-viral properties of γ-IFN reflect its ability to induce α-IFN and β-IFN (Hughes and Baron, 1987; Gessani *et al.*, 1989; Cederblad and Alm, 1991).

Recombinant preparations of the α-2 variant of α-IFNs are now the most commonly used preparation in clinical practice. Named α-2a-, α-2b-, or α-2c-IFN, they are not glycosylated and differ in AA sequence at positions 23 and 34. All three are similar to the human natural form.

In 1981, a novel synthetic α-IFN was synthesized and called consensus IFN. It is a wholly synthetic Type I-IFN developed by scanning several α-IFNs subtypes and assigning the most frequently observed AA in each position. Consensus IFN contains 166 AA residues and has approximately 30% sequence identity with β-IFN and 60% with ω-IFN. Compared to naturally occurring Type I-IFNs, consensus IFN shows similar anti-viral, anti-proliferative, and immuno-modulatory activity. However, specific activity is higher, probably because of a higher affinity for the Type I-IFN receptor (Blatt *et al.*, 1996).

There are two recombinant forms of β-IFN (rec-IFN) used in clinical practice (see Table A.2). β-IFN-1a is generated in Chinese Hamster Ovary cells, is glycosylated, and has the same amino acid sequence as human natural β-IFN. β-IFN-1b is generated in Escherichia coli, is not glycosylated, and lacks an N-terminal methionine residue removed by bacterial ribosomal machinery. Furthermore, the cysteine residue at position 17 has been replaced by a serine residue to avoid inappropriate formation of disulfide bonds with one of the two other cysteine residues in the molecule. These differences of

Table A.1 Comparative properties of Type I and Type II IFNs

	Type I α-IFNs	β-IFN	Type II γ-IFN
Gene location	Short arm of chromosome 9	1	Chromosome 12
Number of genes	>= 18	1	1
Number of AA	165–187	166	143
Glycosylation	Some of the subtypes	Yes	Yes
Superstructure	Monomeric	Monomeric	Homodimeric
Molecular weight	17–25 kD	23 kD	20 or 25 kD
Physical properties	Stable at pH 2, labile at 56°C	6. 8–7. 8	Acid labile, stable at 56°C
Isoelectric point	5. 7–7. 0		8. 6–8. 7
Former names	α₁ or leukocyte-IFN	Fibroblast-IFN	Immune-IFN
Receptor	Unique IFN₁R coded on chromosome 21	IFN₁₁R coded on chromosome 9	

AA: amino acid.

Table A.2   Comparative properties of the different forms of β-IFNs

	Natural human β-IFN	Rec β-IFN-1a	Rec β-IFN-1b
Source	–	*Escherichia coli*	Chinese hamster ovarian cell
Number of AA	166	166	165
Glycosylation	Yes	Yes	No
AA Sequence	–	As natural human β-IFN	Lacks methionine #1 Serine instead of cysteine #17
Molecular weight	23 kD	23 kD	18. 5 kD

AA: amino acid.

primary structure are probably the reason why the specific activity of natural β-IFN and β-IFN-1a is higher than that of β-IFN-1b (Chernajovsky *et al.*, 1984; The IFNB Multiple Sclerosis Study Group, 1993).

IFNs are usually measured by their anti-viral activity in cell culture. However, comparison of the anti-viral activity of different IFNs preparations is quite deceiving, despite the efforts made to define international standards (Pestka *et al.*, 1987). In interpreting data, one must note that, revaluation, in 1993, of the titer of the β-IFN-1b preparation resulted in an approximately five-fold decrease in specific activity (i.e., 45 MU (old units, NIH standards) is now titered at 8 MIU (new units, WHO standards)). In this article, we will use the new units standard, unless otherwise mentioned.

3 Induction and regulation of Type I-IFN synthesis

α-IFNs (formerly leukocyte-IFNs) are induced preferentially in leukocytes by foreign, virus-infected or tumor cells, by bacteria and their products, and by viral envelopes. β-IFN (formerly fibroblast-IFN) is best induced in fibroblasts, epithelial cells, and macrophages by viruses, viral and other foreign nucleic acids, bacteria, mycoplasmae, and protozoa. β-IFN is also induced by interleukin(IL)-2 released by activated T cells, as well as IL-1 and Tumor Necrosis Factor-α (TNF-α) released by activated macrophages (Lowenthal *et al.*, 1989; Osborn *et al.*, 1989). However, most human cells can produce both α-IFN and β-IFN, whereas only certain lymphocytes secrete γ-IFN. Double-stranded (ds) RNA is a potent inducer of both α-IFN and β-IFN, and is thought to be the side-product or mediator responsible for IFN induction during viral infection (Sen and Lengyel, 1992). Polyinosinic polycytidylic acid (Poly I:C), a synthetic analogue of dsRNA, induces β-IFN, α-IFN less, and γ-IFN still less (Arnason and Reder, 1994).

The control of IFN production can be exerted both at transcriptional and post-transcriptional levels. Induction is transient even if the inducing signal is prolonged. The rate of turnover of mRNA is regulated in a protein synthesis-dependent manner. Indeed, induction can be prolonged (super-induction) by protein synthesis inhibitors. Transcriptional regulation depends on regulatory regions extending 200 base pairs 5' from the transcription initiation site. For β-IFN there are two negative regulatory domains numbered NRD-I and NRD-II, and four 'virus responsive' positive regulatory domains (PRD-I to PRD-IV). Two transcription factors belonging to the IFN regulatory factors family, IRF-1 and IRF-2, bind specifically to PRD-I. IRF-2 acts as a transcription repressor and IRF-1 as an activator perhaps through displacement of IRF-2 from DNA (Harada *et al.*, 1989). Interestingly, though IRF-2 transcription is constitutive, IRF-1 transcription is induced by IFNs and is probably important for priming. Priming is the process by which Type I-IFNs are able to prime uninfected cells to produce IFN in response to stimuli that otherwise fail to result in IFN production (Isaacs and Burke, 1958; Stewart *et al.*, 1971). The PRD-II site resembles NF-κB transcription factor binding site and many agents that can activate NF-κB (i.e. viruses, dsRNA, phorbol 12-myristate 13-acetate, IL-1, TNF-α, or HTLV-1 tax protein) promote β-IFN induction through PRD-II. The regulation of α-IFN transcription includes also a virus-responsive PRD-I like region but no NF-κB binding site. Differences in the sequence of nucleotides in their regulatory regions account for some of the variations in the virus activability among the different α-IFN genes.

4 Type I-IFN receptor and signal transduction

During the last years, major advances have been made in the characterization of the membrane receptor and molecular pathways underlying the actions of Type I-IFNs.

4.1 The Type I-IFN receptor

α-IFNs and β-IFN share, and even compete for, the same receptor (IFNIR). This receptor is composed of three subunits detected by affinity cross-linking (Van den Broecke and Pfeffer, 1988; Benoit *et al.*, 1993). Of the three, two have been purified and their cDNA cloned (Uze *et al.*, 1990; Novick *et al.*, 1994). Their genes are localized on chromosome 21. The respective role of each subunit is under extensive study (Langer and Pestka, 1988; Pfeffer and Constantinescu, 1997). As α-IFN and β-IFN induce partially different effects in the same cells, major efforts have been made to isolate a second receptor but only one receptor has been identified so far. Another explanation may be receptor heterogeneity leading to α-IFN or β-IFN preferential binding and differential intracellular signaling. This heterogeneity may consist in conformational, glycosylation, or subunit recruitment variability. It is also possible that the binding of either α-IFN or β-IFN to the common receptor results in conformational changes responsible for specific intracellular signals (Fig. A.1, Part A). For example, it has already been demonstrated that β-IFN, but not α2-IFN or α8-IFN, induces the tyrosine phosphorylation of a IFNIR associated protein (Abramovich *et al.*, 1994; Platanias *et al.*, 1994).

IFNIR are displayed on nearly all human cell lines and tissues, and are species-specific. After binding with their ligand, they are down-regulated and do not recycle to an appreciable extent (Arnason and Reder, 1994; Pfeffer and Constantinescu, 1997).

4.2 Intracellular signal transduction

IFNIR occupation results in activation of at least two intracellular pathways. The first one involves two Janus protein kinases, Jak1 and Tyk2. It results in activation of early IFNs-stimulated genes (ISG) transcription. The second path involves protein kinase C (PKC) and may be important for post-transcriptional regulation (Sen and Lengyel, 1992;

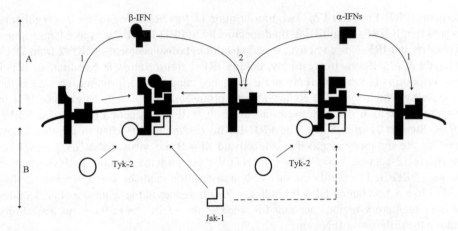

Fig. A.1 Hypothetical scheme of Type I-IFNs engagement on their common receptor and early intracellular consequences. Part A: (1) Receptor heterogeneity may lead to α-IFN or β-IFN preferential binding; or (2) the engagement of either α-IFN or β-IFN on the common receptor results in conformational changes responsible for specific intracellular signals. Part B: β-IFN engagement on IFNIR better activates Jak-1 than α-IFNs do.

Arnason and Reder, 1994; David, 1995; Platanias, 1995; Pfeffer and Constantinescu, 1997).

Janus protein kinases pathway

Janus protein kinases are activated by various cytokine receptors. Ligand-specific responses are probably obtained through the binding of Jak1 or Tyk2 to the occupied receptors; this binding permitting only ligand specific substrates to be phosphorylated by the bound kinase. It may explain why α-IFN or β-IFN engagement differentially activate Jak1 and Tyk2. At least in some cell lines, β-IFN activates Jak1 more than α-IFN does (Fig. A.1, Part B). Moreover, cells defective in Tyk2 retain partial sensitivity to β-IFN but not to α-IFN. The β-IFN-Jak1 pathway is believed to be closer to the ancestral IFN signaling system. Recruitment of Tyk2 would then represent evolutionary diversification as does multiplicity of α-IFNs.

Jak1 and Tyk2 are already activated a few seconds after occupation of IFNIR. This activation leads to the tyrosine phosphorylation of intracellular proteins called signal transducers and activators of transcription (STATs). Phosphorylated STATs form multisubunit complexes with other cytoplasmic proteins, which penetrate the nucleus to regulate ISG transcription. STAT1a (formerly STAT-91 in reference to its molecular weight), STAT1b (STAT-84), and STAT2 (STAT-113) associate with a 48-kD protein (p48) to form the IFN-stimulated gene factor 3 (ISGF-3). p48 is able to bind with low affinity to the IFN stimulus–response element (ISRE), which is a promoter element of ISG, but the association of p48 with the phosphorylated STATs dramatically increase its ISRE affinity and modify slightly its DNA sequence specificity. ISGF-3 is indeed the activating transcription factor for α-IFN and β-IFN stimulated genes.

However, STAT1a is also able to form homodimers associated or not with p48. This complex is designated α-IFN activation factor (AAF) and has in fact indistinguishable properties from the γ-IFN activation factor (GAF). GAF is rapidly activated after binding of γ-IFN to its unique receptor (IFNIIR) and activates the other IFN response element, the γ-IFN activation site (GAS). Genes including this promoter were believed to be purely γ-IFN responsive. Nevertheless, two α-IFN activated transcription factors, AAF and AAF2 (thought to be a dimer of phosphorylated STAT3, another member of the STAT protein family), are also able to activate GAS. Conversely, γ-IFN is also able to potentiate Type I-IFNs response element (ISRE) activation, by inducing p48 and STAT1 synthesis. In addition, γ-IFN also inhibits the repression of already induced ISG, prolonging by this way the effect of Type I-IFNs gene induction.

Protein kinase C mediated effects

In Type I-IFNs responsive cell lines, α-IFN rapidly activates selectively, calcium independent, β and ε subspecies, of PKC through the production of diacylglycerol, a lipid derived second messenger. Experiments on cell lines have shown that, though Janus Kinases and PKC activation is rapid, levels of ISG mRNA increase linearly for 12 h after IFN addition. Moreover, IFN induced ISG transcription remains high for more than 20 h. Stauroporine, a protein kinase inhibitor, blocks STAT phosphorylation and inhibits induction and accumulation of ISG. H7, a selective inhibitor of PKC, does not affect STATs activation. However, in H7 treated cell lines, ISG transcription is transient and ISG mRNA level peaks after 2 h. Similarly, in Type I-IFNs resistant cell lines, α-IFN treatment results in STAT activation, transient ISG transcription, but no PKC activation. These results suggest that PKC activation is important for maintenance of the response to Type I-IFNs. The process involved occurs after the ISG transcription initiation and may be mRNA stabilization.

Janus protein kinases and PKC pathways interact in different ways. First, IRF-1 induction is PKC dependent. As ISGF-3, IRF-1 is able to bind to ISRE. It is proposed that IRF-1 participates in maintaining an elevated transcription rate initiated by ISGF-3. As described before, IRF-1 also activates the transcription of the Type I-IFNs genes and may be so able to prime and amplify the cellular responses to Type I-IFNs. Moreover, PKC is responsible for the serine phosphorylation of STAT1 and STAT3, thus increasing their transcription activation potential.

Other pathways involved

Multiple pathways are involved in the Type I-IFNs induced-ISG activation. The extracellular signal regulated-kinase-2, ERK2, one of the mitogen-activated-protein serine kinases (MAPK), has been found to be tyrosine phosphorylated and thus activated after IFNIR engagement. β-IFN induced-ERK2 activation causes STAT1 and ERK2 to co-precipitate. Furthermore, expression of dominant negative MAPK inhibited α-IFN induced-ISG early transcription, suggesting that MAPK may regulate early ISG transcription by modifying the Jak-STAT cascade (David *et al.*, 1995). The β-IFN induced activation of ERK2 is partially blocked by the inhibition of the serine kinase component of the phosphatidylinositol 3-kinase (PI3'-kinase). PI3'-kinase belongs to another pathway potentially important for Type I-IFNs intracellular signaling. PI3'-kinase is a multisubunit complex that possesses serine kinase and lipid kinase activities. Serine kinase activity of PI3'-kinase is rapidly induced by α/β-IFNs and causes serine phosphorylation of the insulin receptor substrate-1 (IRS-1). IRS-1 plays a critical role in the signal transduction of insulin and insulin-like growth factor-1

(IGF-1) and its function is essential for insulin- and IGF-1-induced proliferation of neoplastic hematopoietic cells. Type I-IFNs may in this way antagonize insulin and IGF-1 signaling pathways through competition for the access to IRS-1 (David *et al.*, 1995; Platanias, 1995; Uddin *et al.*, 1997).

Type I-IFNs also induce rapid tyrosine phosphorylation of the vav guanine nucleotide exchange factor (p95vav). Although the exact function of p95vav is unknown, its structure suggests it may be involved in the transcriptional regulation of the protooncogenes c-myc (Einat *et al.*, 1985; Platanias and Sweet, 1994).

5 Type I-IFNs biological effects

Anti-viral, anti-proliferative and immuno-regulatory effects of Type I-IFNs have been described and partially characterized. Most of these effects are mediated through the synthesis of more than 30 proteins coded by the ISG. Two main mechanisms are involved in the anti-viral and anti-proliferative effects of Type I-IFNs. Some of the proteins induced by Type I-IFNs directly interfere with viral replication or cell cycle through intracellular mechanisms. Other Type I-IFNs induced proteins modify the intercellular signaling system and are so able to potentiate the anti-viral or anti-proliferative reactions of the immune system. Type I-IFNs also inhibit protozoan and bacterial replication and spreading through their immuno-stimulatory capacities (Weinstock Guttman *et al.*, 1995).

5.1 Anti-viral effects of Type I-IFNs

The intracellular anti-viral effects of Type I-IFNs are mediated through inhibition of viral penetration and replication, synthesis of mRNA, translation of viral proteins, and viral assembly and release. For a given virus in a specific cell line, one step may be predominant, but more than one step is usually involved. The proteins involved in some of these inhibitions have been identified, while the mechanisms underlying others remains undetermined. Some viruses, principally DNA viruses, are relatively resistant to IFNs. Other viruses are able to counter the effects of IFNs through the selective inhibition of IFNs inducible proteins. Moreover, adenoviruses and hepatitis virus B are able to impair the transcription activation of ISG by IFNs (Sen and Lengyel, 1992; Sen and Ransohoff, 1993; Arnason and Reder, 1994; Decker, 1997).

The 2′,5′-oligoadenylate synthetase

In human cells, Type I-IFNs induce the synthesis of different isoforms of the 2′–5′-oligoadenylate synthetase (2–5-OAS), which oligomerize adenylate. Their activation requires the binding of certain species of cellular or viral dsRNA. Oligoadenylate, in turn, activates another Type I-IFNs inducible enzyme, the oligoadenylate-dependent RNAase (RNAase L). The activated RNAase L then degrades mRNA transcribed from both viral and cellular genes. Inhibition of RNAase L does not only block the anti-viral effects of Type I-IFNs against some viruses but also the anti-proliferative effects on murine transformed cells. Little is known about the physiological roles of 2–5-OAS and RNAase L. Anyway the selective degradation of mRNA transcribed from cellular genes involved in growth control may be sufficient to mediate some of the Type I-IFNs induced anti-proliferative effects.

The dsRNA dependent protein kinase

The dsRNA dependent protein kinase (pKR) is another example of Type I-IFNs induced enzyme, whose activation depends on the binding of dsRNA. The dsRNA binding causes pKR auto-phosphorylation and consecutive activation. Activated pKR then selectively phosphorylates the α subunit of the eukariotic peptide chain initiation factor 2 (eIF-2α) preventing its recycling to an active form and thus inhibiting initiation of translation. The importance of pKR in the anti-viral effects of Type I-IFNs is further demonstrated by the numerous counter-mechanisms viruses have developed. Some viruses (EBV, Adenovirus) produce RNA that inhibits dsRNA binding to the pKR without activating it. Others can synthesize or induce the cell to synthesize inhibitors of the pKR. Vaccinia virus even encodes an analogue of eIF2-α which competes with eIF2-α for phosphorylation by the pKR.

As for RNAase L, pKR also has anti-proliferative effects in addition to its anti-viral properties. Selective inhibition of the pKR abolishes the anti-proliferative effects of IRF1. pKR may also play a role in the immuno-modulatory effects of Type I-IFNs through its ability to inactivate the NFkB inhibitor, IkB.

Other mechanisms involved in anti-viral effects of Type I-IFNs

Other mechanisms, such as inhibition of viral penetration and replication, have been demonstrated in Type I-IFNs induced viral resistance but the processes involved are barely understood. For example, the Type I-IFNs induced Mx proteins inhibit viral replication but the mechanism of action remains unknown. Conversely, the roles of many Type I-IFNs induced proteins are still under investigation.

Clinical uses of the anti-viral properties of Type I-IFNs

α-IFNs have been shown to be effective therapy for up to 40% of adult-acquired chronic hepatitis B viral infections. Many patients with chronic hepatitis C viral infection also benefit from α-IFNs therapy but the relapse rate remains high (Main and Handley, 1992; Gutterman, 1994).

α-IFNs are also widely used for the treatment of condyloma acumata and juvenile laryngeal papillomatosis, and encouraging results have been obtained with systemic or intralesional α/β-IFNs treatment of human papilloma virus-associated cervical intraepithelial neoplasms (Gutterman, 1994; Penna *et al.*, 1994).

α/β-IFNs have been shown to have clinical effects in various other viral infections, such as genital warts, genital and muco-cutaneous HSV infections, localized herpes zoster, CMV infections of renal transplants, and prophylaxis of rhinovirus colds (Hayden *et al.*, 1986; Birch *et al.*, 1992). However, IFNs treatment is generally associated with excessive side-effects and/or inferior clinical benefits, when compared to conventional anti-viral therapies (Main and Handley, 1992).

Despite proven antiretroviral effects in HIV-infected persons, the combination of α/β-IFNs with zidovudine in advanced HIV infection is associated with only transient benefit and excessive hematologic toxicity. Nevertheless, α-IFNs are effective for the treatment of HIV-related thrombocytopenia resistant to zidovudine therapy (Ellis *et al.*, 1987; Marroni *et al.*, 1994) and may be more potent if administered early in the course of HIV infection (Gutterman, 1994). α/β-IFNs therapy of malignant complications of HIV and HTLV-1 infection is discussed in the next chapter.

Intraventricular α-IFN is the best available treatment to date for subacute sclerosing panencephalitis, the persistent infection of the central nervous system (CNS) by measles (Anlar *et al.*, 1997).

5.2 Anti-proliferative effects of Type I-IFNs

The anti-proliferative effects of Type I-IFNs are mediated through three different kinds of mechanisms. As for anti-viral effects, direct intracellular mechanisms and immunity activation mediate the anti-proliferative effects of Type I-IFNs. In addition, some of the Type I-IFNs anti-proliferative properties involve the regulation of paracrine secretion of tumor growth factors.

Intracellular and paracrine pathways

Intracellular pathways involved in Type I-IFNs induced cell-cycle lengthening are less well known than those involved in their anti-viral effects. In addition to the inhibition of both RNAase L and pKR described before, α/β-IFNs also blocks the induction of ornithine decarboxylase, an enzyme critical for synthesis of growth-promoting polyamines. Interestingly, α-IFNs have been shown to inhibit the expression of cellular protooncogenes, such as c-myc and c-fos, and to reverse the phenotype of c-Harvey-ras-transformed cells. As previously mentioned, these effects may be, at least for c-myc, mediated through the phosphorylation of p95vav (Platanias, 1995). Protooncogenes are critical for cell cycle regulation but further experiments are needed to confirm their role in the anti-proliferative effects of Type I-IFNs.

Malignant cells may be able to stimulate adjacent tumoral cell growth through the paracrine secretion of growth factors. This process, called paracrine growth loop, can be inhibited by α-IFNs in hairy cell leukemia and chronic lymphocytic leukemia. α-IFNs have also been demonstrated to disrupt the paracrine IL-6 growth loop in myeloma cells. Surprisingly, endogenous IL-6 secretion after α-IFNs treatment is not inhibited but even enhanced. The growth inhibition seems to result from a dramatic decrease of the IL-6 receptor α and β chains (Schwabe *et al.*, 1994; Platanias, 1995). Similarly, in human bone marrow stromal cells, α-IFNs inhibit the production of certain growth factor and increase the production of the IL-1 receptor antagonist, IL-1ra (Aman *et al.*, 1994).

Disappearance of the clones bearing chromosomal abnormalities during α-IFNs treatment have been observed in chronic myelogenic leukemia (CML) and in the idiopathic hypereosinophilic syndrome (Roth and Foon, 1986; Malbrain *et al.*, 1996). This clonal deletion may be caused by stimulation of the immune-specific cytotoxic activity or by the induction of programed cell death, namely apoptosis (Knight *et al.*, 1993). During α-IFN treatment of CML, Thiele *et al.*, observed partial normalization of the morphology of the bone marrow cells, which was associated with an increased number of cells undergoing apoptosis (Thiele *et al.*, 1996). Recent experiments showed that α-IFNs inhibit colony formation of CML bone marrow stem cells. Furthermore, this inhibition may be related to the up-regulation of FAS-receptor on these cells by α-IFNs and, thus, be mediated by FAS-receptor dependent apoptosis (Selleri *et al.*, 1997). However, α-IFNs effects on apoptosis are cell-type dependent. α-IFNs did not activate apoptosis on freshly isolated chronic-phase CML cells (Zinzani *et al.*, 1994b) and on cultured human renal cell carcinoma cells (Nonomura *et al.*, 1996), but α-IFNs have shown anti-apoptotic effects on myeloma cells (Egle *et al.*, 1996), on B cell chronic lymphocytic leukemia cells (Jewell,

1996), on Burkitt lymphoma cells (Milner *et al.*, 1993), on T cell clones from allergic patients (Kaneko *et al.*, 1997), and on a Th2 clone from a patient with the idiopathic hypereosinophilic syndrome (Schandene, personal communication). Interestingly, α-IFNs induce apoptosis in squamous cell skin cancer cell lines. However, this effect is limited to the cell lines sensitive to the cytotoxic effects of α-IFNs (Rodriguez Villanueva and McDonnell, 1995). The pathways involved in α-IFNs regulation of apoptosis remains undefined. Despite α-IFNs induced-up-regulation of FAS receptor on myeloma cells and on B cell chronic lymphocytic leukemia cells, these cells became resistant to FAS mediated apoptosis after α-IFNs treatment (Panayiotidis *et al.*, 1995; Egle *et al.*, 1996). The anti-apoptotic effects of α-IFNs correlated with up-regulation of bcl-2 in B cell chronic lymphocytic leukemia cells (Jewell, 1996) and with up-regulation of STAT2 in T cell clones (Kaneko *et al.*, 1997).

As previously mentioned, Type I-IFNs may inhibit the insulin and IGF-1 signaling pathway at the IRS-1 level. It has also been reported that α-IFNs may down-regulate the expression of the IGF-1 receptor tyrosine kinase (Thulasi *et al.*, 1996). The IGF-1 signaling pathway appears to play an important role in the growth of various hematologic and solid malignancies, including breast cancer, rhabdomyosarcomas, osteosarcomas, and Wilms' tumors (Platanias, 1995).

Angiogenesis is an essential process for vascular and also non-vascular tumor growth and metastasis. α/β-IFNs may inhibit angiogenesis through the down-regulation of the expression of the angiogenic basic fibroblast growth factor in human carcinomas (Singh *et al.*, 1995). However, β-IFN, but not α-IFNs, inhibits the growth of cultured smooth muscular cells induced by platelet derived growth factor, IL-1 and TNF-α. As these cytokines are also able to induce β-IFN production in these cells, β-IFN is a potential auto-regulatory factor in smooth muscular cells (Palmer and Libby, 1992).

Despite difficulties in comparing Type I-IFNs specific activities, some studies suggest differences between α- and β-IFNs anti-proliferative effects. Thus, β-IFN exerts greater *in vitro* anti-proliferative activity on embryonal carcinoma and melanoma cells, whereas α-IFNs show greater activity on hematopoietic malignant cells (Roth and Foon, 1986; Pfeffer and Constantinescu, 1997). Type I-IFNs have direct anti-proliferative effects on many other malignant cells, which have justified therapeutic trials.

Clinical uses of the anti-proliferative properties of Type I-IFNs

Although α-IFNs antitumor activity has been seen both *in vitro* and *in vivo* in some solid malignancies, the most impressive responses have occurred in the hematologic malignancies. More than 90% of patients with hairy cell leukemia have a sustained recovery of their peripheral blood cell counts with alpha interferon therapy. Approximately 50% of patients with low-grade non-Hodgkin's lymphoma and cutaneous T cell lymphoma demonstrate a response to alpha interferon. More than 80% of patients CML have a response to alpha interferon, and in one study, nearly half of the patients with response had complete suppression of the Philadelphia chromosome clone on at least one examination (Roth and Foon, 1986; Olsen and Bunn, 1995). In contrast, undifferentiated acute myeloid leukemias and myelodysplasic syndromes are resistant to α-IFNs therapy. Similarly, α-IFNs therapy is only effective in patients with early stage B cell chronic lymphocytic leukemia and not in patients with advanced disease (Foon *et al.*, 1985; McSweeney *et al.*, 1993). These clinical results confirm experimental data on cell lines showing that α-IFNs are able to reverse the phenotype of only partially transformed cells (Gutterman, 1994), suggesting that α-IFNs may be more potent when used early in the disease course.

The combination of zidovudine and α-IFN has clinical activity in HTLV-1-related adult T cell leukemia-lymphoma (Gill *et al.*, 1995).

A 20–40% major tumor response rate has been seen with various α-IFNs in the treatment of patients with early-stage, acquired immuno-deficiency syndrome-related Kaposi sarcomas (Miles *et al.*, 1990). Recent studies strongly support the role of human herpes virus-8 (HHV-8) as the cause of Kaposi sarcomas (Foreman *et al.*, 1997). As HHV-8 replication is sensible to different anti-viral drugs (Kedes and Ganem, 1997), the effects of α-IFNs on Kaposi sarcomas are probably not only related to the previously described ability of α-IFNs to inhibit angiogenesis. α-IFN treatment can also induce dramatic regression in children with life-threatening pulmonary hemangiomas (Folkman and Shing, 1992).

In patients suffering from carcinoid tumor, α-IFNs therapy causes improvement of symptoms in a majority of patients and tumor regression in a smaller fraction (Oberg, 1992).

In collected studies, an overall response rate of 15% was obtained with various schedules of α-IFNs alone in metastatic or unresectable renal cell carcinomas and in diffuse malignant melanomas. β-IFN and combination regimens with conventional chemotherapy and other biologics, such as IL-2, are being investigated. A 45% response rate in ovarian carcinomas has been reported but α-IFNs remains less active than conventional cytotoxics. Trials of α-IFNs in patients with breast, colon, and lung cancers indicate that it has little activity against them (Koeller, 1989; Balmer, 1990). However, the experience of CML suggest that α/β-IFNs therapy may be more potent when used sooner in the evolution of the diseases. Interestingly, α-2b-IFN treatment of primary high risk malignant melanomas delays recurrence and prolongs survival after surgery (Kirkwood *et al.*, 1996).

Because the rec-α-IFNs were the first rec-IFNs available for clinical trials, they were the first to be studied. Despite the previously mentioned differential anti-proliferative effects of α- and β-IFNs, and the better tolerance of β-IFN at high dose regimens, clinical trials in human cancers using β-IFN instead of α-IFNs have not yet proved greater activity of β-IFN. β-IFN is even less effective than α-2b-IFN in CML (Aulitzky *et al.*, 1993).

5.3 Immuno-modulatory effects of α/β-IFNs

Surprisingly, the immuno-modulatory effects of Type I-IFNs were neglected for a long time after their discovery. However, α-IFNs were the first cytokines ever described, purified, cloned, and finally clinically used with clear-cut beneficial results (Belardelli and Gresser, 1996). In addition to their anti-viral and anti-proliferative properties, Type I-IFNs display a wide range of immuno-modulatory effects, which can be roughly divided into Th1-Th2 response regulatory effects, autoimmunity promoting effects, pro-inflammatory effects, and, finally, anti-inflammatory effects. Indeed, immuno-modulatory effects of α/β-IFNs are now used or explored for the treatment of several disorders of immune origin (Belardelli and Gresser, 1996; Tilg, 1997).

Type I-IFNs and the induction of Th1 or Th2 responses

Experiments in mice have shown that T helper (Th) cells can display two different profiles of cytokine secretion. Th1 responses are characterized by IL-2 and γ-IFN production but little or no secretion of IL-4 and IL-5, and result in macrophage activation, delayed type hypersensitivity (DTH) and IgG2a synthesis. Conversely, Th2 responses are characterized by IL-4 and IL-5 production, and result in eosinophilia, and IgE and IgG1 synthesis. Long-term, established human CD4+ T cell clones exhibit a Th1- or Th2-like cytokine secretion profile probably reminiscent of the mouse responses. In addition, human CD4+ T-cell clones with an intermediate cytokine profile, known as Th0, have been described (Romagnani, 1992, 1994). Shift from one to another type of cytokine profile does not lead to increased or decreased inflammatory responses but results in different types of immune responses, and that is why the Type I-IFNs effects on these responses are described separately.

Several *in vitro* and *in vivo* experiments are in accord with the hypothesis of Romagnani that α-IFNs and IL-12 are important inducers of Th0-like or Th1-like instead of Th2 responses in human (Romagnani, 1994). First, IL-4-induced IgE production by normal human lymphocytes is suppressed by α-IFNs (Pene *et al.*, 1988). In addition, T cell clones generated in the presence of α-IFNs display predominantly Th0- or Th1-like responses (Parronchi *et al.*, 1992, 1996; Demeure *et al.*, 1994). Moreover, α/β-IFNs inhibit IL-5 production by human CD4+ T cells (Schandene *et al.*, 1996; Schandene *et al.*, unpublished). However, this effect is selective and, in the same experiments, α/β-IFNs did not modulate or even up-regulated the secretion of the other Th2 cytokine, IL-4. α-IFNs and IL-12 secreted by macrophages are essential for the poly I:C induced Th1 responses (Manetti *et al.*, 1995).

However, in mice, α/β-IFNs inhibit *in vitro* splenic leukocytes IL-12 and γ-IFN production (Cousens *et al.*, 1997). Recent experiments in our laboratory showed suppression of the IL-12 secretion by dendritic cells generated from the blood of healthy humans in the presence of β-IFN. Cultured dendritic cells usually stimulate T cells to produce Th1 cytokines, but in our experiments dendritic cells generated, in presence of β-IFN, induced Th2 instead of Th1 responses (Bartholomé, *et al.*, unpublished). This may help to explain the conflicting results obtained concerning the effects of α/β-IFNs on γ-IFN secretion. In addition to the previously described effects of α-IFNs on the development of Th1-like clones, α/β-IFNs increased the number of γ-IFN secreting cells in short term culture *in vitro* (Brinkmann *et al.*, 1993) and *in vivo*, but only during the first three months of treatment of MS patients (Dayal *et al.*, 1995). However, other experiments demonstrated *in vitro* and *in vivo* β-IFN-induced inhibition of γ-IFN secretion from stimulated T cells (Panitch *et al.*, 1987; Noronha *et al.*, 1993a; Milo and Panitch, 1995; Crucian *et al.*, 1996; Rep *et al.*, 1996). APCs are indeed an important factor in the generation of Th1- or Th2-like responses. Some experiments suggest that APCs may also influence the type of Th response through differential expression of two co-stimulatory molecules, B7–1 (CD80) and B7–2 (CD86), expression (Freeman *et al.*, 1995; Kuchroo *et al.*, 1995). B7–1 expression preferentially leads to Th1-like responses, whereas B7–2 leads to Th2-like responses. Recent experiments showed that β-IFN therapy of MS patients reduces the number of circulating B7–1-positive B cells and increases the number of B7–2-positive monocytes (Genc *et al.*, 1997). Thus, discrepancy between *in vitro* effects on purified T cells and *in vivo* effects may results from the *in vivo* involvement of non T cells such as APCs.

α/β-IFNs stimulate *in vitro* and *in vivo* IL-10 production of T and non-T cells (Byskosh and Reder, 1995; Porrini *et al.*, 1995; Aman *et al.*, 1996; Calabresi *et al.*, 1996; Rep *et al.*, 1996; Rudick *et al.*, 1996; Corssmit *et al.*, 1997). IL-10 is mainly an anti-inflammatory and immuno-suppressive cytokine, and α/β-IFNs-induced secretion of IL-10 may mediate some of the α/β-IFNs anti-inflammatory and Th2 promoting effects (Goldman *et al.*, 1997). β-IFN also increases the secretion of another mainly immuno-suppressive cytokine, TGF-β in stimulated T cells (Noronha *et al.*, 1993b).

Autoimmunity and the immuno-modulatory effects of α/β-IFNs

The most striking evidence of the importance of the immuno-modulatory effects of α/β-IFNs has been provided by the exacerbation or occurrence, during α-IFNs treatment, of diseases involving altered immune functions (Arnason and Reder, 1994; Vial and Descotes, 1995; Belardelli and Gresser, 1996). The diseases reported are numerous and are listed in Table A.3. However, these unwanted effects are rare, which is probably the reason why they have seldom been reported during treatment with the less used β-IFN (Durelli *et al.*, 1997). Conversely, an acid-labile form of IFN has been extracted from the serum of patients with a variety of autoimmune disorders, such as lupus patients, as well as in the serum of patients with advanced AIDS (Francis *et al.*, 1992; Skurkovich *et al.*, 1993; Vial and Descotes, 1995).

The mechanisms underlying the exacerbation of autoimmune disorders by α-IFNs remain undefined. During at least three months of α-IFNs treatment for hairy cell leukemia or hepatitis C viral infection, the new occurrence or the increase in titre of a wide range of auto-antibodies has been demonstrated in at least four prospective studies (Mayet *et al.*, 1989; Kalkner *et al.*, 1990; Saracco *et al.*, 1990; Fattovich *et al.*, 1992; Vial and Descotes, 1995). The titer of previously positive auto-antibodies, mainly antinuclear antibodies (ANA), liver kidney microsomal antibodies (LKM), and smooth muscles antibodies (SMA), usually increased. Induced antibodies were mostly ANA, SMA, parietal cell antibodies, thyroid microsomal antibodies, and thyroglobulin antibodies. Development, during α-IFNs therapy, of functionally relevant anti-phospholipid antibodies have been reported (Becker *et al.*, 1994). During β-IFN treatment in MS patients,

Table A.3 Diseases whose occurrence or exacerbation have been reported during α-IFNs therapy

Auto-immune diseases	Diseases involving altered cell-mediated immune functions
Thyroiditis	Psoriasis
Auto-immune thrombocytopenic purpura	Cutaneous leucocytoplasic vasculitis
Auto-immune hemolytic anemia	Lichen planus
Insulin-dependent diabetes mellitus	Minimal-change nephropathy
Systemic lupus erythematosus	Interstitial nephritis
Rheumatoid-like arthritis	Membrano-proliferative glomerulonephritis
Mixed connective tissue disease	Interstitial pneumonitis
Auto-immune hepatitis	Sarcoidosis
Biliary cirrhosis	Ulcerative colitis
Bullous pemphigus and pemphigoid	

similar induction or increase in titer of ANA, LKM, SMA, and anti-thyroid antibodies have been recently reported (Durelli *et al.*, 1997).

The up-regulation of the production of auto-antibodies may be due to a direct effect of α/β-IFNs on the human B-lymphocytes (Harfast *et al.*, 1981) or be secondary to the activation of auto-reactive T helper-cells, which in turn stimulate B cell immunoglobulin synthesis (Rep *et al.*, 1996).

T cell activation is probably also an important step in the induction by α-IFNs of diseases involving altered cell-mediated immune functions (see Table A.3). Interestingly, strong expression of HLA-DR (class II) molecules have been found on thyrocytes of patients suffering from thyroid disorders induced by α-2a-IFN plus rec-IL-2 therapy (Pichert *et al.*, 1990). Similarly, on autopsy, pancreases of children who die at presentation of insulin-dependent diabetes mellitus, the earliest defined immunological event appears to be expression of α-IFNs by the insulin-containing β cells. Secretion of α-IFNs is associated with hyper-expression of HLA class I molecules (HLA-I) on all the endocrine cells and with aberrant expression of HLA class II molecules (HLA-II) specifically on β cells (Foulis, 1996). Moreover, α-IFNs induced-diabetes in transgenic mice has been proven to be dependent on the over-expression of a costimulatory molecule, B7–2, on the auto-reactive Th1-cells (Chakrabarti *et al.*, 1996). Activation of auto-reactive Th cells or T cytotoxic cells may be due to an abnormally efficacious antigenic presentation of auto-antigens due to the up-regulation of the expression of HLA-I, the aberrant expression of HLA-II on usually HLA-II negative cells, and the up-regulation of co-stimulatory molecules on T cells.

In the particular case of IDDM, α/β-IFNs may aggravate the disease through the inhibition of the insulin intracellular signaling pathway at the level of IRS-1 (discussed before) and thus enhance insulin resistance. Furthermore, recent experiments have proven that the IFNs induced-transcription factor, IRF-1, plays a central role in the regulation of the expression of HLA-I and HLA-II genes *in vivo* (Hobart *et al.*, 1997). The observation that mice lacking IRF-1 display reduced incidence and severity of antigen-induced autoimmune diseases provides new insight into the mechanisms involved in IFNs-induced autoimmunity (Tada *et al.*, 1997).

Pro-inflammatory effects of Type I-IFNs

Type I- and Type II-IFNs enhance the expression of HLA-I on a wide variety of cell Types (Basham and Merigan, 1983). Type I- and Type II-IFNs also enhance HLA-II expression on human monocytes *in vitro* (Steeg *et al.*, 1982; Basham and Merigan, 1983; Basham *et al.*, 1984; Sztein *et al.*, 1984). However, γ-IFN is much more effective than α/β-IFNs in enhancing HLA-I and HLA-II expression (Basham *et al.*, 1984). We recently demonstrated that β-1a-IFN enhances HLA-II expression on other potent antigen presenting cells (APCs), dendritic cells generated from the blood of healthy volunteers (Bartholomé, *et al.*, unpublished). γ-IFN, but not β-IFN, is able to enhance HLA-II expression on adult or fetal cultured human astrocytes and on astrocytoma cell lines. Moreover, α/β-IFNs are able to inhibit *in vitro* γ-IFN-enhanced expression of HLA-II on cultured astrocytes (Barna *et al.*, 1989; Ransohoff *et al.*, 1991; Satoh *et al.*, 1995) and on human monocytes (Panitch *et al.*, 1989). Antagonism of Type I-IFNs to γ-IFN-induced HLA-II up-regulation happens most likely at the level of transcription (Fertsch Ruggio *et al.*, 1988; Ransohoff *et al.*, 1991; Devajyothi *et al.*, 1993). Due to the differential effects of α/β-IFNs on HLA-II expression in the presence or absence of γ-IFN, it is difficult to infer the resulting *in vivo* effects of α/β-IFNs therapy. This effect may be different from one tissue to another and from one disease to another, depending on the level of γ-IFN in the micro-environment. On human monocytes, α/β-IFNs therapy enhances *in vivo* HLA-II expression, at least at short term (Hawkins *et al.*, 1984; Spear *et al.*, 1987; Schiller *et al.*, 1990).

Moreover, β-1b-IFN therapy seems to regulate differentially the three subtypes of HLA-II, namely HLA-DP, HLA-DR, and HLA-DQ. *In vivo*, β-IFN preferentially increases HLA-DQ expression on monocytes (Spear *et al.*, 1987), whereas *in vitro* β-IFN selectively inhibits γ-IFN-induced HLA-DQ, but not HLA-DR or HLA-DP expression on monocytes (Soilu Hanninen *et al.*, 1995). It is an important issue since T suppressor (Ts) cells have been said to recognize antigen in a HLA-DQ-restricted manner (Hirayama *et al.*, 1987; Salgame *et al.*, 1991). However, the results of the different studies of the effects of Type I-IFNs on Ts cell activity are conflicting. Some experiments in mice and healthy humans have shown α/β-IFNs-induced *in vitro* inhibition of Ts cell generation and activity (Fradelizi and Gresser, 1982; Knop *et al.*, 1982, 1987), whereas others have demonstrated *in vitro* activation of Ts cells by α/β-IFNs (Schapner *et al.*, 1983; Noronha, Toscas and Jensen, 1990; Noronha, Toscas and Jensen, 1992). *In vivo*, β-1b-IFN, but not α-IFNs, increased Ts cell function in MS patients (Hirsch and Johnson, 1986; O'Gorman, Oger and Kastrukoff, 1987; Noronha *et al.*, 1994). Similarly, γ-IFN has been shown to stimulate Ts cell induction or to have no effect on Ts cell functions (Noronha *et al.*, 1992; Noma and Dorf, 1985). These contrasting effects may be due to heterogeneity of Ts cells and to differences in the tests used to evaluate Ts cell activity. In fact, there is growing evidence suggesting that the so-called suppressive functions may not be ascribed to a phenotypically defined T cell subset but is supported by various cells that share the ability to secrete anti-inflammatory cytokines, such as TGF-β, IL-4, or IL-10 under specific circumstances (Karpus and Swanborg, 1991; Fontana *et al.*, 1992; Arnason and Reder, 1994; Durelli *et al.*, 1995).

Type I-IFNs are able to increase NK activity *in vivo* and *in vitro* (Perussia *et al.*, 1980). The Type I-IFNs-induced increase in NK activity appears to be due to both the recruitment of previously non-functional NK cells and to the potentiation of the cytolytic activity of functional NK cells above the endogenous levels (Targan and Dorey, 1980). NK activity plays a role in the primary host defences against tumors and viruses (Biron, 1997), and increase in NK activity in the blood of patients treated with α-IFNs was correlated with the clinical response in HCL (Foon *et al.*, 1986), but not in multiple myeloma (Einhorn *et al.*, 1982). Interestingly, NK activity is decreased in untreated patients with HCL (Ruco *et al.*, 1983) and HCL is probably the hematological disease that is most responsive to α-IFNs therapy (Roth and Foon, 1986).

Finally, several experiments demonstrated that Type I-IFNs are important for the generation of specific anti-tumoral responses mediated by cytotoxic T lymphocytes (Belardelli and Gresser, 1996). During *in vitro* cloning of T cells, the cytolytic activity of the generated clones correlates with the secretion of γ-IFN by these clones. α-IFNs may thus influence the cytolytic activity of T cells through its ability to regulate the induction of Th1 or Th2 responses by these T cells (Parronchi *et al.*, 1992).

Anti-inflammatory effects of Type I-IFNs

α/β-IFNs have been shown to:

(1) down-regulate the secretion of major pro-inflammatory cytokines, IL-1, TNF-α, and IL-8;
(2) induce their specific inhibitors; and finally
(3) to up-regulate the secretion of two anti-inflammatory cytokine: IL-10 and TGF-β.

Several experiments have shown α-IFNs-induced inhibition of spontaneous, and both phorbol myristate acetate (PMA)- and lipopolysaccharide (LPS)-induced secretion of IL-1 *in vitro* (Aman *et al.*, 1994; Huang *et al.*, 1995; Dinarello, 1996). Moreover, α/β-IFNs induce *in vitro* and *in vivo* secretion of IL-1 receptor antagonist (IL-1ra), a specific IL-1 inhibitor (Tilg *et al.*, 1993; Huang *et al.*, 1995). Interestingly, in a trial in CML patients in which β-IFN was clinically less effective than α-2b-IFN, β-IFN also induced lower serum levels of IL-1ra than α-2b-IFN, though neopterin and β2-microglobulin induction was similar (Aulitzky *et al.*, 1993).

α-IFNs also inhibits IL-1α-induced TNF-α synthesis *in vitro* (Tilg *et al.*, 1995; Rep *et al.*, 1996) and spontaneous TNF-α gene expression and protein synthesis *in vitro* and *in vivo* (Abu Khabar *et al.*,1992; Bongioanni *et al.*, 1996; Brod *et al.*, 1996; Larrea *et al.*, 1996). In addition, high levels of soluble TNF receptors, specific inhibitors of TNF-α were induced by α-IFNs treatment in patients with chronic hepatitis C viral infection (Tilg *et al.*, 1995) and in healthy humans (Corssmit *et al.*, 1997).

Gene expression of another pro-inflammatory cytokine, IL-8, is inhibited *in vitro* (Oliveira *et al.*, 1992; Aman *et al.*, 1993) and *in vivo* in CML patients (Aman *et al.*, 1993). The stimulating effects of α/β-IFNs on the secretion of two mainly anti-inflammatory cytokines, IL-10 and TGF-β have already been discussed.

The observation that α-IFNs treatment prevents LPS-induced mortality in mice provides further evidence that Type I-IFNs can display relevant *in vivo* anti-inflammatory effects (Tzung *et al.*, 1992).

In addition, α/β-IFNs have been demonstrated to down-regulate the surface expression of two adhesion molecules: the very late activation molecule (VLA)-4 and the intercellular adhesion molecule (ICAM)-1 (Garcia-Monzon *et al.*, 1993; Soilu Hanninen *et al.*, 1995). Moreover, serum levels of the soluble form of the vascular cell adhesion molecule (VCAM)-1, a competitive inhibitor of surface-expressed VCAM-1, are increased during β-1b-IFN therapy in MS patients (Calabresi *et al.*, 1997). *In vitro* experiments have also demonstrated β-IFN-induced inhibition of the activity of matrix metalloproteinases (MMPs), which are considered to be important mediators of cell migration through the extra-cellular matrix (Leppert *et al.*, 1996; Stuve *et al.*, 1996). All these Type I-IFNs effects may lead to inhibition of effector cell access to the inflammatory focus. Indeed, a-IFNs are able to inhibit antigen-induced eosinophil and CD4+ T cell recruitment into tissue in a murine model of airway late phase reaction (Nakajima *et al.*, 1994).

Finally, Type I-IFNs control different steps of allergic inflammation in which eosinophils play a central role. First, as mentioned before, α-IFNs inhibit the secretion of IL-5, which is a key mediator for differentiation and activation of eosinophils. Second, α-IFNs might also exert direct effects on eosinophils and their precursors. As a matter of fact, α-IFNs were also shown to inhibit the proliferation of granulocyte-macrophage progenitor cells (CFU-GM) and their engagement in the eosinophilic lineage, at least in part by inhibiting the action of IL-3 (Broxmeyer *et al.*, 1983; Sillaber *et al.*, 1992). Moreover, there is evidence that α-IFNs inhibits the release of the eosinophilic cationic protein (ECP) and the eosinophil-derived neurotoxin (EDN) by activated eosinophils, as well as their cytotoxic potential *in vitro* (Aldebert *et al.*, 1996). The decrease in ECP serum levels observed during α-IFNs treatment in patients with the HES (Desreumaux *et al.*, 1993) suggests that the direct effects of α-IFNs on eosinophils are also operative *in vivo*. α-IFNs have also been shown to decrease eosinophil-mediated cytotoxicity against parasites, chemotaxis, production of hydrogen peroxyde in response to stimuli, and to inhibit release of granule protein and IL-5 (Saito *et al.*, 1987; Aldebert *et al.*, 1996). In addition, α-IFNs decreases viability of eosinophils that have been generated *in vitro* through induction of their apoptosis (Morita *et al.*, 1996). Finally, α-IFNs not only inhibit the differentiation and effector functions of T cells and eosinophils involved in allergic inflammation, but might also interfere with their homing properties. Indeed, as previously mentioned, α-IFNs are able to inhibit antigen-induced eosinophil and CD4+ T cell recruitment into the airway of sensitised mice (Nakajima *et al.*, 1994).

Clinical uses of the immuno-modulatory effects of Type I-IFNs

It is difficult to predict the resulting *in vivo* effects of the different immuno-modulatory properties of Type I-IFNs. Moreover, *in vivo* Type I-IFNs immuno-modulatory effects seems to differ from one disease to another probably because of the different immune mechanisms involved in the pathogenesis of these diseases.

α/β-IFNs as a treatment of MS

β-1b-IFN at a dose of 8 MIU s.c. given e.o.d. (every other day) to patients with the relapsing-remitting form of MS, lessens the overall frequency of MS attacks by 35%, the frequency of major attacks by 50%, and the number of MS-related hospitalizations by 40% (The IFNB Multiple Sclerosis Study Group, 1993). Benefit persists for at least 5 years (The IFNB Multiple Sclerosis Study Group and The University of British Columbia MS/MRI Analysis Group, 1995). b-IFN-1a at a dose of 6 MIU i.m. given once a week produced similar results (Jacobs *et al.*, 1996). Treatment of MS patients with IFNs other than β-IFN have shown either conflicting results for α-IFNs (Durelli *et al.*, 1994; Jacobs and Johnson, 1994), or even deteriorating effects for γ-IFN (Panitch *et al.*, 1987b). Chronic rec-β-IFN administration is the first treatment that convincingly demonstrated a beneficial influence on the course and activity of MS during randomized, double-blinded, placebo-controlled studies. However, β-IFN treatment is not curative and, at best, only delays the progression of the disease.

Multiple Sclerosis (MS) is a disabling neurological disease affecting more than one million persons world wide (Dean, 1994). Beginning between 20 and 40 years of age, its clinical course is unpredictable, with recurrent attacks that are usually followed by insidious progression. The sum of the neurological sequels engenders growing disability and considerable socio-economic consequences. The exact cause of MS remains undefined, but there is a body of evidence suggesting a pathological autoimmune response directed against myelin antigens in a DTH manner, in which normally silenced auto-reactive T cells are triggered, cross the blood–brain barrier, recognize their myelin auto-antigen, attract followers, and all together cause brain tissue damage. In the relapsing-remitting form of MS, the DTH reaction finally resolves and the repair processes may occur until the next attack (Arnason and Reder, 1994; Weinstock Guttman *et al.*, 1995; Arnason, 1996).

The β-IFNs effects leading to clinical improvement in MS remain unknown. Production of γ- and/or α-IFNs in MS patients has been reported to be low by some (Neighbour and Bloom, 1979; Salonen *et al.*, 1982; Vervliet *et al.*, 1984; Vervliet *et al.*, 1985), though others found it normal (Santoli *et al.*, 1981; Tovell *et al.*, 1983; Haahr *et al.*, 1986). Thus, replacement of a deficient production of Type I-IFNs by β-IFN therapy does not seem to be the crucial process.

The anti-viral properties of β-IFN may be responsible, at least in part, of its beneficial effects in MS. Indeed a viral infection has been hypothesised as the original cause of MS (Cook and Dowling, 1980) and viral infections are established triggers for MS attacks and T cell activation (Sibley *et al.*, 1985). However, there is no evidence that viral illnesses are fewer during β-IFN treatment of MS patients (Panitch, 1994).

In fact, all the previously described anti-inflammatory effects of β-IFN may be beneficial in MS, whereas the pro-inflammatory properties may temper β-IFN efficacy. Since Th1-like responses promote DTH and γ-IFN, the Th1 promoting effect of β-IFN may be deleterious in MS. However, the inhibitory effects of α/β-IFNs on γ-IFNs secretion and its effects have also been described in β-IFN-treated patients with MS. The many α/β-IFNs immuno-modulatory effects already observed in MS patients are listed with references in the Table A.4.

Finally, the β-IFN-induced up-regulation of IL-10 and TGF-β may be relevant effects. Indeed, the secretion of IL-10 and TGF-β in the lesions coincides in time with remission in MS patients and in the animal model of MS, the experimental autoimmune encephalomyelitis (Beck *et al.*, 1991; Kennedy *et al.*, 1992; Carrieri *et al.*, 1996).

The reasons why α-IFNs have been disappointing in MS therapy are unknown and may be due to inappropriate study design, since the most recent clinical trial has shown a very impressive 83% reduction of exacerbation rate during chronic systemic high dose rec-α-2a-IFN therapy of patients with the relapsing-remitting form of MS (Durelli *et al.*, 1994). A better comprehension of the mechanism underlying the effects of IFNs in MS would help to define better treatment regimen in the future.

α-IFNs in the treatment of HES

α-IFNs have been recommended as second-line therapy for refractory HES. Since 1990, quite a few authors have reported successful treatment of HES patients with α-IFNs (Malbrain *et al.*, 1996). In most cases, α-IFNs were used to treat patients with the myeloproliferative variant of the HES, who failed to respond to the classical therapeutic regimen. Maintenance therapy appears to be necessary, as interruption of α-IFNs was often followed by clinical and biological relapse in the cases reported. α-IFNs has been used alone or in association with prednisone or hydroxyurea. Duration of response to treatment is difficult to assess, because of short follow-up in most reported cases. However, several authors have observed prolonged remissions with α-IFNs (Fruehauf *et al.* 1993; Malbrain *et al.*, 1996).

Administration of α-IFNs to patients with the HES is followed by a decrease in circulating eosinophil levels and substantial clinical improvement. In patients initially presenting elevated soluble IL-2 receptor levels, response to treatment with α-IFNs correlated with regression of this disease marker (Prin *et al.*, 1991). Two HES patients with cytoge-

Table A.4 Immuno-modulatory effects of Type I-IFNs in MS patients

Type I-IFNs effect	References
Anti-inflammatory effects:	
Down-regulation of TNF-α secretion	(Bongioanni et al., 1996; Brod et al., 1996)
Up-regulation of IL-10 secretion	(Byskosh and Reder, 1995; Porrini et al., 1995; Rudick et al. 1996; Calabresi et al., 1996)
	(Noronha et al., 1993)
Up-regulation of TGF-β secretion	(Calabresi et al., 1997)
Up-regulation of soluble VCAM-1 secretion	(Leppert et al., 1996; Stuve et al., 1996)
Inhibition of matrix metalloproteinases	(Noronha et al., 1990, 1992)
Activation of T suppressor cell activity *in vitro*	(Hirsch and Johnson, 1986; O'Gorman et al., 1987; Noronha et al., 1994)
Activation of T suppressor cell activity *in vivo*	
Pro-inflammatory effects:	
Inhibition of γ-IFN-enhanced HLA-II expression on monocytes	(Panitch et al., 1989)
Up-regulation of NK cells number or activity	(Arnason and Reder, 1994; Neighbour, 1984; Bongioanni et al., 1996)
Conflicting results on γ-IFN regulation:	(Dayal et al., 1995)
Up-regulation of γ-IFN secretion	(Panitch et al., 1987; Noronha et al., 1993; Milo and Panitch, 1995; Bongioanni et al., 1996; Crucian et al., 1996)
Down-regulation of γ-IFN secretion	
Th2 promoting effects:	
Up-regulation of B7—2 expression and down-regulation of B7—1	(Genc et al., 1997)

netic abnormalities (trisomy 8 and translocation between chromosomes 5 and 9) presented clinical, hematological, and cytogenetic remission under α-IFNs (Canonica *et al.*, 1995; Malbrain *et al.*, 1996).

α-IFNs will probably be of benefit both in all subgroups of HES patients. Morever, the experience gained in CML therapy suggests that HES patients with cytogenetic abnormalities be treated with combined chemotherapy and α-IFNs from the start. Early initiation of aggressive treatment could possibly prevent malignant transformation in such cases.

Other clinical uses of the immuno-modulatory effects of α/β-IFNs

The inhibitory effects of α/β-IFNs on IL-1 and TNF-a secretion may be responsible of their beneficial effects in AIDS since these cytokines play a major role in the pathogenesis of AIDS. A similar process is likely in Kaposi sarcomas, as IL-1 appears to be a paracrine growth factor for Kaposi sarcomas (Tilg, 1997).

Opposite effects of β-IFNs have been described on chronic active ulcerative colitis, a supposed Th2-linked disease in which α-IFNs proved clinical efficacy, and on Crohn's disease, a supposed Th1-linked disease, in which α-IFNs effects are controversial (Tilg, 1997). These effects have been linked to the Th1 promoting effects, but such reasoning would have predicted deleterious effects of β-IFN in MS.

6 Pharmacokinetics and pharmacodynamics of α/β-IFN

Natural and recombinant α-IFNs and β-IFNs are now available for clinical use, but there are no major differences between recombinant and natural preparations in terms of pharmacokinetics and pharmacodynamics.

There is no direct relationship between serum levels of α/β-IFNs and the duration of the biological effects. After intravenous injections of β-IFN, serum concentrations can be measured within minutes and peak at approximately 5 min. After intramuscular (i.m.) or subcutaneous (s.c.) injection, peak serum levels occur later (after 1–6 h). Clearance of b-IFN is high leading to its rapid disappearance from the serum. Hence, consecutive daily s.c. injections of β-IFN do not result in increased peak serum levels. Patients receiving 8 MIU β-IFN-1b s.c. every other day (e.o.d.) showed sustained serum level between 100 and 500 IU/ml (Khan *et al.*, 1996). After i.m. or s.c. injections, absorption of α-IFNs exceeds 80% leading to relatively higher plasma levels. As the plasma half-life of α-IFNs is about 2 h, compared to 1 h for rec-β-IFNs, α-IFNs plasma levels return to baseline after only 18–36 h. Elimination of α/β-IFNs from the blood is due to distribution into the tissues and cellular uptake. Catabolism takes place in the kidney and the liver. Urinary excretion is negligible (Wills, 1990; Witt, 1997).

Biological responses to α/β-IFNs measured in pharmacodynamic studies usually include increased 2–5-OAS activity in peripheral blood mononuclear cells (PBMC) and β2-microglobulin and neopterin levels in serum. Similar biological effects are obtained after i.v., s.c., or i.m. injection. These effects are sustained for at least 72 h (Liberati *et al.*, 1988). Daily injections of β-IFN do not result in increased responses (Chiang *et al.*, 1993). Thus, every other day or once a week injections were selected in clinical trials with MS. Natural or recombinant α/β-IFNs do not readily cross the blood–brain barrier (Wills, 1990). In mice, biological effects are detectable in the central nervous system after systemic injection of IFN. Conversely, intrathecal injection of β-IFN increased 2,5-OAS activity in spleen as well. For the first studies in MS, β-IFN was given intrathecally (Jacobs *et al.*, 1981). However, s.c. or i.m. β-IFN is effective in MS and the site of action of β-IFN in MS (peripheral or in the central nervous system) remains undetermined (Witt, 1997).

Dose-dependent increase in the biological response has been observed for most of the effects of α/β-IFNs (Borden *et al.*, 1990; Wills, 1990). Different regimens of β-IFN-1b (up to 16 MIU β-IFN-1b s.c., e.o.d.) were compared in MS, and higher doses correlated with greater clinical effectiveness, but also more severe side-effects. β-IFN is now used for treatment of MS in countries where local agreement has been obtained at a dose of 6 MIU i.m. once a week for β-IFN-1a (Jacobs *et al.*, 1996). β-IFN-1b is used at the dose of 8 MIU s.c., e.o.d. (The IFNB Multiple Sclerosis Study Group, 1993). Maximum tolerated dose for s.c., e.o.d. injections of β-IFN-1b is 18 MIU (Goldstein *et al.*, 1989).

Optimal dosage and route of administration for lower adverse effects and higher clinical response remain controversial. As pharmacodynamics depends on the parameter of activity measured, a better understanding of the mechanism of action of α/β-IFNs is needed to develop tools able to measure α/β-IFNs bio-effectiveness during treatment of a particular disease.

7 α/β-IFNs side-effects and contraindications

The most common α/β-IFNs side-effects are acute flu-like syndrome, local reactions at injection sites, CNS effects, abnormal laboratory findings, and autoimmune complications (Vial and Descotes, 1995; Lublin *et al.*, 1996). Because of its importance, the development of neutralizing antibodies directed against IFNs during therapy will be discussed separately.

7.1 α/β-IFNs side-effects and their management

S.c. or i.m. injection of α/β-IFNs doses of more than 1–2 MIU causes an acute flu-like syndrome beginning as early as 4 h after injection and usually resolving within 12 h. Symptoms include fever, chills, headache, arthralgias, myalgias, tachycardia, nausea, vomiting, and diarrhoea. These symptoms can be reduced by pretreatment with various antipyretics, and tolerance gradually develops in most patients within a few months of institution of chronic therapy. The flu-like syndrome does not appear to be a direct effect of IFNs but probably results from the acute release of fever-promoting factors from the hypothalamus.

Injection-site reactions, ranging from local redness to necrosis have been observed after i.m. or s.c. injections. Lesions are usually self-healing but impose rotation of injection sites.

Confusion, somnolence, emotional lability, and depersonalization are occasionally observed during α/β-IFNs therapy. Encephalopathies associated with slowing of encephalographic activity have been observed with α-IFNs but not β-IFN, maybe because of the broader use of α-IFNs to date.

The occurrence of one suicide and four attempted suicides in the β-1b-IFN treated group during the MS therapy clinical trial has raised great concern about depression and the use of IFNs (The IFNB Multiple Sclerosis Study Group and The University of British

Columbia MS/MRI Analysis Group, 1995). However, depression and suicide are relatively common in MS patients and the frequency of depression was equivalent between the treatment groups and the placebo group in the same trial. If active and severe depression is now accepted as a contraindication to β-IFN treatment in MS, it may be considered in non-depressed patients with a history of depression or mildly depressed patients, provided a careful follow-up and a good support system are available. Under more severe conditions, such as a history of attempted suicide, the decision should be discussed in conjunction with the patient's psychiatrist.

Abnormal laboratory findings are usually mild and self-limiting at the doses of β-IFN used in MS but can be the dose-limiting toxicity for α-IFNs in cancer patients (Sherwin *et al.*, 1982). Definite interruption of therapy is only recommended in patients with persisting elevations of serum hepatic enzymes greater than ten times the upper limit of normal, and of serum bilirubin greater than five times the upper limit of normal. The combination with other hepatotoxic drugs may potentiate the effects of α/β-IFNs. Conversely, α/β-IFNs reduces the metabolism of various drugs by the hepatic cytochrome P450 system and significantly increase levels of drugs such as theophylline. Bone marrow suppression with granulocytopenia and thrombocytopenia is dose related and α/β-IFNs can thus increase the bone marrow toxicity of myelotoxic drugs such as zidovudine.

As previously discussed, α-IFNs treatment can cause the exacerbation or occurrence of several types of auto-antibodies or auto-immune diseases (see Table A.3). Immunological side-effects have been seldom reported with β-IFN but the extent of clinical experience is relatively limited (Vial and Descotes, 1995). Nevertheless, it is still not clearly understood whether α-IFNs therapy aggravate previous autoimmune disorders, unmask silent autoimmune processes, or induce de novo auto-immunity. However, predisposed patients have been identified as asymptomatic patients bearing HLA haplotypes strongly associated with a particular autoimmune disease, asymptomatic patients with previously positive auto-antibodies and patients presenting symptoms of autoimmune disease before treatment (Vial and Descotes, 1995).

7.2 Antibodies against α/β-IFNs

Since the first report of the occurrence of antibodies to β-IFN during therapy (Vallbracht *et al.*, 1981), various types of assays have been developed to measure antibodies to α/β-IFNs. Enzyme immunoassay, enzyme-linked immunosorbent assay, and radio-immunoassay are used as screening methods because they reveal all types of antibodies. Neutralization assays test the ability of the antibodies to interfere with one function of IFNs. Anti-viral neutralization assays have been the golden standard to date but anti-proliferative neutralization assays are under evaluation (Prummer *et al.*, 1994). A recently developed assay tests the ability of the antibodies to inhibit the α- or β-IFN induced production of MxA in human cells (Towbin *et al.*, 1992). The antibodies to α/β-IFNs detected with immunoassays are not all neutralizing ones, and there is great variability in sensibility and specificity among the different tests.

Antibodies to α-IFNs can develop in patients that have been treated with either natural or recombinant α-IFN preparations. However, high-titer neutralizing IFN antibodies are more common in patients treated with rec-α-2a-IFN (Grander *et al.*, 1990; Antonelli *et al.*, 1991; Von Wussow *et al.*, 1994). In many studies, the development of neutralizing antibodies, but probably not of non-neutralizing antibodies, is associated with a higher frequency of relapse or secondary resistance to further therapy with the same IFN (Vial and Descotes, 1995). This was observed in cancer therapy (Quesada *et al.*, 1985, 1987; Leavitt *et al.*, 1987; Von Wussow *et al.*, 1987, 1991; Steis *et al.*, 1988; Freund *et al.*, 1989; Oberg *et al.*, 1989; Berman *et al.*, 1990; Prummer, 1993), as well as in chronic hepatitis C therapy (Millela *et al.*, 1993; Gianelli *et al.*, 1994). Other studies, including large numbers of patients and using sensitive means of detection, failed to prove any clinical deleterious effect of the development of neutralizing antibodies (Figlin *et al.*, 1986; Itri *et al.*, 1987). Usually antibodies to α-2a-IFN cross-react with α-2b-IFN but not with natural α-IFNs. Thus, some antibody-positive patients, which show clinical resistance to rec-α-IFNs therapy, can be successfully treated with natural α-IFN preparations (Freund *et al.*, 1988; Steis *et al.*, 1988; Von Wussow *et al.*, 1991; Ronnblom *et al.*, 1992).

Because of relatively limited clinical use, much less information is available on antibodies to β-IFNs. Chronic s.c. β-IFN treatment of malignant melanoma resulted in an incidence of neutralizing antibodies of up to 95% with the natural β-IFN preparation and of only 28% with the recombinant β-1b-IFN (Dummer *et al.*, 1991; Fierlbeck *et al.*, 1994). The occurrence of neutralizing antibodies correlated with a decrease in β2-microglobulin serum level and 2–5-OAS activity. These studies failed to prove any difference in clinical outcome between antibody-positive and antibody-negative patients. During clinical trials on MS therapy, neutralizing antibodies to β-IFN developed in 35% of the patients treated with β-1b-IFN and in 22% of the β-1a-IFN treated patients (Jacobs *et al.*, 1996; The IFNB Multiple Sclerosis Study Group and The University of British Columbia MS/MRI Analysis Group, 1995). Separate analysis of the β-1b-IFN trial proved that treatment benefit was lost in antibody-positive treated patients whose relapse rate reverted to the placebo level (The IFNB Multiple Sclerosis Study Group and The University of British Columbia MS/MRI Analysis Group, 1996).

Development of neutralizing antibodies to α/β-IFNs is not a rare phenomenon and, at least for certain patients, results in reduction or abolition of clinical efficacy. Different parameters, such as the nature of the underlying disease, dosage, and type of IFN and route of administration, may influence the development of these antibodies. Comparisons of the incidence of neutralizing antibodies are often difficult because of the various tests used and the differences in specific activity. In the same test, for the same dosage in term of unity, a preparation with low specific activity may need more antibodies to be inhibited than a more active preparation containing a lower amount of IFN in terms of weight. Change in the type of preparation of α-IFN has proven clinically beneficial but such attempts have not been documented to date for β-IFNs. Interestingly, cross-reactivity has been found between natural β-IFN and rec-β-1a-IFN (Fierlbeck and Schreiner, 1994), but not between rec-α-2a-IFN and rec-β-IFN (Ikeda *et al.*, 1989). Moreover, neutralizing antibodies to α- and β-IFNs have been demonstrated in human IgG preparations and in the sera of healthy blood donors and of myasthenia gravis patients with thymoma (Ross *et al.*, 1990, 1995; Meager *et al.*, 1996). These results suggest that endogenous natural α/β-IFNs are able to trigger the development of auto-antibodies against them.

Neutralizing or non-neutralizing antibodies may modify α/β-IFNs effects by prolonging their presence in the serum. In mice, injection of cytokine-anti-cytokine complexes have been surprisingly able to prolong the effects of IL-4, IL-3, and IL-7 (Finkelman *et al.*, 1993).

Discrepancy between studies on the clinical relevance of neutralizing antibodies to α/β-IFNs may be due to the fact that antibodies able to neutralize the anti-viral effects of α/β-IFNs may not inhibit the other effects (Imam *et al.*, 1995). A better understanding of the mechanisms of action of the α/β-IFNs in the different clinical situations may help to develop tools to asses the relevance of the antibodies developed during treatment. However, neutralizing antibody apparition should be monitored during α/β-IFNs therapy and treatment adaptation or discontinuation should be considered if sustained secondary clinical failure coincides with the development of high titers of neutralizing antibody.

7.3 α/β-IFNs contraindications

The only absolute contraindications of α/β-IFNs are:

(1) hypersensitivity to any component of the product; and
(2) active and severe depression.

Pregnant and nursing women, and those who are actively attempting to become pregnant, should not be treated with α/β-IFNs. Safety during pregnancy has not been established in well-controlled studies and spontaneous abortion has occurred. Moreover, it is not known whether α/β-IFNs are excreted in human milk (Lublin *et al.*, 1996).

8 Concluding remarks

Type I-IFNs display a wide range of effects, which have been exploited for the therapy of many different diseases. However, the mechanisms involved in their beneficial effects in a particular disease remain often unknown. Therefore, a better understanding of these mechanisms would help to improve the clinical use of Type I-IFNs. It would also help to reduce side-effects and to elaborate tools able to predict Type I-IFNs efficacy and to measure biorelevance of antibodies raised against them. Finally, it may help to develop combination therapy able to promote the beneficial effects of Type I-IFNs and/or to temper the deleterious ones.

9 Acknowledgement

F. E. Roufosse and E. J. Bartholomé, are research assistants of the Belgium National Fund for Scientific Research (Télévie grant and Smith Kline Beecham fellowship respectively). This work was supported by a grant of the Fondation Charcot, Belgium.

We regret that space limitations may have precluded citing the publications of many individuals who have made important contributions to the field.

References

Abramovich, C., L. M. Shulman, E. Ratovitski, S. Harroch, M. Tovey, P. Eid, and M. Revel (1994). Differential tyrosine phosphorylation of the IFNAR chain of the Type I interferon receptor and of an associated surface protein in response to IFN-alpha and IFN-beta. *EMBO J.*, **13**, 5871.

Abu Khabar, K. S., J. A. Armstrong, and M. Ho (1992). Type I interferons (IFN-alpha and -beta) suppress cytotoxin (tumor necrosis factor-alpha and lymphotoxin) production by mitogen-stimulated human peripheral blood mononuclear cell. J. *Leukoc. Biol.*, **52**, 165.

Adolf, G. R. (1987). Antigenic structure of human interferon omega 1 (interferon alpha II1): comparison with other human interferons. J. *Gen. Virol.*,. **68**, 1669.

Aldebert, D., B. Lamkhioued, C. Desaint, A. S. Gounni, M. Goldman, A. Capron *et al.* (1996). Eosinophils express a functional receptor for interferon alpha: inhibitory role of interferon alpha on the release of mediators. *Blood*, **87**, 2354.

Allen, G. and M. O. Diaz (1994). Nomenclature of the Human Interferon Proteins. *J. Interferon. Res.*, **14**, 223.

Aman, M. J., G. Rudolf, J. Goldschmitt, W. E. Aulitzky, C. Lam, C. Huber *et al.* (1993). Type I interferons are potent inhibitors of interleukin-8 production in hematopoietic and bone marrow stromal cells. *Blood*, **82**, 2371.

Aman, M. J., U. Keller, G. Derigs, M. Mohamadzadeh, C. Huber, and C. Peschel (1994). Regulation of cytokine expression by interferon-alpha in human bone marrow stromal cells: inhibition of hematopoietic growth factors and induction of interleukin-1 receptor antagonist. *Blood*, **84**, 4142.

Aman, M. J., T. Tretter, I. Eisenbeis, G. Bug, T. Decker, W. E. Aulitzky *et al.* (1996). Interferon-alpha stimulates production of interleukin-10 in activated CD4+ T cells and monocytes. *Blood*, **87**, 4731.

Anlar, B., K. Yalaz, F. Oktem, and G. Kose (1997). Long-term follow-up of patients with subacute sclerosing panencephalitis treated with intraventricular alpha-interferon. *Neurology*, **48**, 526.

Antonelli, G., M. Currenti, O. Turriziani, and F. Dianzani (1991). Neutralizing antibodies to interferon-alpha: relative frequency in patients treated with different interferon preparations. *J. Infect. Dis.*, **163**, 882.

Arnason, B. G. (1996). Interferon beta in multiple sclerosis. *Clin. Immunol. Immunopathol.*, **81**, 1.

Arnason, B. G. and A. T. Reder (1994). Interferons and Multiple Sclerosis. *Clin. Neuropharmacol.*, **17**, 495.

Aulitzky, W. E., C. Peschel, D. Despres, J. Aman, P. Trautman, H. Tilg *et al.* (1993). Divergent *in vivo* and *in vitro* antileukemic activity of recombinant interferon beta in patients with chronic-phase chronic myelogenous leukemia. *Ann. Hematol.*, **67**, 205.

Balmer, C. M. (1990).Clinical use of biologic response modifiers in cancer treatment: an overview. Part I. The interferons. *DICP*, **24**, 761.

Barna, B. P., S. M. Chou, B. Jacobs, B. Yen Lieberman, and R. M. Ransohoff (1989). Interferon-beta impairs induction of HLA-DR antigen expression in cultured adult human astrocytes. *J. Neuroimmunol.*, **23**, 45.

Basham, T. Y. and T. C. Merigan (1983). Recombinant Interferon-gamma increases HLA-DR synthesis and expression. *J. Immunol.*, **4**, 1492.

Basham, T., W. Smith, L. Lanier, V. Morhenn, and T. Merigan (1984). Regulation of expression of class II major histocompatibility antigens on human peripheral blood monocytes and langerhans cells by interferon. *Human. Immunology*, **10**, 83.

Beck, J., P. Rondot, P. Jullien, J. Wietzerbin, and D. A. Lawrence (1991). TGF-b-like activity produced during regression of exacerbations in multiple sclerosis. *Acta. Neurol. Scand.*, **84**, 452.

Becker, J. C., B. Winkler, S. Klingert, and E. B. Brocker (1994). Antiphospholipid syndrome associated with immunotherapy for patients with melanoma. *Cancer*, **73**, 1621.

Belardelli, F. and I. Gresser (1996). The neglected role of Type I interferon in the T-cell response: implications for its clinical use. Immunol. *Today*, **17**, 369.

Benoit, P., D. Maguire, I. Plavec, H. Kocher, M. Tovey, and F. Meyer (1993). A monoclonal antibody to recombinant human IFN-alpha receptor inhibits biologic activity of several species of human IFN-alpha, IFN-beta, and IFN-omega. Detection of heterogeneity of the cellular Type I IFN receptor. *J. Immunol.*, **150**, 707.

Berman, E., G. Heller, S. Kempin, T. Gee, L. L. Tran, and B. Clarkson (1990).Incidence of response and long-term follow-up in patients with hairy cell leukemia treated with recombinant interferon alpha-2a. *Blood*, **75**, 839.

Birch, C. J., D. P. Tyssen, G. Tachedjian, R. Doherty, K. Hayes, A. Mijch *et al.* (1992). Clinical effects and *in vitro* studies of trifluorothymidine combined with interferon-alpha for treatment of drug-resistant and sensitive herpes simplex virus infections. *J. Infect. Dis.*, **166**, 108.

Biron, C. A. (1997). Activation and function of natural killer cell responses during viral infections. *Curr. Opin. Immunol.*, **9**, 24.

Blatt, L. M., J. M. Davis, S. B. Klein, and M. W. Taylor (1996). The biologic activity and molecular characterization of a novel synthetic interferon-alpha species, consensus interferon. *J. Interferon. Cytokine. Res.*, **16**, 489.

Bongioanni, M. R., L. Durelli, B. Ferrero, D. Imperiale, A. Oggero, E. Verdun *et al.* (1996). Systemic high-dose recombinant-alpha-2a-interferon therapy modulates lymphokine production in multiple sclerosis. *J. Neurol. Sci.*, **143**, 91.

Borden, E. C., J. J. Rinehart, B. E. Storer, D. L. Trump, D. M. Paulnock, and A. P. Teitelbaum (1990).Biological and clinical effects of interferon-beta ser at two doses. *J. Interferon. Res.*, **10**, 559.

Brinkmann, V., T. Geiger, S. Alkan, and C. H. Heusser (1993). Interferon alpha increases the frequency of interferon gamma-producing human CD4+ T cells. *J. Exp. Med.*, **178**, 1655.

Brod, S. A., G. D. Marshall, Jr., E. M. Henninger, S. Sriram, M. Khan, and J. S. Wolinsky (1996). Interferon-beta 1b treatment decreases tumor necrosis factor-alpha and increases interleukin-6 production in multiple sclerosis. *Neurology*, **46**, 1633.

Broxmeyer, H. E., L. Lu, E. Platzer, C. Feit, L. Juliano, and B. Y. Rubin (1983). Comparative analysis of the influences of human gamma, alpha and beta interferons on human multipotential (CFU-GEMM), erythroid (BFU-E) and granulocyte-macrophage (CFU-GM) progenitor cells. *J. Immunol.*, **3**, 1300.

Byskosh, P. and A. T. Reder (1995). Interferon-b-1b effects on cytokine mRNA in multiple sclerosis. *Ann. Neurol.*, **38**, 340. (Abstract.)

Calabresi, P. A., L. R. Tranquill, L. A. Stone, E. P. Cowan, and H. F. McFarland (1996). Cytokine mrna expression changes in CSF cells from multiple sclerosis patients treated with betaseron. *Neurology*, **46**, A165. (Abstract.)

Calabresi, P. A., L. R. Tranquill, J. M. Dambrosia, L. A. Stone, H. Maloni, C. N. Bash *et al.* (1997). Increases in soluble VCAM-1 correlate with a decrease in MRI lesions in multiple sclerosis treated with interferon b-1b. *Ann. Neurol.*, **41**, 669.

Canonica, G. W., G. Passalacqua, C. Pronzato, L. Corbetta, and M. Bagnasco (1995). Effective long-term alpha-interferon treatment for hypereosinophilic syndrome. *J. Allergy Clin. Immunol.*, **96**, 131.

Carrieri, P. B., A. Maiorino, A. Perrella, and O. Perrella (1996). Evaluation of interleukin 10 and interferon-a in the cerebrospinal fluid and serum of patients with multiple sclerosi. *Eur. J. Neurol.*, **3**, 544.

Cederblad, B. and G. V. Alm (1991). Interferons and the colony-stimulating factors IL-3 and GM-CSF enhance the IFN-alpha response in human blood leucocytes induced by herpes simplex virus. *Scand. J. Immunol.*, **34**, 549.

Chakrabarti, D., B. Hultgren, and T. A. Stewart (1996). IFN-alpha induces autoimmune T cells through the induction of intracellular adhesion molecule-1 and B7. 2. *J. Immunol.*, **157**, 522.

Charlier, M., D. Hue, M. Boisnard, J. Martal, and P. Gaye (1991). Cloning and structural analysis of two distinct families of ovine interferon-alpha genes encoding functional class II and trophoblast (oTP) alpha-interferons. *Molecular and Cell Endocrinology*, **76**, 161.

Chernajovsky, Y., Y. Mory, L. Chen, Z. Marks, D. Novick, M. Rubinstein *et al.* (1984). Efficient constitutive production of human fibroblast interferon by hamster cells transformed with the IFN-beta 1 gene fused to an SV40 early promoter. *DNA*, **3**, 297.

Chiang, J., C. A. Gloff, C. N. Yoshizawa, and G. J. Williams (1993). Pharmacokinetics of recombinant human interferon-beta ser in healthy volunteers and its effect on serum neopterin. *Pharm. Res.*, **10**, 567.

Cook, S. D. and P. C. Dowling (1980).Multiple sclerosis and viruses: an overview. *Neurology*, **30**, 80.

Corssmit, E. P., R. Heijligenberg, C. E. Hack, E. Endert, H. P. Sauerwein, and J. A. Romijn (1997). Effects of interferon-alpha (IFN-alpha) administration on leucocytes in healthy humans. *Clin. Exp. Immunol.*, **107**, 359.

Cousens, L. P., J. S. Orange, H. C. Su, and C. A. Biron (1997). Interferon-alpha/beta inhibition of interleukin 12 and interferon-gamma production *in vitro* and endogenously during viral infection. *Proc. Natl. Acad. Sci. USA*, **94**, 634.

Cross, J. C. and R. M. Roberts (1991). Constitutive and trophoblast-specific expression of a class of bovine interferon genes. *Proc. Natl. Acad. Sci. USA*, **88**, 3817.

Crucian, B., P. Dunne, H. Friedman, R. Ragsdale, S. Pross, and R. Widen (1996). Detection of altered T helper 1 and T helper 2 cytokine production by peripheral blood mononuclear cells in patients with multiple sclerosis utilizing intracellular cytokine detection by flow cytometry and surface marker analysis. *Clin. Diagn. Lab. Immunol.*, **3**, 411.

David, M. (1995). Transcription factors in interferon signaling. Pharmacol. Ther., 65, 149.

David, M., E. Petricoin, C. Benjamin, R. Pine, M. J. Weber, and A. C. Larner (1995). Requirement for MAP kinase (ERK2) activity in interferon alpha- and interferon beta-stimulated gene expression through STAT proteins. *Science*, **269**, 1721.

Dayal, A. S., M. A. Jensen, A. Lledo, and B. G. Arnason (1995). Interferon-gamma-secreting cells in multiple sclerosis patients treated with interferon beta-1b. Neurology, 45, 2173.

Dean, G. (1994). How many people in the world have multiple sclerosis? *Neuroepidemiology*, **13**, 1.

Decker, T. (1997). The molecular biology of Type I interferons (Interferon-a/b) (Gene activation, promoters, proteins induced). In Interferon therapy of multiple sclerosis, (ed. A. T. Reder), p. 41. Marcel Dekker, Inc. New York.

Demeure, C. E., C. Y. Wu, U. Shu, P. V. Schneider, C. Heusser, H. Yssel *et al.* (1994). *In vitro* maturation of human neonatal CD4 T lymphocytes. II. Cytokines present at priming modulate the development of lymphokine production. *J. Immunol.*, **152**, 4775.

Desreumaux, P., A. Janin, S. Dubucquoi, M. C. Copin, G. Torpier, A. Capron *et al.* (1993). Synthesis of interleukin-5 by activated eosinophils in patients with eosinophilic heart diseases. *Blood*, **82**, 1553.

Devajyothi, C., I. Kalvakolanu, G. T. Babcock, H. A. Vasavada, P. H. Howe, and R. M. Ransohoff (1993). Inhibition of interferon-gamma-induced major histocompatibility complex class II gene transcription by interferon-beta and Type beta 1 transforming growth factor in human astrocytoma cells, definition of cis-element. *J. Biol. Chem.*, **268**, 18794.

Dinarello, C. A. (1996). Biologic basis for interleukin-1 in disease. *Blood*, **87**, 2095.

Dummer, R., W. Muller, F. Nestle, J. Wiede, J. Dues, W. Lechner *et al.* (1991). Formation of neutralizing antibodies against natural interferon-beta, but not against recombinant interferon-gamma during adjuvant therapy for high-risk malignant melanoma patients. *Cancer*, **67**, 2300.

Durelli, L., M. R. Bongioanni, R. Cavallo, B. Ferrero, R. Ferri, M. F. Ferrio *et al.* (1994). Chronic systemic high-dose recombinant interferon alfa-2a reduces exacerbation rate, MRI signs of disease activity, and lymphocyte interferon gamma production in relapsing-remitting multiple sclerosis. *Neurology*, **44**, 406.

Durelli, L., M. R. Bongioanni, B. Ferrero, E. Verdun, A. Riva, M. Geuna *et al.* (1995). Chronic alpha interferon (IFN-alpha) treatment for multiple sclerosis (MS) modulates cytokine production rather than antigen presentation. *Neurology*, **45**, A234.

Durelli, L., G. Saracco, M. Rizzetto, R. Pagni, E. Verdun, M. R. Bongioanni, and B. Bergamasco (1997). Autoimmune side-effect profile during chronic interferon (IFN) therapy for multiple sclerosis. *Neurology*, **48**, A245. (Abstract.)

Egle, A., A. Villunger, M. Kos, G. Bock, J. Gruber, B. Auer, and R. Greil (1996). Modulation of Apo-1/Fas (CD95)-induced programmed cell death in myeloma cells by interferon-alpha 2. Eur. *J. Immunol.*, **26**, 3119.

Einat, M., D. Resnitzky, and A. Kimchi (1985). Close link between reduction of c-myc expression by interferon and G0/G1 arrest. *Nature*, **313**, 597.

Einhorn, S., A. Ahre, H. Blomgren, B. Johanson, H. Mellstedt, and H. Strander (1982). Interferon and natural killer activity in multiple myeloma. Lack of correlation between interferon-induced enhancement of natural killer activity and clinical response to human interferon-alpha. Int. J. *Cancer*, **30**, 167.

Ellis, M. E., K. R. Neal, C. L. S. Leen, and A. C. Newland (1987). Alpha-2a recombinant interferon in HIV associated thrombocytopenia. *BMJ*, **295**, 1519.

Fattovich, G., C. Betterle, L. Brollo, G. Giustina, B. Pedini, and A. Alberti (1992). Induction of autoantibodies during alpha interferon treatment in chronic hepatitis B. *Arch. Virol.*, **4** (supplement), 291.

Fertsch Ruggio, D., D. R. Schoenberg, and S. N. Vogel (1988). Induction of Ia antigen expression by rIFN-gamma and down-regulation by IFN-alfa/beta and dexamethasone are regulated transcriptionally. *J. Immunol.*, **141**, 1582.

Fierlbeck, G. and T. Schreiner (1994). Incidence and clinical significance of therapy-induced neutralizing antibodies against interferon-beta. *J. Interferon. Res.*, **14**, 205.

Fierlbeck, G., T. Schreiner, B. Schaber, A. Walser, and G. Rassner (1994). Neutralizing interferon beta antibodies in melanoma patients treated with recombinant and natural interferon beta. *Cancer Immunol. Immunother.*, **39**, 263.

Figlin, R. A., J. B. deKernion, E. Mukamel, E. F. Schnipper, A. V. Palleroni, L. A. DeVenezia *et al.* (1986). Recombinant leukocyte A interferon (rIFN-alpha-A) antibody development in advanced renal cell carcinoma (RCC). *Proc. Am. Soc. Clin. Oncol.*, **5**, 222.

Finkelman, F. D., K. B. Madden, S. C. Morris, J. M. Holmes, N. Boiani, I. M. Katona *et al.* (1993). Anti-cytokine antibodies as carrier proteins. *J. Immunol.*, **151**, 1235.

Folkman, J. and Y. Shing (1992). Angiogenesis. *J. Biol. Chem.*, **267**, 10931.

Fontana, A., D. B. Constam, K. Frei, U. Malipiero, and H. W. Pfister (1992). Modulation of the immune response by transforming growth factor beta. *Int. Arch. Allergy Immunol.*, **99**, 1.

Foon, K. A., G. C. Bottino, P. G. Abrams, M. F. Fer, D. L. Longo, C. S. Schoenberger *et al.* (1985). Phase II trial of recombinant leukocyte A interferon in patients with advanced chronic lymphocytic leukemia. *Am. J. Med.*, **78**, 216.

Foon, K. A., A. E. Maluish, P. G. Abrams, S. Wrightington, H. C. Stevenson, A. Alarif *et al.* (1986). Recombinant leukocyte A interferon therapy for advanced hairy cell leukemia. *Am. J. Med.*, **80**, 351.

Foreman, K. E., P. E. Bacon, E. D. Hsi, and B. J. Nickoloff (1997). In ssitu polymerase chain reaction-based localization studies support role of human herpesvirus-8 as the cause of two AIDS-related neoplasms: Kaposi's sarcoma and body cavity lymphoma. *J. Clin. Invest.*, **99**, 2971.

Foulis, A. K. (1996). The pathology of the endocrine pancreas in Type 1 (insulin-dependent) diabetes mellitus. *APMIS*, **104**, 161.

Fradelizi, D. and I. Gresser (1982). Interferon inhibits the generation of allospecific suppressor T lymphocytes. *J. Exp. Med.*, **155**, 1610.

Francis, M. L., M. S. Meltzer, and H. E. Gendelman (1992). Interferons in the persistence, pathogenesis, and treatment of HIV infection. *AIDS Res. Hum. Retroviruses*, **8**, 199.

Freeman, G. J., V. A. Boussiotis, A. Anumanthan, G. M. Bernstein, X. Y. Ke, P. D. Rennert *et al.* (1995). B7–1 and B7–2 do not deliver identical costimulatory signals, since B7–2 but not B7–1 preferentially costimulates the initial production of IL-4. *Immunity*, **2**, 523.

Freund, M., P. Von Wussow, J. Knuver Hopf, M. Mohr, U. Pohl, G. Exeriede *et al.* (1988). Treatment with natural human interferon alpha of a CML-patient with antibodies to recombinant interferon alpha-2b. *Blut*, **57**, 311.

Freund, M., P. Von Wussow, H. Diedrich, R. Eisert, H. Link, H. Wilke *et al.* (1989). Recombinant human interferon (IFN) alpha-2b in chronic myelogenous leukaemia: dose dependency of response and frequency of neutralizing anti-interferon antibodies. *Br. J. Haematol.*, 72, 350.

Fruehauf, S., C. Fiehn, R. Haas, H. Doehner, and W. Hunstein (1993). Sustained remission of idiopathic hypereosinophilic syndrome following alpha-interferon therapy. Acta Haematol., 89, 91.

Garcia-Monzon, C., L. Garcia-Buey, A. Garcia-Sanchez, J. M. Pajares, and R. Moreno-Otero (1993). Down-regulation of intercellular adhesion molecule 1 on hepatocytes in viral hepatitis treated with interferon alfa-2b. Gastroenterol., 105, 462.

Genc, K., D. L. Dona, and A. T. Reder (1997). Increased CD80+ B cells in active multiple sclerosis and reversal by interferon b-1b therapy. *J. Clin. Invest.*, **99**, 2664.

Gessani, S., F. Belardelli, A. Pecorelli, P. Puddu, and C. Baglioni (1989). Bacterial lipopolysaccharide and gamma interferon induce transcription of beta interferon mRNA and interferon secretion in murine macrophages. *J. Virol.*, **63**, 2785.

Gianelli, G., G. Antonelli, G. Fera, S. Del Vecchio, E. Riva, C. Broccia *et al.* (1994). Biological and clinical signifiance of neutralizing and binding antibodies to interferon-alpha (IFN-alpha) during therapy for chronic hepatitis C. *Clin. Exp. Immunol.*, **97**, 4.

Gill, P. S., W. J. Harrington, M. H. Kaplan, R. C. Ribeiro, M. F. Ferrio, H. A. Liebman *et al.* (1995). Treatment of adult-T-cell leukemia-lymphoma with a combination of interferon alpha and zidovudine. *New Engl. J. Med.*, **332**, 1744.

Goldman, M., T. Velu, and M. Pretolani (1997). Interleukin-10. Actions and therapeutic potential. *Biodrugs*, **7**, 6.

Goldstein, D., K. M. Sielaff, B. E. Storer, R. R. Brown, S. P. Datta, P. L. Witt *et al.* (1989). Human biologic response modification by interferon in the absence of measurable serum concentrations: a comparative trial of subcutaneous and intravenous interferon-beta serine. *J. Natl. Cancer Inst.*, **81**, 1061.

Grander, D., K. Oberg, M. L. Lundqvist, E. T. Janson, B. Eriksson, and S. Einhorn (1990). Interferon-induced enhancement of 2',5'-oligoadenylate synthetase in mid-gut carcinoid tumours. *Lancet*, **336**, 337.

Gutterman, J. U. (1994). Cytokine therapeutics: lessons from interferon alpha. *Proc. Natl. Acad. Sci. USA*, **91**, 1198.

Haahr, S., A. Moller-Larsen, J. Justesen, and E. Pedersen (1986). Interferon induction, 2'-5' oligo A synthetase and lymphocyte subpopulations in out-patients with multiple sclerosis in a longitudinal study. *Acta. Neurol. Scand.*, **73**, 345.

Harada, H., T. Fujita, M. Miyamoto, Y. Kimura, M. Maruyama, A. Furia *et al.* (1989). Structurally similar but functionally distinct factors, IRF-1 and IRF-2, bind to the same regulatory elements of IFN and IFN-inducible genes. *Cell*, **58**, 729.

Harfast, B., J. R. Huddlestone, P. Casali, T. C. Merigan, and M. B. A. Oldstone (1981). Interferon acts directly on human B lymphocytes to modulate immunoglobulin synthesis. *J. Immunol.*, **127**, 2146.

Hawkins, M. J., S. E. Krown, E. C. Borden *et al.* (1984). American Cancer Society phase I trial of naturally produced beta-interferon. *Cancer Res.*, **44**, 5934.

Hayden, F. G., J. K. Albrecht, D. L. Kaiser, and J. M. Gwaltney (1986). Prevention of natural colds by contact prophylaxis with intranasal alpha2-interferon. *New Engl. J. Med.*, **314**, 71.

Hirayama, K., S. Matsushita, I. Kikuchi, M. Iuchi, N. Ohta, and T. Sasazuki (1987). HLA-DQ is epistatic to HLA-DR in controlling the immune response to schistosomal antigen in humans. *Nature*, **327**, 426.

Hirsch, R. L. and K. P. Johnson (1986). The effects of long-term administration of recombinant alpha-2 interferon on lymphocytes subsets, proliferation, and suppressor cell function in multiple sclerosis. *J. Interferon. Res.*, **6**, 171.

Hobart, M., V. Ramassar, N. Goes, J. Urmson, and P. F. Halloran (1997). IFN Regulatory factor-1 plays a central role in the regulation of the expression of class i and class II MHC genes *in vivo*. *J. Immunol.*, **158**, 4260.

Huang, Y., L. M. Blatt, and M. W. Taylor (1995). Type 1 interferon as an antiinflammatory agent: inhibition of lipopolysaccharide-induced interleukin-1 beta and induction of interleukin-1 receptor antagonist. *J. Interferon. Cytokine. Res.*, **15**, 317.

Hughes, T. K. and S. Baron (1987). A large component of the antiviral activity of mouse interferon gamma may be due to its induction of interferon-alpha. *J. Biol. Regul. Homeost. Agents*, **1**, 29.

Ikeda, Y., K. Miyake, G. Toda, H. Yamada, M. Yamanaka, and H. Oka (1989). Detection of anti-interferon-alpha 2a antibodies in chronic liver disease. *J. Gastroenterol. Hepatol.*, **4**, 411.

Imakawa, K., R. V. Anthony, M. Kazemi, K. R. Marotti, H. G. Polites, and R. M. Roberts (1987). Interferon-like sequence of ovine trophoblast protein secreted by embrionic trophectoderm. *Nature*, **330**, 377.

Imam, H., E. T. Janson, A. Gobl, G. Alm, and K. Oberg (1995). Induction of MxA mRNA in patients with neuroendocrine tumors after interferon treatment. Lack of correlation with antitumor response. *Anticancer Res.*, **15**, 2191.

Isaacs, A. and D. C. Burke (1958). Mode of action of interferon. *Nature*, **182**, 1073.

Isaacs, A. and J. Lindenmann (1957). Virus interference. I. The interferon. *Proc. Roy. Soc. Lond.*, **147**, 258.

Itri, L. M., M. Campion, R. A. Dennin, A. V. Palleroni. J. U. Gutterman, J. E. Groopman *et al.* (1987). Incidence and clinical signifiance of neutralizing antibodies in patients receiving recombinant interferon alfa-2a by intramuscular injection. *Cancer*, **59**, 668.

Jacobs, L. and K. P. Johnson (1994). A brief history of the use of interferons as treatment of multiple sclerosis. *Arch. Neurol.*, **51**, 1245.

Jacobs, L., J. A. O'Malley, A. Freeman, and R. Ekes (1981). Intrathecal interferon reduces exacerbations of multiple sclerosis. *Science*, **214**, 1026.

Jacobs, L. D., D. L. Cookfair, R. A. Rudick, R. M. Herndon, J. R. Richert, A. M. Salazar *et al.* (1996). Intramuscular interferon beta-1a for disease progression in relapsing multiple sclerosis. The Multiple Sclerosis Collaborative Research Group (MSCRG). *Ann. Neurol.*, 39, 285.

Jarpe, M. A., H. M. Johnson, F. W. Bazer, T. L. Ott, E. V. Curto, N. Rama Krishna *et al.* (1994). Predicted structural motif of IFN tau. *Protein Eng.*, **7**, 863.

Jewell, A. P. (1996). Interferon-alpha, Bcl-2 expression and apoptosis in B-cell chronic lymphocytic leukemia. *Leuk. Lymphoma*, **21**, 43.

Kalkner, M., H. Hagberg, and A. Karlsson Parra (1990). Autoantibody occurence in hairy-cell leukemia during prolonged interferon treatment. *Eur. J. Haematol.*, **45**, 233.

Kaneko, S., N. Suzuki, H. Koizumi, S. Yamamoto, and T. Sakane (1997). Rescue by cytokines of apoptotic cell death induced by IL-2 deprivation of human antigen-specific T cell clones. *Clin. Exp. Immunol.*, **109**, 185.

Karpus, W. J. and R. H. Swanborg (1991). CD4+ suppressor cells inhibit the function of effector cells of experimental autoimmune encephalomyelitis through a mechanism involving transforming growth factor-beta. *J. Immunol.*, **146**, 1163.

Kedes, D. H. and D. Ganem (1997). Sensitivity of Kaposi's sarcoma-associated herpesvirus replication to antiviral drugs. *J. Clin. Invest.*, **99**, 2082.

Kennedy, M. K., D. S. Torrance, K. S. Picha, and K. M. Mohler (1992). Analysis of cytokine mRNA expression in the central nervous system of mice with experimental autoimmune encephalomyelitis reveals that IL-10 mRNA expression correlates with recovery. *J. Immunol.*, **149**, 2496.

Khan, O. A., Q. Xia, C. T. Bever, Jr., K. P. Johnson, H. S. Panitch, and S. S. Dhib Jalbut (1996). Interferon beta-1b serum levels in multiple sclerosis patients following subcutaneous administration. *Neurology*, **46**, 1639.

Kirkwood, J. M., M. H. Strawderman, M. S. Ernstoff, T. J. Smith, E. C. Borden, and R. H. Blum (1996). Interferon alfa-2b adjuvant therapy of high-risk resected cutaneous melanoma: the Eastern Cooperative Oncology Group Trial EST 1684. *J. Clin. Oncol.*, **14**, 7.

Klemann, S. W., K. Imakawa, and R. M. Roberts (1990, Sequence variability among ovine trophoblast interferon cDNA. *Nucleic Acid Research*, **18**, 6724.

Knight, C. R., R. C. Rees, A. Platts, T. Johnson, and M. Griffin (1993). Interleukin-2-activated human effector lymphocytes mediate cytotoxicity by inducing apoptosis in human leukaemia and solid tumour target cells. *Immunology*, **79**, 535.

Knop, J., R. Stremmer, C. Neumann, E. DeMaeyer, and E. Macher (1982). Interferon inhibits the suppressor T cell response of delayed-type hypersensitivity. *Nature*, **296**, 757.

Knop, J., B. Taborski, and J. DeMaeyer Guignard (1987). Selective inhibition of the generation of T suppressor cells of contact sensitivity *in vitro* by interferon. *J. Immunol.*, **138**, 3684.

Koeller, J. (1989). Biologic response modifiers: The interferon alfa experience. *Am. J. Hosp. Pharm.*, **46**, S11.

Kuchroo, V. K., M. P. Das, J. A. Brown, A. M. Ranger, S. S. Zamvil, H. L. Sobel *et al.* (1995). B7–1 and B7–2 co-stimulatory molecules activate differentially the Th1/Th2 develomental pathways: application to autoimmune disease therapy. *Cell,* **80,** 707.

Langer, J. A. and S. Pestka (1985). Structure of interferons. *Pharmacol. Ther.,* **27,** 371.

Langer, J. A. and S. Pestka (1988). Interferon receptors. *Immunol. Today,* **9,** 393.

Larrea, E., N. Garcia, C. Qian, M. P. Civeira, and J. Prieto (1996). Tumor necrosis factor a gene expression and the response to interferon in chronic hepatitis C. *Hepathology,* **23,** 210.

Leavitt, R. D., V. Ratanatharathorn, H. Ozer, J. E. Ultmann, C. Portlock, J. W. Myers *et al.* (1987). Alfa-2b Interferon in the treatment of Hodgkin's disease and non-Hodgkin's lymphoma. *Semin. Oncol.,* **14,** 18.

Leppert, D., E. Waubant, M. R. Burk, J. R. Oksenberg, and S. L. Hauser (1996). Interferon beta-1b inhibits gelatinase secretion and *in vitro* migration of human T cells: a possible mechanism for treatment efficacy in multiple sclerosis. *Ann. Neurol.,* **40,** 846.

Liberati, A. M., M. Fizzotti, M. G. Proietti, R. Di Marzio, M. Schippa, B. Biscottini *et al.* (1988). Biochemical host response to interferon-beta. *J. Interferon. Res.,* **8,** 765.

Lowenthal, J. W., D. W. Ballard, E. B"hnlein, and W. C. Greene (1989). Tumor necrosis factor a induces proteins that bind specifically to kB-like enhancer elements and regulate interleukin 2 receptor a-chain gene expression in primary human T lymphocytes. *Proc. Natl. Acad. Sci. USA,* **86,** 2331.

Lublin, F. D., J. N. Whitaker, B. H. Eidelman, A. E. Miller, B. G. Arnason, and J. S. Burks (1996). Management of patients receiving interferon beta-1b for multiple sclerosis: report of a consensus conference. *Neurology,* **46,** 12.

Main, J. and J. Handley (1992). Interferon: current and future clinical uses in infectious disease practice. Int. J. STD. *AIDS,* **3,** 4.

Malbrain, M. L., H. Van den Bergh, and P. Zachee (1996). Further evidence for the clonal nature of the idiopathic hypereosinophilic syndrome: complete haematological and cytogenetic remission induced by interferon-alpha in a case with a unique chromosomal abnormality. *Br. J. Haematol.,* **92,** 176.

Manetti, R., F. Annunziato, L. Tomasevic, V. Gianno, P. Parronchi, S. Romagnani *et al.* (1995). Polyinosinic acid: polycytidylic acid promotes T helper Type 1-specific immune responses by stimulating macrophage production of interferon-alpha and interleukin-12. *Eur. J. Immunol.* **25,** 2656.

Marroni, M., P. Gresele, G. Landonio, A. Lazzarin, M. Coen, R. Vezza *et al.* (1994). Interferon-alpha is effective in the treatment of HIV-1-related, severe, zidovudine-resistant thrombocytopenia. A prospective, placebo-controlled, double-blind trial. *Ann. Intern. Med.,* **121,** 423.

Martal, J., M. C. Lacroix, C. Loudes, M. Saunier, and S. Winterberger Torres (1979). Trophoblastin, an antiluteolytic protein present in early pregnancy in sheep. *J. Reprod. Fert.,* **56,** 63.

Mayet, W. J., G. Hess, G. Gerken, S. Rossol, R. Voth, M. Manns *et al.* (1989). Treatment of chronic Type B hepatitis with recombinant alpha-interferon induces autoantibodies not specific for autoimmune chronic hepatitis. *Hepathology,* **10,**

McSweeney, E. N., F. J. Giles, C. P. Worman, A. P. Jewel, C. P. Tsakona, A. V. Hoffbrand *et al.* (1993). Recombinant interferon alfa 2a in the treatment of patients with early stage B chronic lymphocytic leukaemia. *Br. J. Haematol.,* **85,** 77.

Meager, A., N. Willcox, and J. Newson-Davis (1996). High-titred neutralizing Anti -IFN-alpha and Anti-IFN-omega autoantibodies in myasthenia gravis patients with thymoma, 9th European Interferon Workshop. *Interferons and Autoimmunity,* **47.**

Miles, S. A., H. J. Wang, E. Cortes, J. Carden, S. Marcus, and R. T. Mitsuyasu (1990). Beta-interferon therapy in patients with poor-prognosis Kaposi sarcoma related to the acquired immunodeficiency syndrome (AIDS). A phase II trial with preliminary evidence of antiviral activity and low incidence of opportunistic infections. *Ann. Intern. Med.*, **112**, 582.

Millela, M., G. Antonelli, T. Santantonio, M. Currenti, L. Monno, N. Mariano *et al.* (1993). Neutralizing antibodies to recombinant alpha-interferon and response to therapy in chronic hepatitis C virus infection. *Liver*, **13**, 146.

Milner, A. E., R. J. Grand, C. M. Waters and C. D. Gregory (1993). Apoptosis in Burkitt lymphoma cells is driven by c-myc. *Oncogene*, **8**, 3385.

Milo, R. and H. Panitch (1995). Additive effects of copolymer-1 and interferon beta-1b on the immune response to myelin basic protein. *J. Neuroimmunol.*, **61**, 185.

Mitsui, Y., T. Senda, T. Shimazu, S. Matsuda, and J. Utsumi (1993). Structural, functional and evolutionary implications of the three-dimensional crystal structure of murine interferon-beta. *Pharmacol. Ther.*, **58**, 93.

Morita, M., B. Lamkhioued, A. Soussi Gounni, D. Aldebert, E. Delaporte, A. Capron *et al.* (1996). Induction by interferons of human eosinophil apoptosis and regulation by interleukin-3, granulocyte/macrophage-colony stimulating factor and interleukin-5. *Eur. Cytokine. Netw.*, **7**, 725.

Nagano, Y. and Y. Kojima (1958). Inhibition de l'infection vaccinale par un facteur liquide dans le tissu infect, par le virus homologue, *C. R. Soc. Biol.*, **152**, 1627.

Nakajima, H., A. Nakao, Y. Watanabe, S. Yoshida, and I. Iwamoto (1994). IFN-alpha inhibits antigen-induced eosinophil and CD4+ T cell recruitment into tissue. J. Immunol., 153, 1264.

Neighbour, P. A. (1984). Studies of Interferon Production and Natural Killing by Lymphocytes from Multiple Sclerosis Patients. Ann. *NY Acad. Sci.*, **436**, 181.

Neighbour, P. A. and B. R. Bloom (1979, Absence of virus-induced lymphocyte suppression and interferon production in multiple sclerosis. *Proc. Natl. Acad. Sci. USA*, **76**, 476.

Noma, T. and M. E. Dorf (1985). Modulation of suppressor T cell induction with interferon-gamma. *J. Immunol.*, **135**, 3655.

Nonomura, N., T. Miki, M. Yokoyama, T. Imazu, T. Takada, S. Takeuchi *et al.* (1996). Fas/APO-1-mediated apoptosis of human renal cell carcinoma. *Biochem. Biophys. Res. Commun.*, **229**, 945.

Noronha, A., A. Toscas, and M. A. Jensen (1990). Interferon beta augments suppressor cell function in multiple sclerosis. *Ann. Neurol.*, **27**, 207.

Noronha, A., A. Toscas, and M. A. Jensen (1992). Contrasting effects of alpha, beta, and gamma interferons on nonspecific suppressor function in multiple sclerosis. *Ann. Neurol.*, **31**, 103.

Noronha, A., A. Toscas, and M. A. Jensen (1993a). Interferon beta decreases T cell activation, and interferon gamma production in multiple sclerosis. *J. Neuroimmunol.*, **46**, 145.

Noronha, A., M. A. Jensen, and A. Toscas (1993b). TGF-β activity in MS: effect of IFN-β. *Neurology*, **43**, 355. (Abstract.)

Noronha, A., A. Toscas, B. G. Arnason, and M. A. Jensen (1994). IFN-beta augments *in vivo* suppressor function in MS. *Neurology*, **44**, A212. (Abstract.)

Novick, D., B. Cohen, and M. Rubinstein (1994). The human interferon alpha/beta receptor: characterization and molecular cloning. *Cell*, **77**, 391.

Oberg, K. (1992). The action of interferon alpha on human carcinoid tumours. *Semin. Cancer Biol.*, **3**, 35.

Oberg, K., G. Alm, A. Magnuson, G. Lundqvist, E. Theodorsson, L. Wide *et al.* (1989). Treatment of malignant carcinoid tumors with recombinant interferon alfa-2b: development of neutralizing interferon antibodies and possible loss of antitumor activity. *J. Natl. Cancer Inst.*, **81**, 531.

O'Gorman, M. R. G., J. Oger, and L. F. Kastrukoff (1987, Reduction of immunoglobulin G secretion *in vitro* following long term lymphoblastoid interferon (Wellferon) treatment in multiple sclerosis patients. *Clin. Exp. Immunol.*, **67**, 66.

Oliveira, I. C., P. J. Sciavolino, T. H. Lee, and J. Vilcek (1992). Downregulation of interleukin 8 gene expression in human fibroblasts: unique mechanism of transcriptional inhibition by interferon. *Proc. Natl. Acad. Sci. USA*, **89**, 9049.

Olsen, E. A. and P. A. Bunn (1995). Interferon in the treatment of cutaneous T-cell lymphoma. Hematol. *Oncol. Clin. North Am.*, **9**, 1089.

Osborn, L., S. Kunkel, and G. J. Nabel (1989, Tumor necrosis factor a and interleukin 1 stimulate the human immunodeficiency virus enhancer by activation of the nuclear factor kB. *Proc. Natl. Acad. Sci. USA*, **86**, 2336.

Palmer, H. and P. Libby (1992). Interferon-beta. A potential autocrine regulator of human vascular smooth muscle cell growth. *Lab. Invest.*, **66**, 715.

Panayiotidis, P., K. Ganeshaguru, L. Foroni, and A. V. Hoffbrand (1995). Expression and function of the FAS antigen in B chronic lymphocytic leukemia and hairy cell leukemia. *Leukemia*, **9**, 1227.

Panitch, H. S. (1994). Influence of infection on exacerbations of multiple sclerosis. *Ann. Neurol.*, **36** (supplement), S25.

Panitch, H. S., R. L. Hirsch, A. S. Haley, and K. P. Johnson (1987a). Exacerbations of multiple sclerosis in patients treated with gamma interferon. *Lancet*, **1**, 893.

Panitch, H. S., J. S. Folus, and K. P. Johnson (1987b). Recombinant beta interferon inhibits gamma interferon production in multiple sclerosis. *Ann. Neurol.*, **22**, 139. (Abstract.)

Panitch, H. S., J. S. Folus, and K. P. Johnson (1989). Beta Interferon Prevents HLA Class II Antigen Induction by Gamma Interferon in MS. *Neurology*, **39**, 171.

Parronchi, P., M. De Carli, R. Manetti, C. Simonelli, S. Sampognaro, M. P. Piccinni *et al.* (1992). IL-4 and IFN (alpha and gamma) exert opposite regulatory effects on the development of cytolytic potential by Th1 or Th2 human T cell clones. *J. Immunol.*, **149**, 2977.

Parronchi, P., S. Mohapatra, S. Sampognaro, L. Giannarini, U. Wahn, P. Chong *et al.* (1996). Effects of interferon-alpha on cytokine profile, T cell receptor repertoire and peptide reactivity of human allergen-specific T cells. *Eur. J. Immunol.*, **26**, 697.

Pene, J., F. Rousset, F. Briere, I. Chretien, J. Y. Bonnefoy, H. Spits *et al.* (1988). IgE production by normal human lymphocytes is induced by interleukine 4 and suppressed by interferons gamma and alpha and prostaglandine E2. *Proc. Natl. Acad. Sci. USA*, **85**, 6880.

Penna, C., M. G. Fallani, R. Gordigiani, L. Sonni, G. L. Taddei, and M. Marchionni (1994). Intralesional beta-interferon treatment of cervical intraepithelial neoplasia associated with human papillomavirus infection. *Tumori.*, **80**, 146.

Perussia, B., D. Santoli, and G. Trinchieri (1980). Interferon modulation of natural killer cell activity. *Ann. NY Acad. Sci.*, **350**, 55.

Pestka, S., J. A. Langer, K. C. Zoon, and C. E. Samuel (1987) Interferons and their actions. *Ann. Rev. Biochem.*, **56**, 727.

Pfeffer, L. M. and S. N. Constantinescu (1997). The molecular biology of interferon-b from receptor binding to transmembrane signaling. In Interferon therapy of multiple sclerosis, (ed. A. T. Reder), p. 1. Marcel Dekker Inc. New York.

Pichert, G., L. M. Jost, L. Zobeli, B. Odermatt, G. Pedio, and R. A. Stahel (1990). Thyroiditis after treatment with interleukin-2 and interferon-alpha-2a. *Br. J. Cancer*, **62**, 100.

Platanias, L. C. (1995). Interferons: laboratory to clinic investigations. *Curr. Opin. Oncol.*, **7**, 560.

Platanias, L. C. and M. E. Sweet (1994). Interferon alpha induces rapid tyrosine phosphorylation of the vav proto-oncogene product in hematopoietic cells. *J. Biol. Chem.*, **269**, 3143.

Platanias, L. C., S. Uddin, and O. R. Colamonici (1994). Tyrosine phosphorylation of the alpha and beta subunits of the Type I interferon receptor. Interferon-beta selectively induces tyrosine phosphorylation of an alpha subunit-associated protein. *J. Biol. Chem.*, **269**, 17761.

Porrini, A. M., D. Gambi, and A. T. Reder (1995). Interferon effects on interleukin-10 secretion. Mononuclear cell response to interleukin-10 is normal in multiße sclerosis patients. *J. Neuroimmunol.*, **61**, 27.

Prin, L., J. Plumas, V. Gruart, S. Loiseau, D. Aldebert, J. C. Ameisen *et al.* (1991). Elevated serum levels of soluble interleukin-2 receptor: a marker of disease activity in the hypereosinophilic syndrome. *Blood*, **78**, 2626.

Prummer, O. (1993). Interferon-alpha antibodies in patients with renal cell carcinoma treated with recombinant interferon-alpha-2A in an adjuvant multicenter trial. The Delta-P Study Group. *Cancer*, **71**, 1828.

Prummer, O., U. Streichan, H. Heimpel, and F. Porzsolt (1994). Sensitive antiproliferative neutralization assay for the detection of neutralizing IFN-alpha and IFN-beta antibodies. *J. Immunol. Methods*, **171**, 45.

Quesada, J. R., A. Rios, D. Swanson, P. Trown, and J. U. Gutterman (1985). Antitumor activity of recombinant-derived interferon alpha in metastatic renal cell carcinoma. *J.Clin. Oncol.*, **3**, 1522.

Quesada, J. R., L. Itri, and J. U. Gutterman (1987). Alpha interferons in hairy cell leukemia (HCL), a five year follow-up in 100 patients. *J. Interferon. Res.*, **7**, 678.

Ransohoff, R. M., C. Devajyothi, M. L. Estes, G. Babcock, R. A. Rudick, E. M. Frohman *et al.* (1991). Interferon-beta specifically inhibits interferon-gamma-induced class II major histocompatibility complex gene transcription in a human astrocytoma cell line. *J. Neuroimmunol.*, **33**, 103.

Rep, M. H., R. Q. Hintzen, C. H. Polman, and R. A. van Lier (1996). Recombinant interferon-beta blocks proliferation but enhances interleukin-10 secretion by activated human T-cells. *J. Neuroimmunol.*, 67, 111.

Rodriguez Villanueva, J., and T. J. McDonnell (1995). Induction of apoptotic cell death in non-melanoma skin cancer by interferon-alpha. *Int. J. Cancer*, **61**, 110.

Romagnani, S. (1992). Induction of Th1 and th2 responses: a key role for the 'natural' immune response? *Immunol. Today*, **13**, 379.

Romagnani, S. (1994). Regulation of the development of Type 2 T-helper cells in allergy. *Curr. Opin. Immunol.*, **6**, 838.

Ronnblom, L. E., E. T. Janson, A. Perers, K. E. Oberg, and G. V. Alm (1992). Characterization of anti-interferon-alpha antibodies appearing during recombinant interferon-alpha 2a treatment. *Clin. Exp. Immunol.*, **89**, 330.

Ross, C., M. B. Hansen, T. Schyberg, and K. Berg (1990). Autoantibodies to crude human leucocyte interferon (IFN), native human IFN, recombinant human IFN-alpha 2b and human IFN-gamma in healthy blood donors. *Clin. Exp. Immunol.*, **82**, 57.

Ross, C., M. Svenson, M. B. Hansen, G. L. Vejlsgaard, and K. Bendtzen (1995). High avidity IFN-neutralizing antibodies in pharmaceutically prepared human IgG. *J. Clin. Invest.*, **95**, 1974.

Roth, M. S. and K. A. Foon (1986). Alpha interferon in the treatment of hematologic malignancies. *Am. J. Med.*, **81**, 871.

Ruco, L. P., A. Procopio, V. Maccallini *et al.* (1983). Severe deficiency of natural killer activity in the peripheral blood of patients with hairy cell leukemia. *Blood*, **61**, 1132.

Rudick, R. A., R. M. Ransohoff, R. Peppler, S. VanderBrug Medendorp, P. Lehmann, and J. Alam (1996). Interferon beta induces interleukin-10 expression: relevance to multiple sclerosis. *Ann. Neurol.*, **40**, 618.

Saito, H., T. Hayakawa, Y. Yui, and T. Shida (1987, Effect of human interferon on different functions of human neutrophils and eosinophils. *Int. Arch. Allergy Appl. Immunol.*, **82**, 133.

Salgame, P., J. Convit, and B. R. Bloom (1991). Immunological suppression by human CD8+ T cells is receptor dependent and HLA-DQ restricted. *Proc. Natl. Acad. Sci. USA*, **88**, 2598.

Salonen, R., J. Ilonen, M. Reunanen, and A. Salmi (1982). Defective production of interferon-a associated with HLA-Dw2 antigen in stable multiple sclerosis. *J. Neurol. Sci.*, **55**, 197.

Santoli, D., W. Hall, L. F. Kastrukoff, R. P. Lisak, B. Perussia, G. Trinchieri *et al.* (1981). Cytotoxic activity and interferon production by lymphocytes from patients with multiple sclerosis. *J. Immunol.*, **126**, 1274.

Saracco, G., A. Touscoz, M. Durazzo, F. Rosina, E. Donegani, L. Chiandussi *et al.* (1990). Autoantibodies and response to alpha-interferon in patients with chronic viral hepatitis. *J. Hepatol.*, **11**, 339.

Satoh, J., D. W. Paty, and S. U. Kim (1995). Differential effects of beta and gamma interferons on expression of major histocompatibility complex antigens and intercellular adhesion molecule-1 in cultured fetal human astrocytes. *Neurology*, **45**, 367.

Schandene, L., G. F. Del Prete, E. Cogan, P. Stordeur, A. Crusiaux, B. Kennes *et al.* (1996). Recombinant interferon-alpha selectively inhibits the production of interleukin-5 by human CD4+ T cells. *J. Clin. Invest.*, **97**, 309.

Schapner, H. W., T. M. Aune, and C. W. Pierce (1983). Suppressor T cell activation by human leukocyte interferon. *J. Immunol.*, **131**, 2301.

Schiller, J. H., B. Storer, D. M. Paulnock *et al.* (1990). A direct comparison of biological response modulation and clinical side effects by interferon-beta-ser, interferon-gamma, or the combination of interferons beta-ser and gamma in humans. *J. Clin. Invest.*, **86**, 1211.

Schwabe, M., A. T. Brini, M. C. Bosco, F. Rubboli, M. Egawa, J. Zhao *et al.* (1994). Disruption by interferon-alpha of an autocrine interleukin-6 growth loop in IL-6-dependent U266 myeloma cells by homologous and heterologous down-regulation of the IL-6 receptor alpha- and beta-chains. *J. Clin. Invest.*, **94**, 2317.

Selleri, C., T. Sato, L. Del Vecchio, L. Luciano, A. J. Barrett, B. Rotoli *et al.* (1997). Involvement of Fas-mediated apoptosis in the inhibitory effects of interferon-alpha in chronic myelogenous leukemia. *Blood*, **89**, 957.

Sen, G. C. and P. Lengyel (1992). The interferon system. A bird's eye view of its biochemistry. *J. Biol. Chem.*, **267**, 5017.

Sen, G. C. and R. M. Ransohoff (1993). Interferon-induced antiviral actions and their regulation. *Adv. Virus Res.*, **42**, 57.

Sherwin, S. A., J. A. Knost, S. Fein, P. G. Abrams, K. A. Foon, J. J. Ochs *et al.* (1982). A multiple-dose phase i trial of recombinant leukocyte A interferon in cancer patients. *JAMA*, **248**, 2461.

Sibley, W. A., C. R. Bamford, and N. Suzuki (1985). Clinical viral infections and multiple sclerosis. *Lancet*, **1**, 1313.

Sillaber, C., K. Geissler, R. Scherrer, R. Kaltenbrunner, P. Bettelheim, K. Lechner *et al.* (1992). Type beta transforming growth factors promote interleukin-3 (IL-3)-dependent differentiation of human basophils but inhibit IL-3-dependent differentiation of human eosinophils. *Blood*, **80**, 634.

Singh, R. K., M. Gutman, C. D. Bucana, R. Sanchez, N. Llansa, and I. J. Fidler (1995). Interferons alpha and beta down-regulate the expression of basic fibroblast growth factor in human carcinomas. *Proc. Natl. Acad. Sci. USA*, **92**, 4562.

Skurkovich, S., B. Skurkovich, and J. A. Bellanti (1993). A disturbance of interferon synthesis with the hyperproduction of unusual kinds of interferon can trigger autoimmune disease and play a pathogenetic role in AIDS: the removal of these interferons can be therapeutic. *Med. Hypotheses*, **41**, 177.

Soilu Hanninen, M., A. Salmi, and R. Salonen (1995). Interferon-beta downregulates expression of VLA-4 antigen and antagonizes interferon-gamma-induced expression of HLA-DQ on human peripheral blood monocytes. *J. Neuroimmunol.*, **60**, 99.

Spear, G. T., D. M. Paulnock, R. L. Jordan, D. M. Meltzer, J. A. Merritt, and E. C. Borden (1987). Enhancement of monocyte class I and II histocompatibility antigen expression in man by *in vivo* beta-interferon. *Clin. Exp. Immunol.*, **69**,

Steeg, P. S., R. N. Moore, H. M. Johnson, and J. J. Oppenheim (1982). Regulation of murine macrophage Ia antigen expression by a lymphokine with immune interferon activity. *J. Exp. Med.*, **156**, 1780.

Steis, R. G., J. W. Smith II, W. J. Urba, J. W. Clark, L. M. Itri, L. M. Evans *et al.* (1988). Resistance to recombinant interferon alpha-2a in hairy-cell leukemia associated with neutralizing anti-interferon antibodies. *New Engl. J. Med.*, **318**, 1409.

Stewart, H. J., S. H. E. McCann, P. J. Barker, K. E. Lee, G. E. Lamming, and A. P. F. Flint (1987). Interferon sequence homology and receptor binding activity of ovine trophoblast antiluteolytic protein. *J. Endocr.*, **115**, R13.

Stewart, H. J., S. H. E. McCann, A. J. Northrop, G. E. Lamming, and A. P. F. Flint (1989). Sheep antiluteolytic interferon: cDNA sequence and analysis of mRNA levels. *J. Mol. Endocrinol.*, **2**, 65.

Stewart, W. E., 2d, L. B. Gosser, and R. Z. Lockart, Jr (1971). Priming: a Nonantiviral Function of Interferon. *J. Virol.*, **7**, 792.

Stuve, O., N. P. Dooley, J. H. Uhm, J. P. Antel, G. S. Francis, G. Williams *et al.* (1996). Interferon beta-1b decreases the migration of T lymphocytes *in vitro*: effects on matrix metalloproteinase-9. *Ann. Neurol.*, **40**, 853.

Sztein, M. B., P. S. Steeg, H. M. Johnson, and J. J. Oppenheim (1984). Regulation of human peripheral blood monocyte DR antigen expression *in vitro* by lymphokines and recombinant interferons. *J. Clin. Invest.*, **73**, 556.

Tada, Y., A. Ho, T. Matsuyama, and T. W. Mak (1997). Reduced incidence and severity of antigen-induced autoimmune diseases in mice lacking interferon regulatory factor-1. *J. Exp. Med.*, **185**, 231.

Targan, S. and F. Dorey (1980). Interferon activation of 'pre-spontaneous killer' (pre-SK) cells and alteration in kinetics of lysis of both 'pre-SK' and active SK cells. *J. Immunol.*, **124**, 2157.

The IFNB Multiple Sclerosis Study Group (1993). Interferon beta-1b is effective in relapsing-remitting multiple sclerosis. I. Clinical results of a multicenter, randomized, double-blind, placebo-controlled trial. *Neurology*, **43**, 655.

The IFNB Multiple Sclerosis Study Group and The University of British Columbia MS/MRI Analysis Group (1995). Interferon beta-1b in the treatment of multiple sclerosis: final outcome of the randomized controlled trial. *Neurology*, **45**, 1277.

The IFNB Multiple Sclerosis Study Group and The University of British Columbia MS/MRI Analysis Group (1996, Neutralizing antibodies during treatment of multiple sclerosis with interferon beta-1b: experience during the first three years. *Neurology*, **47**, 889.

Thiele, J., T. K. Zirbes, H. M. Kvasnicka, J. Lorenzen, N. Niederle, L. D. Leder *et al.* (1996). Effect of interferon therapy on bone marrow morphology in chronic myeloid leukemia: a cytochemical and immunohistochemical study of trephine biopsies. *J. Interferon. Cytokine. Res.*, **16**, 217.

Thulasi, R., P. Dias, P. J. Houghton, and J. A. Houghton (1996, Alpha 2a-interferon-induced differentiation of human alveolar rhabdomyosarcoma cells: correlation with down-regulation of the insulin-like growth factor Type I receptor. *Cell Growth Differ.*, **7**, 531.

Tilg, H. (1997). New insight into the mechanisms of interferon alpha: an immunoregulatory and anti-inflammatory cytokine. *Gastroenterol.*, **112**, 1017.

Tilg, H., J. W. Mier, W. Vogel, W. E. Aulitzky, C. J. Wiedermann, E. Vannier *et al.* (1993). Induction of circulating IL-1 receptor antagonist by IFN treatment. *J. Immunol.*, **150**, 4687.

Tilg, H., W. Vogel, and C. A. Dinarello (1995). Interferon-alpha induces circulating tumor necrosis factor receptor p55 in humans. *Blood*, **85**, 433.

Tovell, D. R., I. A. McRobbie, K. G. Warren, and D. L. J. Tyrrell (1983). Interferon production by lymphocytes from multiple sclerosis and non-MS patients. *Neurology*, **33**, 640.

Towbin, H., A. Schmitz, D. Jakschies, P. Von Wussow, and M. A. Horisberger (1992). A whole blood immunoassay for the interferon-inducible human Mx protein. *J. Interferon. Res.*, **12**, 67.

Tzung, S. P., T. C. Mahl, P. Lance, V. Andersen, and S. A. Cohen (1992). Interferon-alpha prevents endotoxin-induced mortality in mice. *Eur. J. Immunol.*, **22**, 3097.

Uddin, S., E. N. Fish, D. A. Sher, C. Gardziola, M. F. White, and L. C. Platanias (1997). Activation of the phosphatidylinositol 3-kinase serine kinase by IFN-alpha. *J. Immunol.*, **158**, 2390.

Uze, G., G. Lutfalla, and I. Gresser (1990). Genetic transfer of a functional human interferon alpha receptor into mouse cells: cloning and expression of its cDNA. *Cell*, **60**, 225.

Vallbracht, A., J. Treuner, B. Flehmig, K. E. Joester, and D. Niethammer (1981). Interferon-neutralizing antibodies in a patient treated with human fibroblast interferon. *Nature*, **289**, 496.

Van den Broecke, D., and L. M. Pfeffer (1988). Characterization of interferon-a binding sites on human cell lines. *J. Interferon. Res.*, **8**, 803.

Vervliet, G., H. Carton, E. Meulepas, and A. Billiau (1984). Interferon production by cultured peripheral leucocytes of MS patients. *Clin. Exp. Immunol.*, **58**, 116.

Vervliet, G., H. Carton, and A. Billiau (1985). Interferon-gamma production by peripheral blood leukocytes from patients with multiple sclerosis and other neurological diseases. *Clin. Exp. Immunol.*, **59**, 391.

Vial, T. and J. Descotes (1995). Immune-mediated side-effects of cytokines in humans. *Toxicology*, **105**, 31.

Von Wussow, P., M. Freund, B. Block, H. Diedrich, H. Poliwoda, and H. Deicher (1987). Clinical signifiance of anti-IFN-alpha antibody titres during interferon therapy. *Lancet*, **2**, 635.

Von Wussow, P., H. Pralle, H. K. Hochkeppel, D. Jakschies, S. Sonnen, H. Schmidt *et al.* (1991). Effective natural interferon-alpha therapy in recombinant interferon-alpha-resistant patients with hairy cell leukemia. *Blood*, **78**, 38.

Von Wussow, P., R. Hehlmann, T. Hochhaus, D. Jakschies, K. U. Nolte, O. Prummer *et al.* (1994). Roferon (rIFN-alpha-2a) is more immunogenic than intron A (rIFN-alpha-2b) in patients with chronic myelogenous leukemia. *J. Interferon. Res.*, **14**, 217.

Weinstock Guttman, B., R. M. Ransohoff, R. P. Kinkel, and R. A. Rudick (1995). The interferons: biological effects, mechanisms of action, and use in multiple sclerosis. *Ann. Neurol.*, **37**, 7.

Wills, R. J. (1990). Clinical pharmacokinetics of interferons. *Clin. Pharmacokinet.*, **19**, 390.

Witt, P. L. (1997). Pharmacokinetics of interferon-b and the biological markers it induces, In *Interferon therapy of multiple sclerosis*, (ed. A. T. Reder), p. 77. Marcel Dekker Inc. New York.

Zinzani, P. L., M. Buzzi, P. Farabegoli, G. Martinelli, P. Tosi, E. Zuffa *et al.* (1994a). Apoptosis induction with fludarabine on freshly isolated chronic myeloid leukemia cells. *Haematologica*, **79**, 127.

Zinzani, P. L., M. Buzzi, P. Farabegoli, P. Tosi, A. Fortuna, G. Visani *et al.* (1994b). Induction of '*in vitro*' apoptosis by fludarabine in freshly isolated B-chronic lymphocytic leukemia cells. *Leuk. Lymphoma*, **13**, 95.

Index